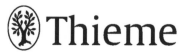

Interventional Oncology

Ripal T. Gandhi
Attending Physician
Vascular and Interventional Radiology
Miami Cardiac and Vascular Institute

Associate Clinical Professor
Herbert Wertheim College of Medicine at Florida International University
Assistant Clinical Professor
University of South Florida School of Medicine
Miami, Florida

Suvranu Ganguli
Associate Chief of Interventional Radiology
Co-Director, Center for Image-Guided Cancer Therapy
Massachusetts General Hospital
Assistant Professor of Radiology
Harvard Medical School
Boston, Massachusetts

1874 illustrations

Thieme
New York • Stuttgart • Delhi • Rio de Janeiro

Executive Editor: William Lamsback
Managing Editor: Elizabeth Palumbo
Director, Editorial Services: Mary Jo Casey
Editorial Assistant: Haley Paskalides
International Production Director: Andreas Schabert
Vice President, Editorial and E-Product Development:
   Vera Spillner
International Marketing Director: Fiona Henderson
International Sales Director: Louisa Turrell
Director of Sales, North America: Mike Roseman
Senior Vice President and Chief Operating Officer:
   Sarah Vanderbilt
President: Brian D. Scanlan

Library of Congress Cataloging-in-Publication Data

Interventional oncology (2015)
  Interventional oncology / [edited by] Suvranu Ganguli, Ripal
T. Gandhi, Salomão Faintuch.
      p. ; cm. – (Practical guides in interventional radiology)
  Includes bibliographical references and index.
  ISBN 978-1-62623-081-1 – ISBN 978-1-62623-082-8
  (electronic)
  I. Ganguli, Suvranu, editor. II. Gandhi, Ripal T., editor.
  III. Faintuch, Salomão, editor. IV. Title. V. Series: Practical
  guides in interventional radiology.
  [DNLM: 1. Neoplasms–radiotherapy. 2. Radiography,
  Interventional–methods. 3. Diagnostic Imaging. QZ 269]
  RC271.R3
  616.99'40642–dc23   2015014982

© 2016 Thieme Medical Publishers, Inc.

Thieme Publishers New York
333 Seventh Avenue, New York, NY 10001 USA
+1 800 782 3488, customerservice@thieme.com

Thieme Publishers Stuttgart
Rüdigerstrasse 14, 70469 Stuttgart, Germany
+49 [0]711 8931 421, customerservice@thieme.de

Thieme Publishers Delhi
A-12, Second Floor, Sector-2, Noida-201301
Uttar Pradesh, India
+91 120 45 566 00, customerservice@thieme.in

Thieme Publishers Rio de Janeiro, Thieme Publicações Ltda.
Edifício Rodolpho de Paoli, 25º andar
Av. Nilo Peçanha, 50 – Sala 2508
Rio de Janeiro 20020-906 Brasil
+55 21 3172-2297 / +55 21 3172-1896

Cover design: Thieme Publishing Group
Typesetting by DiTech Process Solutions

Printed in India by Replika Press Pvt. Ltd.   5 4 3 2 1

ISBN 978-1-62623-081-1

Also available as an e-book:
eISBN 978-1-62623-082-8

Important note: Medicine is an ever-changing science undergoing continual development. Research and clinical experience are continually expanding our knowledge, in particular our knowledge of proper treatment and drug therapy. Insofar as this book mentions any dosage or application, readers may rest assured that the authors, editors, and publishers have made every effort to ensure that such references are in accordance with **the state of knowledge at the time of production of the book.**

Nevertheless, this does not involve, imply, or express any guarantee or responsibility on the part of the publishers in respect to any dosage instructions and forms of applications stated in the book. **Every user is requested to examine carefully** the manufacturers' leaflets accompanying each drug and to check, if necessary in consultation with a physician or specialist, whether the dosage schedules mentioned therein or the contraindications stated by the manufacturers differ from the statements made in the present book. Such examination is particularly important with drugs that are either rarely used or have been newly released on the market. Every dosage schedule or every form of application used is entirely at the user's own risk and responsibility. The authors and publishers request every user to report to the publishers any discrepancies or inaccuracies noticed. If errors in this work are found after publication, errata will be posted at www.thieme.com on the product description page.

Some of the product names, patents, and registered designs referred to in this book are in fact registered trademarks or proprietary names even though specific reference to this fact is not always made in the text. Therefore, the appearance of a name without designation as proprietary is not to be construed as a representation by the publisher that it is in the public domain.

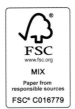

To my parents, without whom none of my achievements would be possible. Thank you for your continuous love and for sacrificing all that you have. You have supported me in every way possible. I will never be able to repay you.

Ripal T. Gandhi, MD

To my parents, who epitomize humanity, sacrifice, and the quest for knowledge, which have been instilled in me and my siblings by their example. To my boys—Ronan, Kieran, and Arik—who make every day an adventure. And to my wife and partner-in-life, Kriston, without whom nothing I have and will accomplish would be possible.

Suvranu Ganguli, MD

Contents

Foreword

I was excited to be asked to write a foreword for Interventional Oncology because *interventional oncology* is the fastest growing part of interventional radiology and, in my opinion, the most important development in clinical care of cancer patients in the last decade. With the growth and evolution of this treatment, patients can now be offered the various and diverse forms of treatments described in this book.

The practice of interventional oncology, which stresses both clinical care and a variety of technical considerations, is not a simple field. In fact, I suspect in a few years it may be considered a separate subspecialty within the confines of interventional radiology.

Drs. Ganguli and Gandhi, who are well known in the interventional community, have selected leaders in the field and experts in the various techniques of interventional oncology. Their superb editing has produced a very easy-to-read and well-organized book on the subject. The specific chapters and the way in which the editors have presented the information allow the reader to look at specific problems of interventional oncology (e.g., treating bone metastasis or colorectal cancer). What makes this book distinct is the concise way in which the chapters are written and organized. The material included is so pertinent to both an academic and general practice interventionalist. The editors have produced a book that is a thorough summary of the salient techniques, results, potential complications, and expectations of success.

Interventional Oncology is a great book to read and a must-have for those interested and practicing in interventional oncology.

Peter R. Mueller, MD
Professor of Radiology
Harvard Medical School
Massachusetts General Hospital
Division Head Interventional Radiology

Series Preface

For decades, practitioners have used classic textbooks of several thousand pages to study interventional radiology. We, however, identified a great need for small, subject-focused, and clinically oriented guides to help practitioners and trainees master key skills on the job. We envisioned portable, printed books that could easily be carried to the clinic, procedure suite, and inpatient ward, as well as new technologies that would enable access on any phone, tablet, or computer.

This Practical Guides in Interventional Radiology Series will be extremely valuable for residents, fellows, practicing physicians, and midlevel practitioners who are currently involved in or look forward to specializing in areas within the interventional radiology spectrum. Book chapters systematically cover indications, contraindications, patient selection and preprocedure workup, procedural technique, postprocedure management and follow-up, side effects and complications, clinical data and outcomes, and key references.

Interventional oncology (IO) has been an area of tremendous growth and interest over the last 20 years —considered by some to be its own subspecialty. I am very pleased to see that both classic IO and the latest advances and procedures are so well represented in our Interventional Oncology volume.

Our editors, Suvranu Ganguli, MD, of Massachusetts General Hospital, Harvard Medical School, and Ripal Gandhi, MD, of Miami Cardiac and Vascular Institute, did a wonderful job working with a stellar group of authors and thought leaders in the field.

We hope that readers find our Practical Guides in Interventional Radiology Series to be a new and improved way to master procedures and clinical care skills in a focused and time-efficient manner.

Salomão Faintuch, MD, MSc
Series Editor–Practical Guides in
Interventional Radiology
Assistant Professor of Radiology
Beth Israel Deaconess Medical Center
Boston, Massachusetts
Harvard Medical School
Clinical Director of Interventional Radiology

Preface

Interventional oncology is an exciting, fast-growing, and rapidly changing area within our specialty of interventional radiology. Interventional oncology uses image-guided techniques to diagnose and treat localized cancers in targeted and minimally invasive ways. The specialty of interventional oncology had its origins in the development of specific treatments for hepatocellular carcinoma, including transarterial chemoembolization and percutaneous alcohol injection, well before the term *interventional oncology* had ever been recognized. Interventional oncology has expanded far beyond its scattered origins, with the mature specialty now comprising a variety of new treatment technologies and incorporating the full clinical care of the oncology patient before, during, and after treatment. Supported by ever-increasing clinical expertise and clinical trial data, interventional oncology is cementing its place as one of the four pillars of comprehensive, multidisciplinary cancer care—medical oncology, radiation oncology, surgical oncology, and interventional oncology.

Given the rapidly advancing field, we envisioned this textbook on interventional oncology to be succinct, clinically focused, and image-rich. We wanted to create a concise resource on interventional oncology that could be used by trainees as well as seasoned interventional radiologists starting or expanding an interventional oncology practice. Each chapter is laid out with a similar format, including indications, contraindications, patient selection, preprocedure workup, technique (including equipment), postprocedure management and follow-up evaluation, side effects and complications, clinical data and outcomes, pearls, and references. The layout makes for high-yield preparation before seeing the oncology patient in clinical consultation before any proposed intervention, as well as knowing what to expect and look for in terms of patient management after the procedure.

We compiled a fabulous and experienced group of authors for the chapters of this book—international leaders and experts in the area. We hope that you find this book a valuable addition and resource for your interventional oncology practice.

Ripal T. Gandhi, MD
Suvranu Ganguli, MD

Contributors

Fereidoun Abtin, MD
Associate Professor
UCLA Department of Radiological Sciences
David Geffen School of Medicine
Los Angeles, California

Muneeb Ahmed, MD
Chief
Division of Vascular and Interventional Radiology
Beth Israel Deaconess Medical Center
Assistant Professor of Radiology
Harvard Medical School
Boston, Massachusetts

Shawn Ahmed, MD, PhD
Clinical Fellow
Vascular and Interventional Radiology
Massachusetts General Hospital
Boston, Massachusetts

Karen Brown, MD
Professor of Radiology
Weill-Cornell Medical College
Cornell University
Attending Physician
Interventional Radiology
MH Member
Memorial Sloan Kettering Cancer Center
New York, New York

Matthew Brown, MD
Resident
Department of Radiology
University of Colorado School of Medicine
Anschutz Medical Campus
Aurora, Colorado

Matthew R. Callstrom, MD, PhD
Professor of Radiology
Mayo Clinic College of Medicine
Rochester, Minnesota

Arash Eftekhari, MD, FRCPC
Department of Radiology
University of British Columbia
Department of Radiology
Vancouver General Hospital
Vancouver, British Columbia
Canada

Salomão Faintuch, MD, MSc—SERIES EDITOR
Assistant Professor of Radiology
Beth Israel Deaconess Medical Center
Boston, Massachusetts
Harvard Medical School
Clinical Director of Interventional Radiology

Ripal T. Gandhi, MD, FSVM—EDITOR
Attending Physician
Vascular and Interventional Radiology
Miami Cardiac and Vascular Institute
Associate Clinical Professor
Herbert Wertheim College of Medicine at Florida
    International University
Assistant Clinical Professor
University of South Florida School of Medicine
Miami, Florida

Suvranu Ganguli, MD– EDITOR
Associate Chief of Interventional Radiology
Co-Director, Center for Image-Guided Cancer Therapy
Massachusetts General Hospital
Assistant Professor of Radiology
Harvard Medical School
Boston, Massachusetts

Scott Genshaft, MD
Assistant Professor
Radiology
UCLA Department of Radiological Sciences
David Geffen School of Medicine
Los Angeles, California

Debra A. Gervais, MD
Division Chief
Abdominal Imaging
Department of Radiology
Massachusetts General Hospital
Boston, Massachusetts

Rajan K. Gupta, MD
Assistant Professor
Department of Radiology
University of Colorado School of Medicine
Anschutz Medical Campus
Aurora, Colorado

Antonio Gutierrez, MD
Assistant Professor, Radiology
UCLA Department of Radiological Sciences
David Geffen School of Medicine
Los Angeles, California

Steven L. Hsu, MD, MBA
Assistant Professor
Radiology
University of Texas Southwestern Medical Center
Dallas, Texas

Sanjeeva P. Kalva, MD, FSIR
Chief
Interventional Radiology
Associate Professor of Radiology
University of Texas Southwestern Medical Center
Dallas, Texas

Darren Klass, MD, PhD
Clinical Assistant Professor
University of British Columbia
Division of Interventional Radiology
Vancouver General Hospital
Vancouver, British Columbia
Canada

Matthew J. Kogut, MD
Assistant Professor
Interventional Radiology
University of Washington
Seattle, Washington

A. Nicholas Kurup, MD
Assistant Professor of Radiology
Mayo Clinic College of Medicine
Rochester, Minnesota

Edward Wolfgang Lee, MD, PhD
Assistant Professor
Interventional Radiology
UCLA Department of Radiological Sciences
David Geffen School of Medicine
Los Angeles, California

Riccardo Lencioni, MD, FSIR, EBIR
Professor and Director
Division of Diagnostic Imaging and Intervention
Pisa University Hospital and School of Medicine
Pisa, Italy

David Liu, MD, FRCPC, FSIR
Clinical Associate Professor
Department of Radiology
University of British Columbia
Vancouver Imaging LLC
Vancouver, British Columbia
Canada

Charles McGraw, MD, MBA
Fellow
Miami Cardiac and Vascular Institute
Miami, Florida

Prasoon P. Mohan, MD, MRCS (Eng.)
Clinical Instructor
Vascular and Interventional Radiology
University of Miami/Miller School of Medicine
Miami, Florida

Govindarajan Narayanan, MD
Chief
Vascular and Interventional Radiology
Associate Professor of Clinical Radiology
Program Director
Vascular Interventional Radiology Fellowship
University of Miami
Miller School of Medicine
Miramar, Florida

Rahmi Oklu, MD, PhD
Assistant Professor of Radiology
Harvard Medical School
Interventional Radiologist
Massachusetts General Hospital
Boston, Massachusetts

Siddharth A. Padia, MD
Associate Professor
Interventional Radiology
University of Washington
Seattle, Washington

Elena N. Petre, MD
Senior Research Scientist
Department of Radiology
Memorial Sloan Kettering Cancer Center
Section of Interventional Radiology
New York, New York

Charles E. Ray Jr., MD, PhD
Professor
Department of Radiology
University of Illinois at Chicago
Chairman of Radiology
University of Illinois Medical Center
Chicago, Illinois

Paul J. Rochon, MD
Assistant Professor, Radiology
University of Colorado School of Medicine
Anschutz Medical Campus
Aurora, Colorado

Constantinos Sofocleous, MD, PhD, FSIR, FCIRSE
Professor of Radiology
Weill-Cornell Medical College
Cornell University
Attending Physician, Interventional Radiology
MH Member
Memorial Sloan Kettering Cancer Center
New York, New York

Robert Suh, MD
Professor, Clinical Radiology
Director, Diagnostic Radiology Training Program
Director, Thoracic Interventional Services
University of California, Los Angeles
UCLA Department of Radiological Sciences
David Geffen School of Medicine
Ronald Reagan UCLA Medical Center
Los Angeles, California

Avnesh S. Thakor, BA, MA, MSc, MD, PhD, MB, BChir, FHEA, FRCR(IR)
Assistant Professor
Division of Interventional Radiology, Department of Radiology
Lucile Packard Children's Hospital and Stanford University Medical Center
Stanford, California

Raul N. Uppot, MD
Assistant Professor
Harvard Medical School
Director, Abdominal Imaging Fellowship
Associate Director, Harvard Medical School Core Radiology Clerkship
Boston, Massachusetts

Aradhana M. Venkatesan, MD
Associate Professor, Term Tenure Track
Section of Abdominal Imaging
Department of Diagnostic Radiology
MD Anderson Cancer Center
Houston, Texas

Bradford J. Wood, MD
Chief
Interventional Radiology
Director
Center for Interventional Oncology, Radiology and Imaging Sciences
NIH Clinical Center and National Cancer Institute
National Institutes of Health
Bethesda, Maryland

Omar Zurkiya, MD, PhD
Instructor
Division of Interventional Radiology
Massachusetts General Hospital
Harvard Medical School
Boston, Massachusetts

Chapter 1

Percutaneous Ablation of Renal Cell Carcinoma

1

1 Percutaneous Ablation of Renal Cell Carcinoma

Shawn Ahmed, Raul N. Uppot, and Debra A. Gervais

1.1 Introduction

Renal cell carcinoma (RCC) accounts for approximately 4% of all adult malignancies, with more than 65,000 estimated new cases projected in the United States in 2015, resulting in nearly 14,000 deaths during the same period of time.[1] The disease is more common in men than in women.[1] Risk factors include hypertension, smoking, obesity, and hemodialysis in patients with end-stage renal disease. Patients with certain genetic syndromes, such as von Hippel–Lindau (VHL) disease,

have a high incidence of multiple and recurrent tumors. The classic presentation is the triad of flank pain, hematuria, and palpable abdominal mass. Other symptoms include loss of appetite, weight loss, anemia, and fatigue. Four dominant RCC subtypes have been identified, with the clear cell variety representing about 75% of cases.[2]

Renal malignancies are staged using the TNM staging system (▶ Table 1.1).[3] Approximately one-fifth of patients present with advanced disease and have associated poor 5-year survival.[1] The increased use of cross-sectional imaging, however,

Table 1.1 TNM classification of renal cell carcinoma

Primary tumor (T)	
TX	Primary tumor cannot be assessed
T0	No evidence of primary tumor
T1	Tumor ≤ 7 cm in greatest dimension, limited to the kidney
T1a	Tumor ≤ 4 cm in greatest dimension, limited to the kidney
T1b	Tumor > 4 cm but ≤ 7 cm in greatest dimension, limited to the kidney
T2	Tumor > 7 cm in greatest dimension, limited to the kidney
T2a	Tumor > 7 cm but ≤ 10 cm in greatest dimension
T2b	Tumor > 10 cm, limited to the kidney
T3	Tumor extends into major veins or perinephric tissues but not into the ipsilateral adrenal gland and not beyond Gerota's fascia
T3a	Tumor grossly extends into the renal vein or its segmental (muscle-containing) branches, or tumor invades perirenal and/or renal sinus fat but not beyond Gerota's fascia
T3b	Tumor grossly extends into the vena cava below the diaphragm
T3c	Tumor grossly extends into the vena cava above the diaphragm or invades the wall of the vena cava
T4	Tumor invades beyond Gerota's fascia (including contiguous extension into the ipsilateral adrenal gland)
Regional lymph nodes (N)	
NX	Regional lymph nodes cannot be assessed
N0	No regional lymph node metastasis
N1	Metastasis to regional lymph node(s)
Distant metastasis (M)	
M0	No distant metastasis
M1	Distant metastasis

has led to earlier detection. Currently, more than half of all renal masses are discovered incidentally,[4] with as many as 80% of patients presenting with localized, low-stage disease.[1] Early detection of small, organ-confined tumors has led to the development of nephron-sparing treatment options. Partial nephrectomy has shown comparable long-term survival when compared to radical nephrectomy in the treatment of organ-confined, stage I and II tumors,[5,6,7] and has thus become the treatment of choice for these patients. Image-guided percutaneous ablation is also fast becoming an accepted treatment option for select patients with small tumors.[8,9,10,11,12,13,14,15,16,17,18,19] These methods offer a number of advantages over surgery. First, percutaneous ablation has been shown to be associated with fewer complications and faster recovery compared to surgery.[8] The procedures can also be repeated when not completely successful or in syndromic patients with recurrent tumors. Importantly, there is some evidence to suggest that renal function in patients with solitary kidneys is better preserved following ablation as compared to partial nephrectomy.[20] Finally, percutaneous ablation may be the only local treatment option in patients who are poor surgical candidates.

Several percutaneous ablative methods have been described, including radiofrequency ablation (RFA), cryoablation, microwave ablation, and high-intensity, focused ultrasound ablation. The largest experience to date has been with RFA and cryoablation, with hundreds of cases reported in the literature.[8,9,10,11,12,13,14,15,16,17,18,19,20,21,22,23,24,25,26,27,28,29,30,31,32,33,34,35,36,37,38,39,40,41,42,43,44,45,46,47,48,49,50,51,52,53,54,55,56,57,58,59,60,61,62,63,64,65,66,67,68] There are comparatively limited data on the effectiveness of percutaneous microwave ablation and high-intensity focused ultrasound.[16,69,70,71,72,73,74,75,76] Several investigators have reported the short-term and mid-term effectiveness of both RFA and cryoablation of small renal masses with favorable results.[8,9,10,11,12,13,14,15,16,17,18,19,20,21,22,23,24,25,26,27,29,30,31,32,33,34,35,36,37,38,39,40,41,42,43,44,45,46,47,48,49,50,51,52,53,54,55,56,57,58,59,60,62,63,65,66,67,77,78] Long-term survival data (> 5 years) following RCC ablation is sparse; however, early studies have shown promise.[13,28,61,64,77] To date, there is no compelling evidence to suggest superiority of one ablative method over another. A recent meta-analysis comparing RFA and cryoablation demonstrated similar clinical efficacy and complication rates.[79] As such, the choice between RFA or cryoablation is often driven by physician preference and local practice patterns.

1.2 Indications

Surgical resection remains the standard of care for RCC treatment given the lack of robust, long-term survival and disease-free survival data with percutaneous ablation procedures. Percutaneous ablation is thus limited to patients who are not ideal surgical candidates. Formal indications for the use of percutaneous ablation in the treatment of RCC have yet to be validated with prospective scientific studies.[33] Percutaneous ablation therapies are, however, considered appropriate for use in elderly patients, in patients with comorbid conditions that preclude surgery, in individuals with a solitary kidney or renal insufficiency, and in patients with multiple or recurrent tumors as with VHL disease. Additionally, ablation is usually performed in patients with a > 1-year life expectancy, because a small RCC is unlikely to cause clinically significant morbidity before 1 year.[14]

In addition to the patient-specific criteria already listed, there are tumor-specific criteria, such as lesion size and location, that are also important in determining the feasibility of percutaneous intervention. Multiple studies have shown decreased effectiveness of RFA with increasing tumor size.[14,15,16,17,19,20,21,23,34,35,36,37,53,55] Zagoria et al[17] reported a technical success rate with RFA ablation of 100% in tumors < 3 cm as compared to 69% with tumors > 3 cm. In a retrospective study of 100 tumors treated with RFA, Gervais et al[14,15] found that tumor size was an independent predictor of RFA success. Ninety-two percent of tumors < 3 cm were successfully ablated in a single session, whereas 44% of tumors measuring 3 to 5 cm required more than one ablative session for complete eradication. Tumors > 5 cm invariably required more than one session.

Tumor location is also important in determining the success of an ablative procedure. Gervais et al showed that a noncentral location is an independent predictor of complete tumor necrosis.[14,15] This is believed to be due in part to insulation of the exophytic tumor by surrounding perirenal fat allowing generation of higher ablative temperatures. Poor treatment outcomes with centrally located tumors in turn may be the result of a "heat sink" effect of blood flow in hilar vessels causing perfusion-mediated tumor cooling.[80] A retrospective study of 115 renal tumors treated with cryoablation reported similar results with regard to tumor size and position.[39] In the study, Atwell et al reported technical success in 112 of 115 tumors (97%). The three technical failures occurred in central tumors, two of which were > 4 cm. Other considerations include the proximity of central tumors to the collecting system, ureter, and central renal vasculature, which increases the risk of complication, including significant hemorrhage and ureteral injury. On the other hand, injury to adjacent organs or bowel is a concern with some exophytic masses.

1.3 Contraindications

Absolute contraindications to percutaneous renal ablation include uncorrected coagulopathy and acute illness.[33] Serious comorbidities (e.g., congestive heart failure, pulmonary hypertension, cardiac arrhythmias) can be considered a relative contraindication necessitating assessment on a case by case basis. High-risk patients may benefit from close monitoring by anesthesiology personnel. Patients with large tumors, as already discussed, may be better served by surgical resection. By the same token, local tumor spread beyond Gerota's fascia or distant metastatic spread may preclude curative intent. Ablation may still be indicated with advanced disease, with the purpose of debulking or for palliation to control pain or hematuria.[81]

1.4 Patient Selection and Preprocedure Workup

All potential ablation patients are evaluated in the interventional radiology clinic in the weeks or months leading up to the procedure. The clinic visit is an opportunity for the physician to develop a rapport with the patient as well as the patient's family. The proposed procedure, including the risks, benefits, and alternatives, is discussed in detail with the patient. A detailed medical history is obtained and a full physical exam performed. Additionally, every patient should undergo contrast-enhanced computed tomography (CT) or magnetic resonance imaging (MRI) for tumor staging, and appropriate laboratory tests should be ordered.

1.4.1 Laboratory Studies

Appropriate blood tests include a complete blood count (CBC), coagulation studies, and renal function tests. Anticoagulants and antiplatelet agents are discontinued far enough in advance of the procedure for coagulation parameters and function to

return to normal.[32] Given the elective nature of the procedure and the hypervascularity of RCCs, it is reasonable to postpone the procedure in the setting of markedly abnormal laboratory findings, such as an international normalized ratio (INR) > 1.5 or a platelet count < 50 × 103/μL. If necessary, fresh frozen plasma and platelets can be administered prior to or during the procedure.

Patients being considered for percutaneous ablation often have abnormal renal function. It is important to assess renal function prior to the procedure with a serum creatinine and estimated glomerular filtration rate (GFR) because this will help to guide the procedural approach and imaging follow-up. Iodinated contrast may be used during CT-guided ablation to define the tumor margins before applicator placement or during the procedure to assess whether the tumor has been successfully ablated. In the case of cryoablation, contrast is not used as frequently because the ice ball is well seen with both unenhanced CT and MRI.[9,11,12,41,42,43,44,45,46,47,48,49,50,51,82]

1.4.2 Preprocedure Biopsy

There is some controversy regarding the need for a biopsy prior to percutaneous ablation. However, given that a substantial fraction of small, solid masses are benign,[83] it seems prudent to obtain a tissue diagnosis in most cases. This not only has the advantage of decreasing unnecessary treatment in patients with benign neoplasms, such as angiomyolipoma or oncocytoma, it also allows tumor subtyping and grading in the case of malignancy, information that can be used to tailor future treatment and surveillance.[84] The timing of the biopsy is also somewhat controversial; some advocate tissue sampling prior to ablation,[85] whereas others favor performing both procedures on the same day.[86] In most circumstances, it seems reasonable to obtain a biopsy in advance of the ablation because this provides the pathologist more time to analyze the specimen with special staining, and, in the case of a benign diagnosis, it obviates the need for an additional clinic visit and further workup.[87] On the other hand, if the probability of renal cancer is extremely high, as in the case of a suspicious mass in a patient with VHL disease, same-day biopsy may be a reasonable approach .

1.4.3 Prophylactic Antibiotics

Periprocedural administration of prophylactic antibiotics is another topic of debate.[32] Some practitioners favor empirical antibiotic use in all patients, whereas others reserve prophylaxis for select, high-risk cases.[88,89] At our institution, antibiotics are given only to patients who are felt to be at increased risk of infection. This includes patients with a history of ileal conduit and ureteral stent placement. Some have advocated that patients with diabetes and those with a history of chronic immunosuppression also warrant consideration for extended antibiotic coverage tailored toward gram-negative enterics.[54]

1.5 Technique

Many ablation procedures can be performed on an outpatient basis using conscious sedation. General anesthesia is usually reserved for high-risk patients. At our institution, patients are required to have nothing by mouth for 8 hours prior to the procedure. A peripheral intravenous (IV) catheter is placed in the outpatient holding area, and prophylactic antibiotics and hydration are instituted if necessary.

A number of factors determine the choice of the ablative therapy and equipment, including equipment availability as well as operator experience and preference. Though other technologies, such as high-intensity focused ultrasound (HIFU) and microwave ablation have been described, RFA and cryoablation are the most widely available and studied. Each has its own advantages though, as mentioned earlier; there is no convincing evidence to suggest superiority of one method over the other. Based on the current available evidence, both cryoablation and RFA are likely to be equally effective in technical adequacy and in oncological control.[79]

1.5.1 Radiofrequency Ablation

Tumor RFA involves the delivery of an electrical current to the tissue, resulting in agitation of intracellular molecules and frictional heating.[33] High tissue temperatures are achieved by placing needle-like electrodes into the tumor. The electrodes are connected to a radiofrequency generator, and the circuit is completed using grounding pads on the patient's thighs. Cell death occurs at temperatures > 45°C with complete tumor necrosis being achieved at 60 to 100°C .

The type of RF electrode chosen for a particular treatment depends on the size of the target tumor and the preference of the operator. Small ablations can be performed using linear electrodes, whereas multitined electrodes are available in various sizes from 2 to 7 cm (▶ Fig. 1.1a–d). Overlapping ablations are used for larger tissue volumes with the general aim of obtaining a 0.5 to 1 cm circumferential treatment margin beyond the tumor edge. Some operators elect to perform track ablation while withdrawing the RFA electrode, which may reduce the risk of track seeding and bleeding complications.

1.5.2 Cryoablation

Cryoablation works by exposing tissues to rapid freeze–thaw cycles resulting in cell death by a combination of cellular dehydration, cell membrane rupture, and vascular thrombosis.[89] Cell death occurs at temperatures between − 20 and − 40°C.[9] The procedure involves the placement of cryoprobes (▶ Fig. 1.2a–d) into the tumor under imaging guidance and takes advantage of the so-called Joule–Thomson effect.[9] The tissue is first cooled when high-pressure argon gas is converted to cold, low-pressure liquid. This is subsequently followed by a thawing cycle when a cold, high-pressure gas, such as helium, is converted to a warm, low-pressure gas.

One advantage of cryoablation is the ability to visualize the ice ball under image guidance. The ice ball has a nonlethal leading edge and a lethal zone 5 mm inside the edge of the visible margin.[89] As such, it is recommended that the ice ball extend at least 5 mm and preferably 1 cm beyond the margin of the tumor to ensure adequate treatment. This is achieved by varying the size, number, and position of the cryoprobes. Small (< 2 cm) tumors may be adequately treated with as few as two appropriately sized cryoprobes, whereas larger tumors often require the use of multiple probes. Cryoablation applicators are placed approximately 1.5 to 2 cm apart for optimal freezing, and a treatment typically consists of two to three freeze–thaw cycles.

As already mentioned, one of the advantages of cryoablation is the ability to visualize the ice ball by ultrasound, CT, and MRI. This increases the potential for complete tumor treatment and minimizes the risk of injury to adjacent structures. Cryoablation applicators can also be individually controlled, allowing the operator to achieve an ice ball that matches the geometry of the tumor. Finally, cryoablation does not require the use of the grounding pads; hence skin burns are not an issue with this procedure.

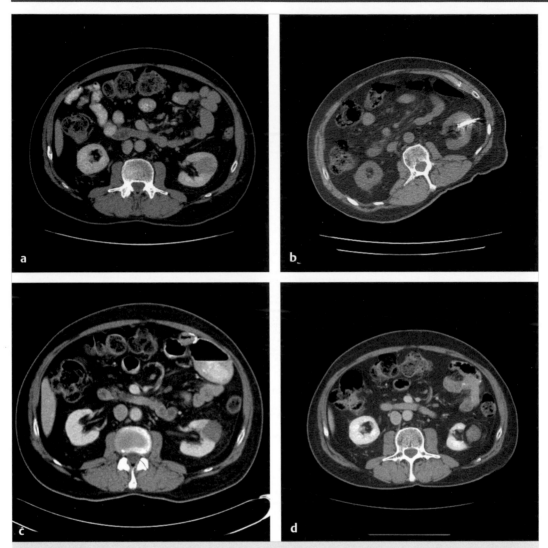

Fig. 1.1 Renal cell carcinoma (RCC) radiofrequency ablation (RFA). **(a)** Axial contrast-enhanced computed tomography (CT) demonstrating a 2 cm enhancing left RCC in a 60-year-old man. **(b)** Intraprocedural nonenhanced CT scan obtained at a slightly oblique position at time of RFA shows a cluster probe within the left renal mass. A total of three 12-minute, overlapping ablations were performed. **(c)** One-month follow-up contrast-enhanced CT showing a nonenhancing lesion at the ablation zone in the left kidney with no evidence of residual tumor. **(d)** Contrast-enhanced CT scan 4 years following RFA showing a small residual nonenhancing soft tissue mass with a surrounding halo of fat in the left kidney giving the classic pseudo-angiomyolipoma (AML) appearance.

1.6 Imaging Guidance

CT, MRI, or ultrasound can be used for image guidance of percutaneous ablation therapy. The choice typically depends on a combination of equipment availability as well as operator experience and comfort. Each modality has its advantages and disadvantages.

CT is the most commonly used modality for ablation guidance. It has the advantage of being widely available and offering good contrast and spatial resolution allowing accurate depiction of the tumor and surrounding structures. An initial noncontrast CT scan is acquired after placement of a radiopaque grid on the skin. This allows the operator to determine the ideal skin entry site,

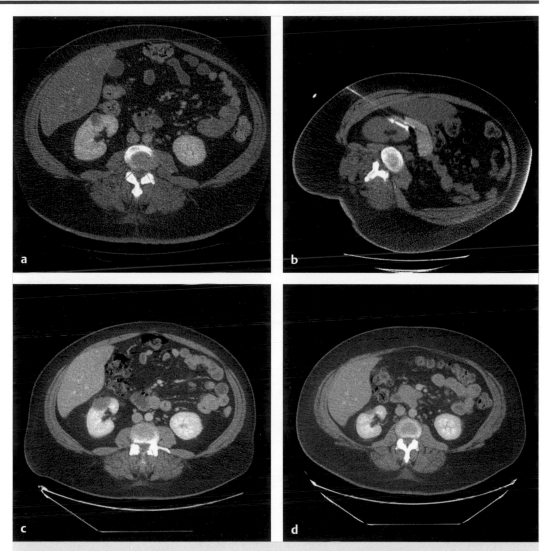

Fig. 1.2 Renal cell carcinoma (RCC) cryoablation. **(a)** Axial contrast-enhanced computed tomography (CT) demonstrating a 1.9 cm heterogeneously enhancing mass in the right kidney In a 44-year-old woman. **(b)** Intraprocedural nonenhanced CT scan with the patient in the contralateral oblique position. A cryoprobe is visualized within the right renal mass. Slightly more anteriorly, a 20-gauge Chiba needle has been inserted, and hydrodissection is being performed with the injection of a mixture of normal saline and Isovue contrast with the intent of displacing the colon and liver away from the ablation zone. The ablation involved two 10-minute freeze cycles separated by an 8-minute thaw. **(c)** Axial contrast-enhanced CT at 1 month postablation showing a small residual nonenhancing mass with no evidence of residual tumor. **(d)** Two-year follow-up contrast-enhanced CT showing a further decrease in size of the right renal ablation zone with no evidence of tumor recurrence.

trajectory, and distance to the tumor. The main limitation of CT is that RFA cannot be monitored. With cryoablation, the growing ice ball can be visualized in soft tissue, but it is not well seen in perinephric fat.[90]

MRI can also be used to guide renal ablations.[44,52,91,92] MRI has the advantage of improved soft tissue contrast, lack of ionizing radiation, and multiplanar and near-real-time imaging capabilities.[89] The effects of both RFA and cryoablation are well visualized on MRI. Specialized temperature-sensitive sequences allow real-time monitoring of ablation zone temperatures with both RFA and cryoablation. With cryoablation, the ice ball is low signal on both T1- and T2-weighted spin-echo sequences.[44,52] The ice ball is also better visualized in the perinephric fat with MRI than with CT. The disadvantages of MRI guidance include its relatively high cost, the need for specialized MRI-compatible equipment, and limitations with electrocardiographic (ECG) monitoring of patients.

Although ultrasound guidance offers some advantages, including rapid probe placement, real-time visualization, and lack of ionizing radiation, the use of this modality is somewhat limited. Small tumors and adjacent structures are often suboptimally visualized with ultrasound. Additionally, acoustic shadowing from tissue gas or ice often prevents visualization of deeper structures.[58] In most cases, CT and MRI provide safer, more accurate tumor targeting and are the favored modalities for image guidance.

1.7 Patient Positioning

Patient positioning is dependent on the location of the tumor. Upper-pole tumors are often best approached with the patient in the ipsilateral decubitus (ipsilateral side down) position. This results in relative deflation of the dependent lung, thereby decreasing the chance of pleural transgression and pneumothorax. The prone and supine positions tend to be the most comfortable for the patient. The prone position often allows easy targeting of lower-pole masses with a subcostal approach, whereas the supine position may be useful for targeting lateral or anterior masses. Occasionally, angling the gantry may facilitate targeting, particularly when a subcostal approach is taken. Oblique positioning with the ipsilateral side up can be useful in treating anterior lesions close to the bowel because the position allows the bowel to fall medially and away from the kidney.[89]

1.8 Postprocedure Management and Follow-up Evaluation

Percutaneous ablations are often performed on an outpatient basis with conscious sedation in low-risk patients. In these cases, the patient is observed in the recovery room for 2 to 3 hours following the procedure, during which time vital signs are monitored. In high-risk patients with associated comorbidities, monitored anesthesia care (MAC) or general anesthesia may be appropriate. Some of these patients are also discharged home the same day; however, if there is any concern, overnight observation may be warranted. Following discharge, patients are typically seen in the Interventional Radiology (IR) clinic between 1 week and 1 month postprocedure. The patient is assessed for pain, signs of infection, and urinary symptoms, including hematuria and difficulty urinating. In addition, a follow-up CT or MRI scan is obtained at the first follow-up appointment.

Posttreatment imaging is vital for assessing the zone of ablation, monitoring for recurrence, and evaluating for complications. The choice of imaging depends on multiple factors, including equipment availability and patient renal function. CT is the most commonly used imaging modality for follow-up evaluation. It is widely available and provides high-resolution depiction of the ablation zone and surrounding tissues. The major disadvantages of CT include the use of ionizing radiation and the nephrotoxic effects of iodinated IV contrast. The main advantage of MRI is the lack of ionizing radiation, which becomes a consideration in these patients because they will require indefinite imaging follow-up. After the initial follow-up examination, we image patients at 3, 6, and 12 months, then yearly thereafter. CT imaging includes noncontrast as well as contrast-enhanced imaging in the nephrogenic and excretory phases. The MRI protocol should include precontrast T1- and T2-weighted as well as multiphasic postcontrast imaging. Subtraction images may also be useful.

Postablation imaging often demonstrates a residual small, nonenhancing mass at the ablation site (► Fig. 1.1c and ► Fig. 1.2c). On CT imaging, there may be hyperdense nonenhancing areas consistent with denatured proteins. Immediate postablation, MRI may demonstrate a smooth thin rim of enhancement representing hyperemia, which may persist for several months.[93] Residual or recurrent tumor is seen as crescentic or nodular enhancement at the periphery of the zone of ablation.[15] Dessication of tissues following both RFA and cryoablation results in T1 and T2 shortening on MRI. Thus ablated tissue is typically T1 hyperintense and T2 hypointense, whereas viable tumor tends to be T2 hyperintense. Rarely, a tumor may undergo liquefactive necrosis that is seen as T2-hyperintense signal. Such cases may complicate the evaluation of treatment response and short-term follow-up, or, ultimately, biopsy may be required to exclude residual or recurrent tumor.[80]

Perirenal and pararenal fat stranding is a common finding on postablation CT and is the normal result of thermally induced fat necrosis. Over time, this may coalesce into a dominant halo aligned parallel with the surface of the kidney, giving a so-called pseudo-angiomyolipoma (AML) appearance (▶ Fig. 1.1**d**).[80] It is important to recognize that this appearance represents an inflammatory reaction with encapsulation of surrounding fat necrosis and not tumor capsule.[80] Benign inflammatory nodules are seen along the ablation tract on follow-up imaging in an estimated 1.9% of cases.[94] This so-called pseudoseeding is considerably more common than true tumor seeding (0.01%) and may have a nodular appearance following RFA or a tram-track appearance after cryoablation.[94] Unfortunately, pseudoseeding and true tumor seeding are not distinguishable by imaging alone, thus necessitating short-interval imaging follow-up or, in some cases, tissue sampling for diagnosis.

1.9 Side Effects and Complications

The most common complications associated with percutaneous ablation procedures involve pain and paresthesias at the probe insertion site.[8,9,10,11, 12,13,14,15,16,17,18,19,20,21,22,23,31,32,33,34,35,36,37,38,39,40,41,42, 43,44,45,46,47,48,49,50,51,52,53,54,55,56,57,58,59,60,61,62,63,64,95]

Other minor complications include transient hematuria, wound infection, and urinary tract infection. Approximately one-third of patients will experience so-called postablation syndrome, which is characterized by flulike symptoms, including low-grade fever, malaise, myalgia, nausea, and/or vomiting.[96] The symptoms are believed to be the result of a cytokine-mediated inflammatory response to tumor necrosis.[96] Symptoms typically present within 24 to 48 hours of the procedure, peak at 3 days, and spontaneously resolve within 5 to 7 days. Persistence of fever beyond day 10 is concerning and warrants evaluation for possible infection.[96]

Hemorrhage is the most common major complication[14,15,97] and may be subcapsular or perarenal, or it may extend into the renal collecting system. Hemorrhage into the trunk musculature is also seen. In a series of 100 tumors treated with RFA, Gervais et al[14] reported hemorrhage in five patients. Central tumors have a higher risk of hemorrhage due to their proximity to large central renal vessels.[15] The incidence of hemorrhage may also be slightly higher in patients treated with cryoablation compared with RFA, likely due to the cautery effects of RFA on blood vessels.[98] In a multi-institutional review of 139 cryoablation cases

and 133 radiofrequency ablation cases, Johnson et al[95] reported two cases of postprocedural hemorrhage, both following cryoablation. Large hemorrhage may require hospitalization, blood transfusion, or, rarely, vascular embolization.

Ureteral injury is the next most common potentially serious complication of ablation, typically presenting as either a small urinoma or hydronephrosis secondary to ureteral stricture.[15,19,55,95] Gervais et al[14] reported one case of ureteral stricture and one case of clinically significant urine leak. Management of a ureteral injury may include placement of a percutaneous nephrostomy tube or ureteral stent to decompress the kidney and placement of a percutaneous drainage catheter to drain any associated urinoma.

Other potential complications include inadvertent injury to adjacent organs, including the duodenum, liver, spleen, pancreas, or colon. Small pneumothoraxes may necessitate chest tube placement. Genitofemoral nerve injury is also an uncommonly reported complication following percutaneous ablation.[99] Patients present with chronic pain and tenderness as well as diminished sensitivity of the skin in the ipsilateral groin. Finally, tumor seeding of the applicator track is exceedingly rare, with very few instances reported in the literature.[19] The incidence of inflammatory nodules (pseudoseeding) is considerably higher, occurring in as many as 1.9% of cases.[94] As such, all nodules along the ablation tract are biopsied or followed closely rather than assumed to represent tumor seeding.[80]

1.10 Clinical Data and Outcomes

Percutaneous renal ablative techniques have been shown to be a good option for RCC treatment in a select patient population. The procedures are associated with less morbidity compared with open surgical or even laparoscopic tumor resection.[8,20, 65] Although long-term oncological data remain sparse, and randomized clinical trials are currently not available, multiple retrospective studies have been conducted looking at short- and intermediate-term outcomes with renal tumor ablation. Outcomes can be measured both by technical success of the procedure and by clinical effectiveness.

Technical success with ablative procedures is determined by the lack of enhancing tumor on early (e.g., 1 month) follow-up imaging. Technical success varies with tumor size and location with small, peripheral, exophytic tumors being more amenable to ablation compared to larger or more centrally located masses. In the report by Gervais et al[14] looking at RFA of 100 tumors, all 52 tumors less than 3 cm in size and all 68 exophytic tumors underwent complete necrosis with a single treatment. Up to 50% of large tumors (> 3 cm) required more than one ablation session to achieve complete necrosis. In a separate retrospective study of 105 renal tumors treated with RFA, 83 tumors (79%) were completely treated in a single session.[60] Twelve of the remaining tumors were successfully retreated for an overall technical success of 90.5%. Technical success in this study was clearly correlated with tumor size with all 73 tumors less than 3.5 cm in diameter successfully ablated in a single setting. Zagoria et al[10] reported similar results with 116 of 125 tumors (93%) completely ablated with RFA. All 95 RCCs less than 3.7 cm were completely ablated with a single session while 21 of 30 tumors > 3.7 cm required repeat sessions. Similar technical success rates have been reported with renal cryoablation. In their retrospective review of 115 renal tumors treated with percutaneous cryoablation, Atwell et al[39] reported a 97% technical success rate. The mean tumor size was 3.3 cm (range, 1.5–7.3 cm), with 29 treated tumors measuring 4 cm or larger. In a prospective, nonrandomized study of 120 renal tumors, Buy et al[63] reported a technical success rate of 94%. The mean tumor size in this study was 26 mm (range, 10–68 mm), including 20 tumors > 40 mm.

Clinical success can be measured by recurrence rates and survival. Current data suggest that renal RFA and cryoablation are effective treatments with acceptable short- to intermediate-term clinical success. In a recent retrospective study of 347 patients, Olweny et al[61] reported comparable 5-year disease-free survival rates with partial nephrectomy and RFA (82.1% and 85.4%, respectively; $p = 0.06$) in patients with T1a stage RCC. Sung et al[20] reported similar 3-year disease-free survival rates in patients with size- and location-matched renal masses following percutaneous RFA and open partial nephrectomy (94.7% and 98.9%, respectively; $p = 0.266$). As with technical success, long-term clinical success appears to be dependent on tumor size. In a retrospective study of 203 renal masses treated with RFA, Veltri et al[78] reported 3- and 5-year overall survival rates of 84% and 75%, cancer-specific survival of 96% and 91%, and disease-free survival of 80% and 75%, respectively. Five-year cancer-specific survival increased to 100% in the 79 patients with T1a disease stage.

Pearls ■

1. *Hydrodissection.* Performed by injecting liquid under image guidance into the tissues surrounding the kidney, with the goal of displacing critical structures away from the zone of ablation.
   - Recommend at least 1 to 1.5 cm of displacement of vital structures from the ablation zone.
   - Use nonionic solution like 5% dextrose in water (D5W) with RFA to prevent electrical current conduction.
   - Add a small amount of iodinated contrast to D5 W for opacification when using CT
   - guidance in order to distinguish D5 W from fluid in the bowel and from the ice ball (▶ Fig. 1.2b).
   - Remove metal needles placed for hydrodissection if performing RF to prevent electrical burns along the needle.
2. *Ureteral stent placement.* Retrograde placement of an end-hole ureteral stent by a urologist allows drip infusion of D5 W, which protects the renal collecting system and ureter with either a heat- or cold-sink effect. This technique is helpful in ablation of central renal tumors.
3. *Use the kidney's mobility to your advantage.*
   - **External manual displacement** With MRI guidance, the radiologist's hand can be used to displace critical structures away from the kidney.
   - **Using the ablation probe as a lever** Use the applicator as a lever to exert torque on the kidney and move the kidney away from adjacent structures.
   - **Using the "stick" function on the cryoprobe** After placing the cryoprobe, activating the "stick" function will result in the kidney being movable by pulling back on the applicator.
4. *Iatrogenic pneumothorax/pleural effusion.* Injecting air or D5 W into the pleural space through a 20-gauge needle can help prevent lung injury when treating upper pole masses.
5. *Review postprocedure imaging yourself.* Review follow-up imaging personally to avoid confusion with pseudo-AML or pseudoseeding.

In a retrospective analysis of 159 tumors treated by RFA, Best et al[62] found that disease-free survival was dependent on tumor size with significantly improved 3- and 5-year disease-free survival for tumors < 3 cm (96% and 95%, respectively) compared to tumors 3 cm or larger (79% and 79%, respectively). Similar results have been reported for cryoablation of renal tumors. In a retrospective analysis of 134 biopsy-proven renal cell carcinomas (median tumor size 2.8 ± 1.4 cm) treated with percutaneous cryoablation, Georgiades and Rodriguez[64] reported an overall 5-year survival of 97.8% and cancer-specific 5-year survival of 100%. Overall, for T1a tumors, oncological outcomes after ablation of renal tumors appear to be slightly inferior to outcomes with partial nephrectomy, but the slightly higher recurrence risk may be acceptable in patients who are not good candidates for surgery.

References

[1] National Cancer Institute. SEER Web site. http://seer.cancer.gov/statfacts/html/kidrp.html. Accessed December 27, 2013

[2] Renal and Urology News. CME articles. http://seer.cancer.gov/statfacts/html/kidrp.html. Accessed June 30, 2015. http://seer.cancer.gov/statfacts/html/kidrp.html. Accessed June 30, 2015.

[3] National Cancer Institute. Renal cell cancer treatment (PDQ). http://www.cancer.gov/cancertopics/pdq/treatment/renal-cell/HealthProfessional/page3. Accessed January 6, 2014

[4] Ahrar K, Wallace MJ, Matin SF. Percutaneous radiofrequency ablation: minimally invasive therapy for renal tumors. Expert Rev Anticancer Ther 2006; 6(12): 1735–1744

[5] Frank I, Blute ML, Leibovich BC, Cheville JC, Lohse CM, Zincke H. Independent validation of the 2002 American Joint Committee on cancer primary tumor classification for renal cell carcinoma using a large, single institution cohort. J Urol 2005; 173(6): 1889–1892

[6] Gill IS, Kavoussi LR, Lane BR et al. Comparison of 1,800 laparoscopic and open partial nephrectomies for single renal tumors. J Urol 2007; 178(1): 41–46

[7] Uzzo RG, Novick AC. Nephron sparing surgery for renal tumors: indications, techniques and outcomes. J Urol 2001; 166(1): 6–18

[8] Hui GC, Tuncali K, Tatli S, Morrison PR, Silverman SG. Comparison of percutaneous and surgical approaches to renal tumor ablation: metaanalysis of effectiveness and complication rates. J Vasc Interv Radiol 2008; 19(9): 1311–1320

[9] Littrup PJ, Ahmed A, Aoun HD et al. CT-guided percutaneous cryotherapy of renal masses. J Vasc Interv Radiol 2007; 18 (3): 383–392

[10] Zagoria RJ, Traver MA, Werle DM, Perini M, Hayasaka S, Clark PE. Oncologic efficacy of CT-guided percutaneous radiofrequency ablation of renal cell carcinomas. Am J Roentgenol 2007; 189(2): 429–436

[11] Gupta A, Allaf ME, Kavoussi LR et al. Computerized tomography guided percutaneous renal cryoablation with the patient under conscious sedation: initial clinical experience. J Urol 2006; 175(2): 447–452, discussion 452–453

[12] Silverman SG, Tuncali K, vanSonnenberg E et al. Renal tumors: MR imaging-guided percutaneous cryotherapy—initial experience in 23 patients. Radiology 2005; 236(2): 716–724

[13] McDougal WS, Gervais DA, McGovern FJ, Mueller PR. Long-term followup of patients with renal cell carcinoma treated with radio frequency ablation with curative intent. J Urol 2005; 174(1): 61–63

[14] Gervais DA, McGovern FJ, Arellano RS, McDougal WS, Mueller PR. Radiofrequency ablation of renal cell carcinoma: part 1, Indications, results, and role in patient management over a 6-year period and ablation of 100 tumors. Am J Roentgenol 2005; 185(1): 64–71

[15] Gervais DA, Arellano RS, McGovern FJ, McDougal WS, Mueller PR. Radiofrequency ablation of renal cell carcinoma: part 2, Lessons learned with ablation of 100 tumors. Am J Roentgenol 2005; 185(1): 72–80

[16] Farrell MA, Charboneau WJ, DiMarco DS et al. Imaging-guided radiofrequency ablation of solid renal tumors. Am J Roentgenol 2003; 180(6): 1509–1513

[17] Zagoria RJ, Hawkins AD, Clark PE et al. Percutaneous CT-guided radiofrequency ablation of renal neoplasms: factors influencing success. Am J Roentgenol 2004; 183(1): 201–207

[18] Su Li, Jarrett TW, Chan DY, Kavoussi LR, Solomon SB. Percutaneous computed tomography-guided radiofrequency ablation of renal masses in high surgical risk patients: preliminary results. Urology 2003; 61(4) Suppl 1: 26–33

[19] Mayo-Smith WW, Dupuy DE, Parikh PM, Pezzullo JA, Cronan JJ. Imaging-guided percutaneous radiofrequency ablation of solid renal masses: techniques and outcomes of 38 treatment sessions in 32 consecutive patients. Am J Roentgenol 2003; 180(6): 1503–1508

[20] Sung HH, Park BK, Kim CK, Choi HY, Lee HM. Comparison of percutaneous radiofrequency ablation and open partial nephrectomy for the treatment of size- and location-matched renal masses. Int J Hyperthermia 2012; 28(3): 227–234

[21] Seklehner S, Fellner H, Engelhardt PF, Schabauer C, Riedl C. Percutaneous radiofrequency ablation of renal tumors: a single-center experience. Korean J Urol 2013; 54(9): 580–586

[22] Schmit GD, Thompson RH, Boorjian SA et al. Percutaneous renal cryoablation in obese and morbidly obese patients. Urology 2013; 82(3): 636–641

[23] Wah TM, Irving HC, Gregory W, Cartledge J, Joyce AD, Selby PJ. Radiofrequency ablation (RFA) of renal cell carcinoma (RCC): experience in 200 tumours. BJU Int 201 4; 113(3): 416–428

[24] Atwell TD, Schmit GD, Boorjian SA et al. Percutaneous ablation of renal masses measuring 3.0 cm and smaller: comparative local control and complications after radiofrequency ablation and cryoablation. Am J Roentgenol 2013; 200(2): 461–466

[25] Schmit GD, Thompson RH, Kurup AN et al. Percutaneous cryoablation of solitary sporadic renal cell carcinomas. BJU Int 2012; 110 11 Pt B: E526–E531

[26] Zhao X, Wang W, Zhang S et al. Improved outcome of percutaneous radiofrequency ablation in renal cell carcinoma: a retrospective study of intraoperative contrast-enhanced ultrasonography in 73 patients. Abdom Imaging 2012; 37(5): 885–891

[27] Nitta Y, Tanaka T, Morimoto K et al. Intermediate oncological outcomes of percutaneous radiofrequency ablation for small renal tumors: initial experience. Anticancer Res 2012; 32(2): 615–618

[28] Zagoria RJ, Pettus JA, Rogers M, Werle DM, Childs D, Leyendecker JR. Long-term outcomes after percutaneous radiofrequency ablation for renal cell carcinoma. Urology 2011; 77 (6): 1393–1397

[29] Atwell TD, Callstrom MR, Farrell MA et al. Percutaneous renal cryoablation: local control at mean 26 months of follow-up. J Urol 2010; 184(4): 1291–1295

[30] Park BK, Kim CK. Percutaneous radio frequency ablation of renal tumors in patients with von Hippel-Lindau disease: preliminary results. J Urol 2010; 183(5): 1703–1707

[31] Mylona S, Kokkinaki A, Pomoni M, Galani P, Ntai S, Thanos L. Percutaneous radiofrequency ablation of renal cell carcinomas in patients with solitary kidney: 6 years experience. Eur J Radiol 2009; 69(2): 351–356

[32] Venkatesan AM, Wood BJ, Gervais DA. Percutaneous ablation in the kidney. Radiology 2011; 261(2): 375–391

[33] Zagoria RJ. Imaging-guided radiofrequency ablation of renal masses. Radiographics 2004; 24 Suppl 1: S59–S71

[34] Pavlovich CP, Walther M, Choyke PL et al. Percutaneous radio frequency ablation of small renal tumors: initial results. J Urol 2002; 167(1): 10–15

[35] Ogan K, Jacomides L, Dolmatch BL et al. Percutaneous radiofrequency ablation of renal tumors: technique, limitations, and morbidity. Urology 2002; 60(6): 954–958

[36] Roy-Choudhury SH, Cast JEI, Cooksey G, Puri S, Breen DJ. Early experience with percutaneous radiofrequency ablation of small solid renal masses. Am J Roentgenol 2003; 180(4): 1055–1061

[37] Gervais DA, McGovern FJ, Wood BJ, Goldberg SN, McDougal WS, Mueller PR. Radio-frequency ablation of renal cell carcinoma: early clinical experience. Radiology 2000; 217(3): 665–672

[38] Rouvière O, Badet L, Murat FJ et al. Radiofrequency ablation of renal tumors with an expandable multitined electrode: results, complications, and pilot evaluation of cooled pyeloperfusion for collecting system protection. Cardiovasc Intervent Radiol 2008; 31(3): 595–603

[39] Atwell TD, Farrell MA, Leibovich BC et al. Percutaneous renal cryoablation: experience treating 115 tumors. J Urol 2008; 179(6): 2136–2140, discussion 2140–2141

[40] Atwell TD, Farrell MA, Callstrom MR et al. Percutaneous cryoablation of large renal masses: technical feasibility and short-term outcome. Am J Roentgenol 2007; 188(5): 1195–1200

[41] Tacke J, Speetzen R, Heschel I, Hunter DW, Rau G, Günther RW. Imaging of interstitial cryotherapy—an in vitro comparison of ultrasound, computed tomography, and magnetic resonance imaging. Cryobiology 1999; 38(3): 250–259

[42] Saliken JC, McKinnon JG, Gray R. CT for monitoring cryotherapy. Am J Roentgenol 1996; 166(4): 853–855

[43] Permpongkosol S, Link RE, Kavoussi LR, Solomon SB. Percutaneous computerized tomography guided cryoablation for localized renal cell carcinoma: factors influencing success. J Urol 2006; 176(5): 1963–1968, discussion 1968

[44] Harada J, Dohi M, Mogami T et al. Initial experience of percutaneous renal cryosurgery under the guidance of a horizontal open MRI system. Radiat Med 2001; 19(6): 291–296

[45] Shingleton WB, Sewell PE, Jr. Percutaneous renal tumor cryoablation with magnetic resonance imaging guidance. J Urol 2001; 165(3): 773–776

[46] Shingleton WB, Sewell PE, Jr. Percutaneous renal cryoablation of renal tumors in patients with von Hippel-Lindau disease. J Urol 2002; 167(3): 1268–1270

[47] Shingleton WB, Sewell PE. Percutaneous cryoablation of renal cell carcinoma in a transplanted kidney. BJU Int 2002; 90 (1): 137–138

[48] Sewell PE, Howard JC, Shingleton WB, Harrison RB. Interventional magnetic resonance image-guided percutaneous cryoablation of renal tumors. South Med J 2003; 96(7): 708–710

[49] Shingleton WB, Sewell PE, Jr. Cryoablation of renal tumours in patients with solitary kidneys. BJU Int 2003; 92(3): 237–239

[50] Kodama Y, Abo D, Sakuhara Y et al. MR-guided percutaneous cryoablation for bilateral multiple renal cell carcinomas. Radiat Med 2005; 23(4): 303–307

[51] Miki K, Shimomura T, Yamada H et al. Percutaneous cryoablation of renal cell carcinoma guided by horizontal open magnetic resonance imaging. Int J Urol 2006; 13(7): 880–884

[52] Tuncali K, Morrison PR, Tatli S, Silverman SG. MRI-guided percutaneous cryoablation of renal tumors: use of external manual displacement of adjacent bowel loops. Eur J Radiol 2006; 59(2): 198–202

[53] Mayo-Smith WW, Dupuy DE, Parikh PM, Pezzullo JA, Cronan JJ. Imaging-guided percutaneous radiofrequency ablation of solid renal masses: techniques and outcomes of 38 treatment sessions in 32 consecutive patients. AJR Am J Roentgenol 2003; 180(6): 1503–1508

[54] Dupuy DE, Goldberg SN. Image-guided radiofrequency tumor ablation: challenges and opportunities—part II. J Vasc Interv Radiol 2001; 12(10): 1135–1148

[55] Gervais DA, McGovern FJ, Arellano RS, McDougal WS, Mueller PR. Renal cell carcinoma: clinical experience and technical success with radio-frequency ablation of 42 tumors. Radiology 2003; 226(2): 417–424

[56] Lewin JS, Nour SG, Connell CF et al. Phase II clinical trial of interactive MR imaging-guided interstitial radiofrequency thermal ablation of primary kidney tumors: initial experience. Radiology 2004; 232(3): 835–845

[57] Boss A, Clasen S, Kuczyk M et al. Magnetic resonance-guided percutaneous radiofrequency ablation of renal cell carcinomas: a pilot clinical study. Invest Radiol 2005; 40(9): 583–590

[58] Park BK, Kim CK, Lee HM. Image-guided radiofrequency ablation of Bosniak category III or IV cystic renal tumors: initial clinical experience. Eur Radiol 2008; 18(7): 1519–1525

[59] Merkle EM, Nour SG, Lewin JS. MR imaging follow-up after percutaneous radiofrequency ablation of renal cell carcinoma: findings in 18 patients during first 6 months. Radiology 2005; 235(3): 1065–1071

[60] Breen DJ, Rutherford EE, Stedman B et al. Management of renal tumors by image-guided radiofrequency ablation: experience in 105 tumors. Cardiovasc Intervent Radiol 2007; 30 (5): 936–942

[61] Olweny EO, Park SK, Tan YK, Best SL, Trimmer C, Cadeddu JA. Radiofrequency ablation versus partial nephrectomy in patients with solitary clinical T1a renal cell carcinoma: comparable oncologic outcomes at a minimum of 5 years of follow-up. Eur Urol 2012; 61(6): 1156–1161

[62] Best SL, Park SK, Youssef RF et al. Long-term outcomes of renal tumor radio frequency ablation stratified by tumor diameter: size matters [published correction appears in J Urol 2012;187(6):2284. Yaacoub, Ramy F corrected to Youssef, Ramy F]. J Urol 2012; 187(4): 1183–1189

[63] Buy X, Lang H, Garnon J, Sauleau E, Roy C, Gangi A. Percutaneous renal cryoablation: prospective experience treating 120 consecutive tumors. Am J Roentgenol 2013; 201(6): 1353–1361

[64] Georgiades CS, Rodriguez R. Efficacy and safety of percutaneous cryoablation for stage 1A/B renal cell carcinoma: results of a prospective, single-arm, 5-year study. Cardiovasc Intervent Radiol 2014; 37(6): 1494–1499

[65] Dominguez-Escrig JL, Sahadevan K, Johnson P. Cryoablation for small renal masses. Adv Urol 2008; 1: 479495

[66] Kunkle DA, Egleston BL, Uzzo RG. Excise, ablate or observe: the small renal mass dilemma—a meta-analysis and review. J Urol 2008; 179(4): 1227–1233, discussion 1233–1234

[67] Kunkle DA, Uzzo RG. Cryoablation or radiofrequency ablation of the small renal mass : a meta-analysis. Cancer 2008; 113(10): 2671–2680

[68] Carrafiello G, Mangini M, Fontana F et al. Single-antenna microwave ablation under contrast-enhanced ultrasound guidance for treatment of small renal cell carcinoma: preliminary experience. Cardiovasc Intervent Radiol 2010; 33(2): 367–374

[69] Liang P, Wang Y, Zhang D, Yu X, Gao Y, Ni X. Ultrasound guided percutaneous microwave ablation for small renal cancer: initial experience. J Urol 2008; 180(3): 844–848, discussion 848

[70] Terai A, Ito N, Yoshimura K et al. Laparoscopic partial nephrectomy using microwave tissue coagulator for small renal tumors: usefulness and complications. Eur Urol 2004; 45(6): 744–748

[71] Klatte T, Marberger M. High-intensity focused ultrasound for the treatment of renal masses: current status and future potential. Curr Opin Urol 2009; 19(2): 188–191

[72] Marberger M. Ablation of renal tumours with extracorporeal high-intensity focused ultrasound. BJU Int 2007; 99 5 Pt B: 1273–1276

[73] Guan W, Bai J, Liu J et al. Microwave ablation versus partial nephrectomy for small renal tumors: intermediate-term results. J Surg Oncol 2012; 106(3): 316 321

[74] Yu J, Liang P, Yu XL et al. US-guided percutaneous microwave ablation of renal cell carcinoma: intermediate-term results. Radiology 2012; 263(3): 900–908

[75] Lin Y, Liang P, Yu XL et al. Percutaneous microwave ablation of renal cell carcinoma is safe in patients with a solitary kidney. Urology 2014; 83(2): 357–363

[76] Li X, Liang P, Yu J et al. Role of contrast-enhanced ultrasound in evaluating the efficiency of ultrasound guided percutaneous microwave ablation in patients with renal cell carcinoma. Radiol Oncol 2013; 47(4): 398–404

[77] Ramirez D, Ma YB, Bedir S, Antonelli JA, Cadeddu JA, Gahan JC. Laparoscopic radiofrequency ablation of small renal tumors: long-term oncologic outcomes. J Endourol 2014; 28 (3): 330–334

[78] Veltri A, Gazzera C, Busso M et al. T1a as the sole selection criterion for RFA of renal masses: randomized controlled trials versus surgery should not be postponed. Cardiovasc Intervent Radiol 2014; 37(5): 1292–1298

[79] El Dib R, Touma NJ, Kapoor A. Cryoablation vs radiofrequency ablation for the treatment of renal cell carcinoma: a meta-analysis of case series studies. BJU Int 2012; 110(4): 510–516

[80] Gervais DA, Kalva S, Thabet A. Percutaneous image-guided therapy of intra-abdominal malignancy: imaging evaluation of treatment response. Abdom Imaging 2009; 34(5): 593–609

[81] Zagoria RJ. Imaging of small renal masses: a medical success story. Am J Roentgenol 2000; 175(4): 945–955

[82] Sandison GA, Loye MP, Rewcastle JC et al. X-ray CT monitoring of iceball growth and thermal distribution during cryosurgery. Phys Med Biol 1998; 43(11): 3309–3324

[83] Frank I, Blute ML, Cheville JC, Lohse CM, Weaver AL, Zincke H. Solid renal tumors: an analysis of pathological features related to tumor size. J Urol 2003; 170(6 Pt 1): 2217–2220

[84] Wood BJ, Khan MA, McGovern F, Harisinghani M, Hahn PF, Mueller PR. Imaging guided biopsy of renal masses: indications, accuracy and impact on clinical management. J Urol 1999; 161(5): 1470–1474

[85] Tuncali K, vanSonnenberg E, Shankar S, Mortele KJ, Cibas ES, Silverman SG. Evaluation of patients referred for percutaneous ablation of renal tumors: importance of a preprocedural diagnosis. Am J Roentgenol 2004; 183(3): 575–582

[86] Heilbrun ME, Zagoria RJ, Garvin AJ et al. CT-guided biopsy for the diagnosis of renal tumors before treatment with percutaneous ablation. Am J Roentgenol 2007; 188(6): 1500–1505

[87] Silverman SG, Gan YU, Mortele KJ, Tuncali K, Cibas ES. Renal masses in the adult patient: the role of percutaneous biopsy. Radiology 2006; 240(1): 6–22

[88] Ryan JM, Ryan BM, Smith TP. Antibiotic prophylaxis in interventional radiology. J Vasc Interv Radiol 2004; 15(6): 547–556

[89] Uppot RN, Silverman SG, Zagoria RJ, Tuncali K, Childs DD, Gervais DA. Imaging-guided percutaneous ablation of renal cell carcinoma: a primer of how we do it. Am J Roentgenol 2009; 192(6): 1558–1570

[90] Fennessy FM, Tuncali K, Morrison PR, Tempany CM. MR imaging-guided interventions in the genitourinary tract: an evolving concept. Radiol Clin North Am 2008; 46(1): 149 166, vii

[91] Lewin JS, Connell CF, Duerk JL et al. Interactive MRI-guided radiofrequency interstitial thermal ablation of abdominal tumors: clinical trial for evaluation of safety and feasibility. J Magn Reson Imaging 1998; 8(1): 40–47

[92] Morrison PR, Silverman SG, Tuncali K, Tatli S. MRI-guided cryotherapy. J Magn Reson Imaging 2008; 27(2): 410–420Cantwell CP, Wah TM, G

[93] Wile GE, Leyendecker JR, Krehbiel KA, Dyer RB, Zagoria RJCT. CT and MR imaging after imaging-guided thermal ablation of renal neoplasms. Radiographics 2007; 27(2): 325–339, discussion 339–340

[94] Lokken RP, Gervais DA, Arellano RS et al. Inflammatory nodules mimic applicator track seeding after percutaneous ablation of renal tumors. Am J Roentgenol 2007; 189(4): 845–848

[95] Johnson DB, Solomon SB, Su LM et al. Defining the complications of cryoablation and radio frequency ablation of small renal tumors: a multi-institutional review. J Urol 2004; 172 (3): 874–877

[96] Wah TM, Arellano RS, Gervais DA et al. Image-guided percutaneous radiofrequency ablation and incidence of post-radiofrequency ablation syndrome: prospective survey. Radiology 2005; 237(3): 1097–1102

[97] Saksena M, Gervais D. Percutaneous renal tumor ablation. Abdom Imaging 2009; 34(5): 582–587

[98] Maybody M, Solomon SB. Image-guided percutaneous cryoablation of renal tumors. Tech Vasc Interv Radiol 2007; 10 (2): 140–148

[99] Boss A, Clasen S, Kuczyk M et al. Thermal damage of the genitofemoral nerve due to radiofrequency ablation of renal cell carcinoma: a potentially avoidable complication. Am J Roentgenol 2005; 185(6): 1627–1631

Chapter 2

Adrenal Malignancy: Ablation

2 Adrenal Malignancy: Ablation

Aradhana M. Venkatesan and Bradford J. Wood

2.1 Introduction

Adrenal masses are a common clinical challenge, and incidental adrenal lesions may be detected on imaging in up to 10% of the general population.[1,2,3] Most adrenal incidentalomas are benign, with the nonfunctioning adrenal adenoma representing 80% of all incidentally detected adrenal neoplasms.[1,2] However, the possibility of malignant disease is the major concern when an incidental mass is identified, making biopsy or definitive diagnosis requisite prior to many ablations.[1,2] Malignancies of the adrenal gland include adrenal metastases as well as primary tumors, such as adrenocortical carcinoma, malignant pheochromocytoma, and neuroblastoma. Because the adrenal gland is the fourth most common site of metastatic disease, metastases to the adrenal gland are readily encountered. Primary tumors with a propensity to metastasize to the adrenal gland include lung, renal, and gastrointestinal cancers and melanoma.[4] Adrenocortical carcinoma, a rare but aggressive malignancy originating in the adrenal cortex, has an incidence of 1 to 2 per million population annually.[5] Early metastases are common, with overall 5-year survival being 20 to 35%.[6] Pheochromocytoma, a neuroendocrine tumor arising from the chromaffin cells of the adrenal medulla, can also pose a challenge for standard surgical or nonsurgical palliative management in patients with metastatic or recurrent disease.[7,8,9] Patients with metastatic pheochromocytoma may present with painful lesions, life-threatening lesions, or symptoms related to these catecholamine-producing neuroendocrine tumors.[7,8,9]

Surgical resection remains the mainstay of therapy for localized primary adrenal malignancies. Adrenal metastases in the setting of disseminated disease are conventionally treated with systemic chemotherapy.[4] There is some evidence to suggest that, in selected cases, surgical resection of isolated adrenal metastases may be associated with improved survival, although this remains an area for ongoing investigation.[4,10,11,12] The need for alternative therapies in nonsurgical adrenal cancer patients and the increased detection of adrenal tumors with cross-sectional imaging has prompted application of percutaneous ablative therapies for the management of adrenal malignancy and metastatic cancers of adrenal origin.[4] Both percutaneous thermal and chemical ablative techniques have been used in the treatment of adrenal malignancy, although chemical ablation has not achieved desirable complete response rates, despite excellent results for treatment of benign functional adrenal tumors.[13] This chapter summarizes the role of percutaneous thermal ablation, including radiofrequency ablation (RFA), microwave ablation (MWA), and cryoablation, in the management of adrenal malignancy, with an emphasis on clinical and technical considerations unique to the adrenal gland.

2.2 Indications

Percutaneous thermal ablation of adrenal malignancy has been performed in patients with adrenal metastases, locally recurrent or metastatic adrenocortical carcinoma, and pheochromocytoma metastases who are considered unresectable or poor surgical candidates, who have undergone previous attempts at surgical debulking, and who refuse surgery.[14,15] Determination of the potential benefit from ablation and its impact on survival or quality of life is ideally determined by multidisciplinary consensus.

2.3 Contraindications

Uncorrectable coagulopathies and hemorrhagic diatheses are relative contraindications to percutaneous ablation for adrenal malignancy. Blood product use may be employed as for surgical procedures.[16] The international normalized ratio should ideally be < 1.5 to 1.8 and the platelet count $\geq 50 \times 10^9$/L prior to the procedure,[15] although some use 75×10^9 instead of 50×10^9/L as a threshold. Ablation should not be performed in those patients who are acutely ill or septic. Comorbid conditions, such as chronic obstructive pulmonary disease and congestive heart failure, are not contraindications to ablation; however, multiple comorbid conditions may increase the risk profile. Prior hypertensive crisis or elevated levels of catecholamines also raise the periprocedural risks but are not absolute contraindications with appropriate precautions.[16]

2.4 Patient Selection and Preprocedure Workup

The management of adrenal malignancies requires a multidisciplinary approach, including involvement from medical, surgical, and radiation oncology; endocrinology; and interventional radiology.[4] The patient's clinical and treatment history, lesion histology, and imaging findings should be reviewed followed by a discussion of available treatment options, including surgery, radiation, chemotherapy, and ablative therapy. Before proceeding with ablation, all specialists should ideally be in agreement regarding the utility of ablation, with or without additional medical or surgical treatments.[4] When appropriate, the risk of hypertensive crisis and specific medical risks in patients with significant comorbidities should be discussed. Preprocedure cross-sectional imaging should be reviewed in detail for tumor size, location, and potential access routes or proximities of adjacent organs.[15] Laboratory data, particularly coagulation parameters, should be reviewed for procedural eligibility. For suspected functioning tumors, appropriate serum or urine assays for cortisol, aldosterone, and catecholamines may be obtained before ablation to assess their interval change after treatment.[15]

In general, preablation tumor biopsy is typically recommended because it can prevent unnecessary treatment and more accurately report ablation efficacy.[14,17] Additional factors in favor of pretreatment biopsy include patient preference for a definitive diagnosis, the fact that ablation does not yield a resection specimen, and the need to inform follow-up imaging planning.[17] When planning biopsy for an unknown adrenal tumor, it is important to be prepared for the risk of hypertensive crisis, particularly if the lesion suspected is a pheochromocytoma, for which intraprocedural anesthesia monitoring and readiness are recommended to enable acute management of hypertension. If clinical history and diagnostic imaging suggest pheochromocytoma, prebiopsy plasma or urinary catecholamines are helpful; positive catecholamines may obviate biopsy or indicate the need for arterial pressure monitoring, administration of alpha (α)- and beta (β)-adrenergic inhibitors, or anesthesia consultation if biopsy is to be pursued.[15] When the clinical diagnosis of an adrenal mass can be made confidently on the basis of clinical history, imaging, and endocrinologic findings, biopsy may be avoided; however, evaluation should be on a case-by-case basis.[14]

Preablation endocrinology consultation is critical in the workup of adrenal tumors. The adrenal gland's unique endocrine properties include the secretion of catecholamines (epinephrine and norepinephrine) by the adrenal medulla.[18] As a result, the interventional oncologist must be mindful of the risk of intraprocedural hypertensive crisis during ablation of intra-adrenal malignancies or metastases from functional adrenal malignancies like pheochromocytoma.[14,15,19,20] Of note, hypertensive crisis has been observed, even during ablation of tumors in proximity to the adrenal gland.[21] Preablation endocrinology consultation ensures appropriate management of functional adrenal tumors to minimize the risk of intraprocedural hypertensive crisis as well as to assist with postprocedure monitoring of hormone levels and replacement therapy, as needed.[15] Preablation antihypertensive regimens may include a combination of α- and β-adrenergic inhibitors, which may be titrated for 7 to 21 days prior to the procedure, depending on patient blood pressures ► Table 2.1. When one is premedicating patients for planned adrenal ablation, it is important to note that β-adrenergic inhibitors should not be administered as a sole agent.[4] To minimize the risk of hypertensive crisis and heart failure secondary to unopposed α-adrenergic stimulation α-adrenergic inhibition with phenoxybenzamine should be initiated before β-adrenergic inhibitors.[4] Following several days of phenoxybenzamine to achieve sufficient α-adrenergic inhibition, β-adrenergic inhibition can be performed with an agent such as oral atenolol or labetalol. In selected cases prior to metastatic pheochromocytoma ablation, our endocrinologists have also recommended administration of the tyrosine hydroxylase inhibitor α-methyl-paratyrosine to inhibit ongoing catecholamine synthesis before the procedure. If there are adjustments to patients' medication regimens in anticipation of ablation, it is important to ensure follow-up during this time by a clinical practitioner, so that patients may be screened for signs and symptoms of orthostasis, and counseled about the risks of dizziness, falls, or other side effects. In select patients, it may be of value to intentionally titrate medications such that the patient is orthostatic preprocedurally, in order to better tolerate catecholamine release during subsequent ablation ► Table 2.1.

Preablation anesthesia consultation is also advisable, given the possibility of intraprocedural catecholamine release and hypertensive crisis during ablation of adrenal malignancy. General endotracheal anesthesia may be warranted, with arterial blood pressure monitoring during pheochromocytoma ablation.[9] Careful attention to pre- and intraprocedural medication management and medical monitoring is especially critical in the context of suspected or confirmed pheochromocytoma. Catastrophic clinical consequences of hypertensive crisis and cardiac arrest have been reported during pheochromocytoma metastasis ablation performed in the absence of preprocedural α-adrenergic inhibition, despite intraprocedural anesthesia monitoring.[22] Anesthesiologist readiness with premixed, ready to inject (or drip) short-acting beta-blocker (e.g., esmolol) plus a titratable antihypertensive (e.g., nitroprusside) is advisable. A bag compression device for rapid administration of nitroprusside without delay may be a worthwhile precaution. Careful communication with the anesthesiologist when turning on or off ablative energies is critical and allows adequate preparation. RFA and MWA can be turned off during ablation in the event of hypertension, and there is often a latency period of approximately 30 to 60 seconds between the termination of RF current and the peak blood pressure. It is unknown whether ice ball thawing during cryoablation corresponds temporally with catecholamine release.

2.5 Technique

2.5.1 Methods of Ablation

Percutaneous ablation of adrenal malignancy has been performed using RFA, MWA, and cryoablation.

Radiofrequency Ablation

RFA typically employs three equipment components[1]: a radiofrequency generator generating an alternating current in the 500 kHz range[2]; single- or multitined needle electrodes, which may be monopolar or bipolar; and, in the case of monopolar needle electrodes,[3] grounding pads, which are placed on the patient's thighs. The needle electrode is placed within the tumor by the operating physician, typically under ultrasound and/or computed tomography (CT), cone beam CT (CBCT), or CT/fluoroscopy guidance. After connecting the needle electrode and grounding pads to the generator, a closed loop circuit is created with the patient's target tumor serving as the end resistor. Radiofrequency energy applied to the needle electrode by the generator results in the generation of ionic agitation at the tip of the needle electrode,

leading to frictional heat and near instantaneous coagulation necrosis of tissue when temperatures between 60 and 100°C are achieved. For adequate destruction of tumor tissue, the targeted volume must be treated with temperatures that are above the 60°C threshold for cell death.[14,23] Ablation zones will typically be limited to the region of tissue immediately surrounding the electrode, with most RFA devices generating an approximately 3 cm single ablation zone. To treat a larger tumor, multiple ablations are overlapped to generate a composite ablation zone of sufficient diameter to encompass the tumor and a surrounding tumor-free margin.[24] Real-time ultrasound visualizes gas within the treated region during ablation, which is an estimate of ablation, although less accurate compared to CT or magnetic resonance imaging (MRI). When employing CT guidance, iodinated contrast may be administered at the end of the treatment to assess the expected nonenhancement of the ablation zone.

The companies in the United States manufacturing RFA devices are AngioDynamics (Queensbury, NY), Boston Scientific (Natick, MA), Covidien (Mansfield, MA), and RFA Medical, Inc. (Fremont, CA).[25] Generators are programmed to generate several ablative cycles. The length of the ablation cycle and number of cycles applied to a tumor are dependent on the desired size of the ablation zone. In general, most systems apply an initial gradual increase in power, and once peak power is achieved, it is held for a 12- to 15-minute ablation cycle until energy output feedback or elevations in tissue impedance stop the generator current flow and ablation.[25] For catecholamine-secreting pheochromocytomas, although the rationale is anecdotal, it has been our practice to slowly increase the electrical current at the beginning of an ablation, in order to better assess the degree of resultant hypertension, rather than immediately applying maximal current. In this way, the RFA can be reduced or switched off during episodes of marked hypertension. This technique may permit safer application of RFA in this setting; however, patience is also required because this approach may prolong overall treatment time.

Microwave Ablation

Microwave ablation involves transmission of microwaves through an antenna inserted into a tumor. With application of an oscillating electromagnetic field of 915 or 2,450 MHz in frequency, ionic agitation of water molecules adjacent to the tip of the microwave antenna results in frictional agitation heat and cell death on the basis of coagulative necrosis.[25] In contrast to RFA, grounding pads are not required, given the inherent nonelectric properties of the electromagnetic wave.[14] As is the case for RFA, real-time imaging with ultrasound may be used, which enables visualization of ultrasound echogenicity secondary to the generation of gas within the treated region during ablation. Iodinated contrast may be administered following treatment to assess the size and geometry of the ablation zone. Analogous to RFA, the targeted volume must be treated with temperatures that are above the 60°C threshold for cell death for adequate destruction of tumor tissue. Real-time intraprocedural information about ablation zone temperatures is obtained from thermocouple readings and the manufacturer's information about probe heating capabilities.[25] Compared to RFA, MWA results in faster heating over a larger volume with less susceptibility to heat sink or local perfusion. Higher temperatures and larger ablation zones are therefore achieved in a shorter period of time.[25,26,27,28] Use of MWA over RFA may be particularly advantageous for large tumors, such as those ≥ 5 cm in diameter.[29]

The MWA systems commercially available in the United States employ either a 915 MHz generator (Evident, Covidien; Avecure, Medwaves) or a 2,450 MHz generator (e.g., Certus 140, Neuwave; Amica, Hospital Service; Acculis MTA, Angiodynamics). The antennae used are straight applicators with active tips, ranging in lengths from 0.6 to 4 cm. The majority of available systems require that the antennae are internally cooled with either room-temperature fluid or carbon dioxide to reduce conductive heating and prevent thermal injury to the skin.[30] Although MWA has been associated with oblong or ellipsoid treatments, including proximal burns along the probe shaft, recent technology makes spherical ablations more possible.

Cryoablation

Cryoablation makes use of the Joule–Thomson effect, which describes the change in temperature of a gas resulting from expansion or compression of that gas.[31] Expansion of argon inside a small chamber within the end of a cryoprobe results in cooling of the gas prior to tissue exposure.[25] Extremely low temperatures are produced when an active cryoprobe is placed into a tumor. The application of a series of alternating freeze–thaw cycles results in the generation of intra- and extracellular ice crystal formation and cell membranolysis. Cell death occurs on the basis of apoptosis, with temperatures of − 20 to − 40°C necessary for cell death. Cryotherapy also results in small-vessel thrombosis, which can contribute to indirect cell destruction.[25] Cryoprobes are placed into the target tumor under ultrasound, CT, CBCT, CT/fluoroscopy, or MRI guidance. If multiple probes are placed within a tumor, they are ideally placed within 1 to 2 cm of each other and within 1 cm of the tumor margin.[25] The ice ball generated during the freeze cycles may be visualized as a well demarcated echogenic near-field region by ultrasound, as an area of hypodensity on CT, or as a region of signal loss on MRI. This finding can be used to estimate adequacy of probe geometry and tumor coverage, although the ablation margin may be ~ 4 mm within the circumference of the ice ball. Visualization of the ice ball generated during treatment may also obviate the need for intraprocedural contrast administration. Analogous to RFA, cryoablation shows relative sparing of damage to larger vessels, which can result in heat-sink (in this case cold-sink) effects, necessitating colder thermal temperatures to cause cell death. Potential complications related to the lack of coagulative necrosis achieved with cryoablation include the potential for increased risk of bleeding compared with hyperthermic technologies. In addition, tumor lysis syndrome or cryoshock can occur, attributed to exposure of ablation zone contents to the systemic circulation.[32] Two companies in the United States currently market commercial cryoablation systems for percutaneous use, the Percryo device, (Healthtronics, Inc.) and the Presice and SeedNet systems, manufactured by Galil Medical.[25] These systems employ argon, helium, or nitrogen gas for cooling. The probes provided with these systems range from 1.4 to 4.9 mm in diameter and can achieve a range of ablation zone sizes.[25]

Technical Considerations

Imaging Guidance

Thermal ablation of adrenal neoplasms may be performed with CT fluoroscopy guidance, CT guidance, CBCT, or with a combination of ultrasound and CT guidance.[33,34] MRI may also be used for intraprocedural imaging, but it has limited widespread availability and requires a special system, often with MRI room modifications. Advantages of CT guidance include visualization of the targeted mass and the location and delineation of vulnerable regional anatomy. Concomitant fluoroscopy is particularly advantageous for real-time visualization of the hemidiaphragms during needle insertion to avoid transpleural transgression. Ultrasound alone may not reliably identify the adrenal gland, although it can have value for real-time monitoring during ablation of large adrenal tumors.[33,34] CBCT with integrated real-time fluoroscopic guidance can combine several advantages, but it may have a limited field of view and may complicate the intraprocedural use of ultrasound.

Patient Positioning

At the onset of percutaneous ablation of a primary or metastatic adrenal tumor, the access or approach to the lesion should be assessed on pre-ablation imaging. The location of vulnerable regional anatomy should be evaluated at this time, and the need for protective maneuvers, such as hydrodissection, should be evaluated. Commonly vulnerable anatomical structures during adrenal ablation include the lung and pleura, kidney, colon, duodenum, stomach, pancreas, liver, and spleen.[4,34] Decubitus positioning of the patient (target side down) during adrenal ablation is particularly useful to gain access to the adrenal gland while avoiding transpleural transgression. In the case of large tumors, prone positioning may facilitate safe access to the target tumor, if transpleural transgression is avoidable (▶ Fig. 2.1). For cases when the adrenal tumor cannot be successfully approached via a posterior approach due to intervening lung parenchyma or the presence of colon, an anterolateral, transhepatic approach may be useful (▶ Fig. 2.2).[15]

Intraprocedural Monitoring and Adjunctive Maneuvers

Careful intraprocedural monitoring is critical for safe adrenal tumor ablation. Hypertension can occur during adrenal ablation as a result of catecholamine release. Preclinical studies have demonstrated that RFA of normal adrenal tissue may cause intraprocedural hypertension, with elevations in both norepinephrine and epinephrine during porcine adrenal RFA and elevations in norepinephrine during canine adrenal RFA.[35,36] In a review of five reports, including more than 40 patients undergoing adrenal RFA for both benign functional adrenal neoplasms and adrenal malignancy, a range of incidences of intraprocedural

hypertension has been described, from 0–66.7%.[34,35,37,38,39] Moreover, a significantly higher rate of intra-procedural hypertension has been described in patients undergoing (nonpheochromocytoma) adrenal tumor ablation (6 of 9, 66.7%) compared to nonadrenal abdominal tumors (1 of 9, 11.1%).[35] In a study of 9 patients undergoing adrenal RFA, intraprocedural systolic blood pressure correlated significantly with serum epinephrine ($R^2 = 0.68$, $P < 0.0001$) and norepinephrine values ($R^2 = 0.72$, $P < 0.0001$), whereas other adrenal hormones (dopamine, cortisol) did not correlate with systolic blood pressure.[35] Although rare, hypertensive crisis has also been reported during RFA of hepatic tumors in proximity to the adrenal gland.[19] Etiologic factors implicated for intraprocedural hypertension during adrenal ablation include pain- and anxiety-mediated release of catecholamines, rapid release of catecholamines during destruction of normal adrenal tissue, and RFA-mediated electrical stimulation resulting in catecholamine release.[35] A prior case report has also described malignant hypertension during cryoablation of an adrenal gland tumor, presumably based on analogous mechanisms.[20]

Significant elevations in intra-arterial systolic blood pressure (> 200 mm Hg) and diastolic blood pressure (> 100 mm Hg) have also been observed, specifically in the setting of thermal ablation of pheochromocytoma metastases.[9] Analogous to physical manipulation of these tumors in the operating room, ablation-related physical and thermal stimuli may potentiate tumor catecholamine release, causing abrupt elevations in patient heart rate and blood pressure.[9] During ablation of pheochromocytoma metastases, close communication with the anesthesiologist is critical, with announcements prior to probe insertion into tumor, application of thermal energy, and probe repositioning and removal. Although unusual, needle removal itself can result in immediate hypertension. Gradual, manual application of thermal energy and incremental increases in the energy delivered have been advocated to allow adequate time to observe hemodynamic changes and for careful titration of medication, as needed.[9] General anesthesia with intra-arterial blood pressure monitoring should be considered prior to thermal ablation of these tumors. A combination of β-adrenergic antagonists (e.g., esmolol, labetalol, metoprolol), phenoxybenzamine, sodium nitroprusside, nitroglycerine, and analgesia/anesthetics (e.g., fentanyl, hydromorphone, midazolam, propofol) has been successfully used for intraprocedural control

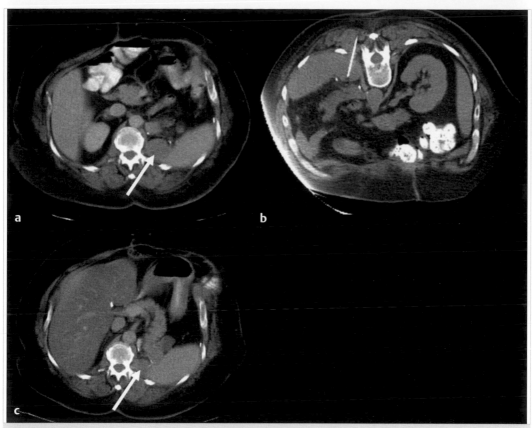

Fig. 2.1 A 65-year-old patient with painful left adrenocortical cancer recurrence in the left adrenalectomy bed. (a) Axial contrast-enhanced computed tomography (CT) demonstrates a 4.5 cm mass in the left adrenalectomy bed (*white arrow*), medial to the spleen. (b) Radiofrequency ablation (RFA) was performed with the patient in the prone position. (c) Contrast-enhanced CT obtained 12 months after ablation shows a reduction of the mass (*white arrow*) and no evidence for residual enhancement. The patient's pain resolved after RFA. (Used with permission from Venkatesan AM et al[14].)

of hypertension, with authors advocating target blood pressures and heart rates within 20% of the patient's baseline hemodynamic profile.[9] ▶ Table 2.1 presents suggested pre- and intraprocedural medications and dosages for pheochromocytoma ablation, although it remains vital for the interventional radiologist to evaluate each patient on a case-by-case basis and in conjunction with consulting endocrinology and anesthesiology services when determining optimal medical management in these cases. Pheochromocytoma ablation can be a challenging procedure for the operating physician due to the rapid or extreme fluctuations in hemodynamics.

Depending on the proximity of the target tumor to vulnerable regional anatomy, hydrodissection may be warranted prior to thermal ablation to ensure safe and successful therapy. It is most useful in protecting the bowel and pancreas and may also facilitate protection of the lung, kidney, or hemidiaphragm and chest wall (including intercostal nerves).[14] Under sonographic guidance a 20- to 22-gauge needle is used to instill a small (~ 50 mL) volume of 5% dextrose in water (D5W) into the targeted location. Ionic solutions like normal saline can conduct electricity, and should not be used for hydrodissection prior to RFA, although they may be used for cryoablation procedures.[14] After confirming initial needle placement and location of the hydrodissection fluid, a needle-sheath catheter is typically inserted into the initially instilled fluid volume (e.g., Yueh centesis catheter, Cook Medical; or Skater centesis catheter, Angiotech). Its needle stylet is then removed, and

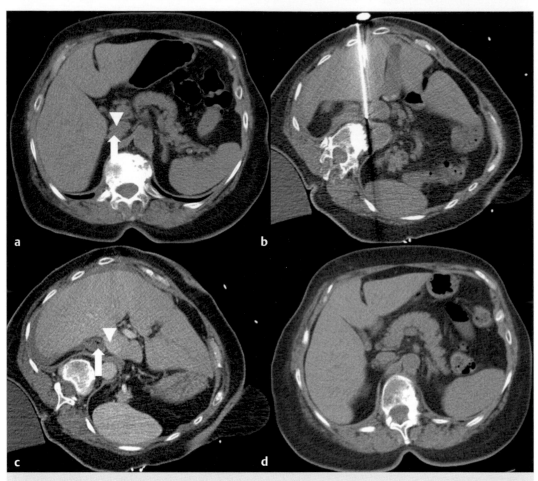

Fig. 2.2 Lung adenocarcinoma metastatic to the right adrenal gland in a 73-year-old woman. (a) Axial noncontrast computed tomographic (CT) image demonstrates progressive 1.8 cm right adrenal metastasis (*arrow*) abutting the inferior vena cava (*arrowhead*). (b) Probe placement during transhepatic radiofrequency ablation of the right adrenal metastasis. (c) Contrast-enhanced CT image obtained immediately after ablation demonstrates complete tumor treatment with no residual contrast enhancement (*arrow*). The adjacent inferior vena cava was unaffected by the ablation treatment (*arrowhead*). (d) Follow-up noncontrast CT image obtained 9 months after ablation demonstrates no interval growth and decreased lesion size consistent with adequate treatment. (Used with permission from Welch BT et al[46].)

additional fluid is hung to gravity with a stopcock in series.[14] Fluid should flow freely if in a peritoneal or retroperitoneal location, with the location and distribution of the fluid and its displacement of regional anatomy assessed with serial CT. Iodinated contrast media (10 mL) may be added to the fluid to improve visualization of the instilled fluid under CT guidance. The total volume of fluid instilled depends on the amount of organ displacement needed to avoid thermal injury to nontarget tissue.[14] If initial attempts at hydrodissection do not adequately protect or displace the anatomical

structure of concern, patient repositioning and additional instillation of fluid may be required, as well as probe repositioning, to ensure a safe and optimal relationship between the ablation probe, tumor, and nontarget anatomy.[14]

Cystic tumor elements can add to procedural complexity. When treating a cystic or mixed cystic and solid adrenal tumor with RFA, the RFA probe may need to be moved multiple times to ablate the solid components and ensure complete treatment.[14] In such cases, MWA may be used to provide optimal heating.[14,26] Longer treatment times

Table 2.1 Suggested pre- and intraprocedural medication regimen and dosages for pheochromocytoma ablation[a]

Suggested preprocedural medication regimen

Medication class	Suggested agent	Dose	Initiation	Duration	Comments
α-adrenergic inhibitor	Phenoxybenzamine	10 mg 2–3 times/d	7–14 + days prior to ablation	Continue up to treatment day	Titrate following ablation depending on hemodynamic response
β-adrenergic inhibitor	Atenolol	12.5 mg twice daily	7–14 + days prior to ablation	Continue up to treatment day	Titrate following ablation depending on hemodynamic response
Dopamine synthesis inhibitor (tyrosine hydroxylase inhibitor)	α-methyl-para-tyrosine	250 mg 2–3 times/d	7–14 + days prior to ablation	Continue up to treatment day	Titrate following ablation depending on hemodynamic response

Suggested intraprocedural medications

Medication class	Agent	Dose	Comments
α-adrenergic inhibitor	Phenoxybenzamine	IV administration	Administration and titration per intraprocedural hemodynamic response
β-adrenergic inhibitor	Labetalol, esmolol, metoprolol	IV administration	Administration and titration per intraprocedural hemodynamic response
Nitric oxide–based vasodilator	Sodium nitroprusside, nitroglycerin	IV administration	Administration and titration per intraprocedural hemodynamic response
Opioid analgesic	Fentanyl, hydromorphone,	IV administration	Administration and titration per intraprocedural hemodynamic response
Hypnotic/amnestic	Propofol	IV administration	Administration and titration per intraprocedural hemodynamic response
Benzodiazepine, short acting	Midazolam	IV administration	Administration and titration per intraprocedural hemodynamic response

Abbreviation: IV, intravenous.

Note: It is critical to note that the agents, their timing, dosage, and duration of administration presented in this table are suggestions only. Interventional radiologists are urged to consult members of their endocrinology and anesthesia services to evaluate patients with pheochromocytoma or who are otherwise at risk for hypertensive crisis during adrenal tumor ablation prior to intended ablation. Preprocedural assessment, intraprocedural monitoring, and postablation evaluation of hemodynamics are critical to safe and successful ablation in this setting. Moreover, it is essential that a patient-specific medical regimen for the mitigation of hypertensive crisis is developed and executed. This plan must take into account an individual patient's medical history and preprocedural, intraprocedural, and postablation hemodynamics to ensure safe, optimal medical management.

[a]General anesthesia with intra-arterial blood pressure monitoring should be considered prior to thermal ablation of these tumors.

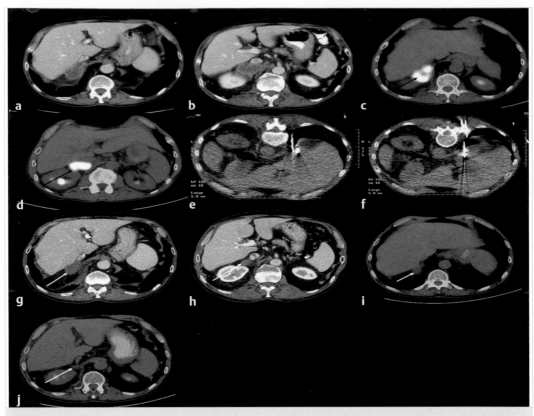

Fig. 2.3 A 65-year-old man with initial stage IIIA non–small cell carcinoma treated with chemotherapy and radiation therapy with a solitary right adrenal metastasis, which remained the sole disease site for 1 year. Preablation (**a, b**) computed tomography (CT) and (**c, d**) positron emission tomographic (PET)-CT demonstrate a fludeoxyglucose avid cystic 6 × 4 cm cystic right adrenal mass (**a, b:** *white arrows;* **c, d:** *black arrows*). Biopsy was consistent with metastatic non–small cell carcinoma. Microwave ablation was chosen given the size and cystic nature of the tumor. (**e, f**) Three 3.7 cm active tip microwave antennae were inserted to cover the mass (Evident, Covidien). A 10-minute treatment was performed at 45 W. (**g, h**) One-month follow-up contrast-enhanced CT shows a decrease in size of the ablation zone and no enhancement *(white arrows)*. (**i, j**) Eight-month follow-up PET-CT demonstrates a complete metabolic response and further decrease in size of the ablation zone *(white arrows)*. (Used with permission from Venkatesan et al[14].)

may be required for cystic lesions, and coagulation may be sudden when it eventually occurs. (▶ Fig. 2.3).

2.6 Postprocedure Management and Follow-up Evaluation

Careful postprocedural monitoring of hemodynamics remains important immediately following completion of ablation and in the hours after treatment, particularly for pheochromocytoma ablation. Marked elevations in systolic (> 200 mm Hg) and diastolic blood pressure (> 100 mm Hg) have been observed following completion of thermal ablation of pheochromocytoma metastases, suggesting that a subset of these patients may benefit from extended monitoring in the postanesthesia care unit (PACU) or postprocedural intensive care unit observation and monitoring of hemodynamics.[9] In some instances, an overnight stay after ablation of pheochromocytoma may be prudent to monitor postprocedural catecholamine-induced changes of blood pressure and heart rate.[9] In one anecdotal case of RFA plus embolization of pheochromocytoma, hemodynamic fluctuations occurred for several days after treatment prior to stabilization. Likewise, rapidly decreasing requirements for α-adrenergic and β-adrenergic inhibitors or additional antihypertensives may require careful titration of medication in the days after ablation.

Following immediate postprocedural recovery and discharge, clinical and imaging follow-up of patients is required. Goals of initial postablation imaging are to document technical success of the procedure, identify procedural complications, and establish a new baseline for future imaging.[4,14,40] Subsequent follow-up imaging surveillance is necessary to screen for primary treatment failure or late tumor recurrence because the treated tumor remains in situ.[14,40] There are no evidence-based guidelines advocating a specific imaging follow-up algorithm following ablation of adrenal malignancy. Generally, a baseline postablation scan (contrast-enhanced CT or MRI) is performed 1 to 3 months postablation, with follow-up imaging performed at 3- to 6-month intervals to enable early detection of recurrence when repeat intervention is still possible.[41,42]

Within the first 6 months after thermal ablation, ablated adrenal tumors may demonstrate internal areas of increased attenuation or increased signal intensity at unenhanced CT and MRI, respectively, corresponding to proteinaceous debris or products of hemorrhage as has been described for other tumors.[14,42] Air bubbles and fat stranding are frequent findings on short-interval follow-up and should not be confused with superinfection.[41] No enhancement should be observed at the level of the ablation zone in the case of successfully treated tumors. Careful evaluation of unenhanced CT or dynamic subtraction (postcontrast–precontrast) MRI on follow-up studies is beneficial to distinguish precontrast hyperdensity or hyperintensity due to proteinaceous debris or hemorrhage from true enhancement associated with residual or locally recurrent tumor. Ablation zone size should decrease over time[4,14,42,43] (▶ Fig. 2.4 and ▶ Fig. 2.5). Areas of contrast enhancement on initial follow-up usually indicate residual viable tumor and primary treatment failure (typically > 10 Hounsfield units [HU] or > 15% with CT and MRI, respectively).[14,42,43] This may be observed subsequent to palliative ablation of large tumors where the treatment goals are focused on addressing patient signs and symptoms rather than complete tumor ablation (▶ Fig. 2.6). Ablation zone enhancement or enlargement on follow-up imaging is considered indicative of tumor recurrence, and patients should be counseled about additional treatments, as appropriate, including repeat ablation, surgery, chemotherapy, or observation.[14] Fludeoxyglucose positron emission tomography

(FDG-PET) is useful in instances where preablation imaging demonstrated FDG avidity of a lesion, and can be used to assess the efficacy of the ablation and the presence of recurrent or residual disease.[14,41]

Clinical and biochemical assessment is particularly important in the follow-up of patients who have undergone ablation of hormonally active adrenal malignancies to ensure complete biochemical response to treatment, to confirm the adequacy of their postablation medication regimen, and to screen for symptoms of either ongoing hormonal excess or postablation hormonal insufficiency.[41,44] Formal endocrinology consultative follow-up and recommendations can be of value in this setting. Patients who have had treatment for adrenocortical carcinoma associated with primary aldosteronism should have serum sodium and potassium levels monitored and may require evaluation for metabolic alkalosis.[4,44] Following tumor treatment, blood pressure and serum potassium levels may decrease, enabling reduction in antihypertensive medications.[4] Patients who have undergone ablation of pheochromocytoma or cortisol-secreting tumors will require metanephrine- and cortisol-level monitoring, respectively, and may be able to decrease their antihypertensive medications following successful therapy.[4]

2.7 Side Effects and Complications

The most commonly described side effect of adrenal thermal ablation is intraprocedural hypertension with a reported incidence of up to 66.7%.[34,35,36,37,38,39] Intraprocedural hypertension has been observed during the application of RFA current and microwave energy as well as during the thaw phase of cryoablation of adrenal tumors, underscoring the importance of operator attention to intra- and postprocedural hemodynamics.[41,45,46] Additional less common complications of thermal ablation for adrenal malignancy that have been described in the literature include pneumothorax, hemothorax, retroperitoneal hematoma (in a thrombocytopenic patient), and postprocedural pain, all of which responded to conservative management.[34,37] Tumor seeding along the probe track is a potential complication. As for ablation in other organs, this risk can be mitigated by ablating the probe track during probe removal. To our knowledge, no published cases of tumor seeding after adrenal malignancy ablation have been described

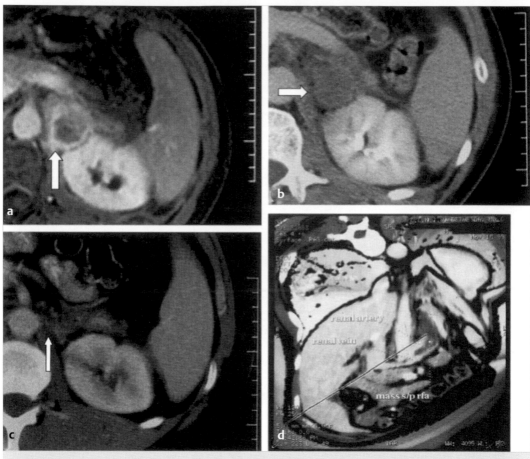

Fig. 2.4 **(a)** Enhanced T1-weighted magnetic resonance image before radiofrequency ablation (RFA) shows the enhancing rim of a recurrent adrenocortical carcinoma (ACC) postsurgery *(arrow)*. The ACC tumor is located in the suprarenal bed, between the aorta and kidney. **(b)** Enhanced computed tomographic (CT) scan immediately after RFA shows devascularized tumor with loss of enhancement *(arrow)*. **(c)** Enhanced CT scan 14 months after RFA shows interval shrinkage of the tumor with a small residual *(arrow)*. **(d)** Three-dimensional shaded surface display from contrast-enhanced CT immediately after RFA. The planes are cut away in the treated region to display the renal artery, renal vein, and intervening treated thermal lesion between these two vessels. S/P, status post. (Used with permission from Wood et al[33].)

to date. Stroke and cardiac syndromes due to catecholamine release are also possible risks, especially with hormonally active tumors and in patients with comorbidities, advanced age, or underlying atherosclerosis. Again, to our knowledge, no published cases of these complications have been described in relation to adrenal malignancy ablation,[4,14,35] although, in our experience, we have observed marked elevation in systolic blood pressures despite α-adrenergic and β-adrenergic inhibitors and rapid infusion of nitroprusside. There has been only one published periprocedural mortality subsequent to ablation of an adrenal malignancy, due to unrecognized bowel

perforation after RFA of four retroperitoneal pheochromocytoma metastases located at the crus of the diaphragm.[47] As the authors themselves emphasize, the nature of this complication was not a result of any intrinsic characteristic of the tumors ablated in this study, in this case metastatic pheochromocytoma, but rather exemplifies the inherent risks of RFA, even in experienced hands.[47]

2.8 Clinical Data and Outcomes

Percutaneous RFA, MWA, and cryoablation have been successfully employed in the treatment of

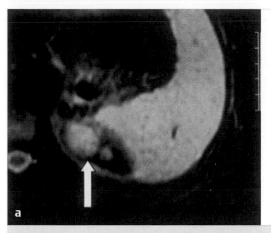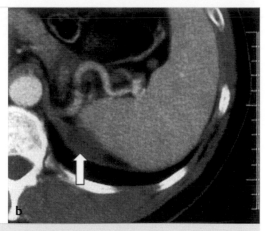

Fig. 2.5 **(a)** T2-weighted magnetic resonance image shows a bilobed tumor *(arrow)* in the adrenal bed adjacent to the spleen before radiofrequency ablation (RFA) was performed. **(b)** Enhanced computed tomographic scan 20 months after RFA demonstrates near-complete involution of the treated tumor with shrinking, nonenhancing residual thermal lesion *(arrow)*, presumably scar tissue. This patient remains disease-free at this location 15 years later. (Used with permission from Wood et al[33].)

primary adrenocortical carcinoma and adrenal metastases. Clinical studies to date indicate that these are effective therapies with acceptable short-term outcomes and low risk in the appropriate setting with attention to pre-, peri-, and postprocedural management.[33,34,39,41,46,48,49] Early data concerning the role of percutaneous ablation for the treatment of metastatic pheochromocytoma has also been promising.[8,47] ▶ Table 2.2 summarizes the results of existing short-term studies (≤ 5-year follow-up) employing thermal ablation to treat adrenal malignancies. Image-guided thermal ablation has also been employed for effective treatment of benign functional adrenal tumors, as summarized within a subset of the results in ▶ Table 2.2. Although a detailed assessment of the results for benign adrenal tumor ablation is beyond the scope of this review, the reader is encouraged to consult several pertinent clinical studies on the subject, which summarize experience with ablation of aldosteronomas, cortisol- and testosterone-secreting adenomas, and organ-confined intra-adrenal pheochromocytomas.[37,38,50]

2.8.1 Adrenal Metastases

The majority of clinical experience with percutaneous thermal ablation for adrenal malignancy has involved treatment of metastases to the adrenal gland. Welch et al treated a total of 37 adrenal metastases, 10 with RFA and 27 with cryoablation.[46] In 32 patients (25 men and 7 women, mean age 66 y, age range 44–88 y) with 37 adrenal tumors, 35 ablation procedures were performed.[46] One patient with an 8.2 cm tumor underwent planned cryoablation debulking. Of the 36 patients treated with curative intent, technical success was achieved in 35 (97%) tumors, with one technical failure during attempted cryoablation of a 3.3 cm left adrenal metastasis that bled during treatment, obscuring its margins. Follow-up imaging was performed on 34 of 37 tumors, excluding patients with intentional debulking (*n* = 1), technical failure (*n* = 1), and absence of follow-up (*n* = 1), with local recurrences in 3 (8.8%) of 34 tumors. Local tumor control was achieved in 31 of 34 lesions at a mean of 22.7 months of follow-up (mean size of tumor treated with cryoablation for curative intent, 3.2 cm; mean size of tumors treated with RFA, 1.8 cm). Recurrence-free survival and overall survival at 36 months were 88% and 52%, respectively, with a median survival of 34.5 months. A Common Terminology Criteria for Adverse Events (CTCAE) version 4.0 grade 3 or 4 complication was observed in three (8.6%) ablation procedures, including hemothorax, pleural effusion, and splenic hemorrhage.[46] Wolf et al treated a total of 23 tumors in 22 patients, with 20 of 23 tumors being adrenal metastases.[39] Of these tumors, 16 were treated with RFA and 4 were treated with MWA. Local tumor progression was found in 3 of 16 tumors treated with RFA (mean size of all treated tumors was 3.9 cm) with a mean 14-month follow-up.[39] Earlier clinical series include studies

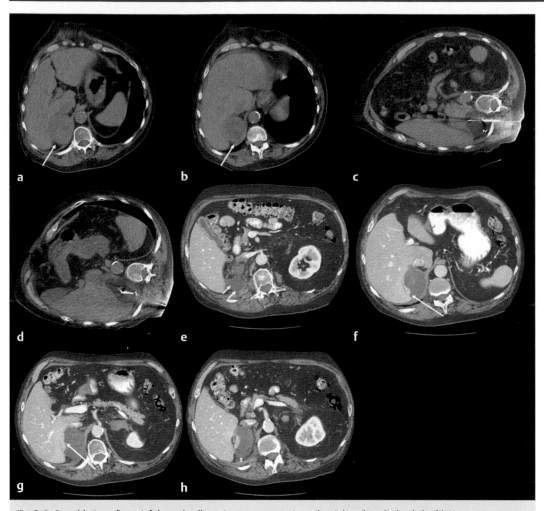

Fig. 2.6 Cryoablation of a painful renal cell carcinoma metastasis to the right adrenal gland. **(a, b)** Noncontrast computed tomography (CT) demonstrates a large heterogeneous right adrenal mass *(arrow)*. **(c, d)** Cryoablation of the patient's right adrenal mass was performed with six cryoprobes using 10-minute freeze, 8-minute thaw, and 10-minute freeze cycles. **(e–h)** Three months follow-up contrast-enhanced CT shows the nonenhancing ablation zone *(small paired white arrows)* and a residual focus of linear enhancement along the lateral margin of the ablation zone *(long white arrow)* consistent with residual tumor. The patient's pain improved significantly following the ablation. (Used with permission from Venkatesan et al[14].)

by Mayo-Smith and Dupuy and Carrafiello et al, demonstrating comparable local control rates and tumor sizes.[34,48] Carrafiello et al describe one case of postablation syndrome and one case of intraprocedural hypertension to 249/140 during right adrenal metastasis ablation, which responded to intravenous esmolol without further clinical sequelae.[48]

Clinical series summarizing the treatment of adrenal metastases with percutaneous MWA have described similar results with regard to local tumor control, albeit in smaller numbers of patients. Li et al treated a total of 10 tumors with MWA, 9 of which were adrenal metastases, with successful treatment of all metastases (mean size, 3.8 cm) and no local tumor progression over a mean 11.3-month follow-up.[45] One patient of this series experienced hypertensive crisis during treatment of a left adrenal lung cancer metastasis, with blood pressure elevation to 243/147 mm Hg accompanied by headache, tachycardia, and ventricular arrhythmia, which responded to

Table 2.2 Results of short-term[a] studies of adrenal tumors treated with percutaneous ablation

Author	Tumor characteristics	Number of tumors/patients	Mean tumor size (range) (cm)	Mean follow-up (range) (mon)	Results
Radiofrequency ablation					
Welch et al (2014)[b46]	37 adrenal metastases 10 metastases treated with RFA	10/36	1.8 (0.8–2.8)	22.7 (1–88)	1. Technical success in 35/36 (97%) tumors 2. Of those available for follow-up, 31/34 successfully treated 3. Local recurrence in 3/34 (8.8%)
Wolf et al (2012)[39]	20 adrenal metastases, 2 pheochromocytoma, 1 aldosteronoma 16 metastases and 3 hyperfunctional tumors treated with RFA	19/18	Adrenal metastases: 3.9 (2–8) Hyperfunctioning tumors: 2.3 (1–4)	Adrenal metastases: 14 (1–67) Hyperfunctioning tumors: 78 (38–91)	1. 13/16 (81%) adrenal metastases successfully treated[c] 2. 2/3 (67%) hyperfunctional tumors successfully treated[d]
McBride et al (2011)[e47]	47 pheochromocytoma and paraganglioma metastases, of which 7/13 adrenal pheochromocytoma metastases treated with RFA	7/3	1.9 (1.4–3.5)	3.7 (2–9.3)	1. Follow-up available in 27 of all treated patients, with successful treatment in 15/27 (56%) 2. Major complications in 2 of 18 (11%) ablation sessions, one case of hypertensive lability after RFA, and one periprocedural death after RFA from complications of bowel perforation
Microwave ablation					
Venkatesan et al (2009)[9]	7 metastases from adrenal pheochromocytoma	7/6	3.4 (2.2–6)	12.3 (2.5–28)	1. 6/7 (%) metastases successfully treated 2. Anesthesia monitoring α- and β-adrenergic and catecholamine synthesis inhibition for all

Table 2.2 continued

Author	Tumor characteristics	Number of tumors/patients	Mean tumor size (range) (cm)	Mean follow-up (range) (mon)	Results
					ablations, with no hypertensive crises 3. Elevated plasma catecholamine levels observed during RFA procedural maneuvers compared to baseline and postablation values
Carrafiello et al (2008)[48]	6 adrenal metastases	6/6[f]	2.9 (1.5–4)	21 (6–36)	1. 5/6 (83%) tumors successfully treated 2. 1 lesion with residual enhancement re-treated 10 days later
Mayo-Smith, Dupuy (2004)[34]	11 adrenal metastases, 1 pheochromocytoma, 1 aldosteronoma	13/12	3.9 (1–8)	11.2 (1–46)	1. 9/11(82%) adrenal metastases successfully treated 2. 2/2 hyperfunctional tumors successfully treated
Wood et al (2003)[33]	Locally recurrent or metastatic adrenocortical carcinoma	15/8	4.3 (1.5–9)	10.3 (1–20)	1. 8/15 (53%) successfully treated 2. 4/15 (27%) did not change in size 3. 3/15 (20%) demonstrated interval growth 4. 8/12 (67%) tumors ≤5 cm successfully treated
Wolf et al (2012)[39]	20 adrenal metastases, 2 pheochromocytoma, 1 aldosteronoma ──── 4 metastases treated with MWA	4/4	Adrenal metastases: 5.1 (4–6)	14.5 (3–28)	4/4 (100%) successfully treated
Li et al (2011)[42,45]	8 metastases, 1 primary adrenocortical carcinoma	10/9	3.8 (2.1–6.1)	11.3 (3–37)	1. 9/10 tumors successfully treated

Table 2.2 continued

Author	Tumor characteristics	Number of tumors/patients	Mean tumor size (range) (cm)	Mean follow-up (range) (mon)	Results
					2. 1 tumor with residual enhancement re-treated 1 month later
Wang et al (2009)[49]	5 adrenal metastases	5/5	3.5 (2.3–4.5)	19.2 (8–31)	5/5 (100%) successfully treated
Author	Tumor Characteristics	Number of Tumors/Patients	Mean Tumor Size (range) (cm)	Mean Follow-Up (range) (mo.)	Results
Cryoablation					
Welch et al (2014)[46]	37 adrenal metastases 27 metastases treated with cryoablation	27/36	3.2 (1.2–8)[9]	22.7 (1–88)	1. Technical success in 35/36 (97%) tumors 2. 1 technical failure during adrenal cryoablation complicated by intraprocedural hemorrhage, requiring subsequent intraprocedural salvage with RFA 3. Of those available for follow-up, 31/34 successfully treated 4. Local recurrence in 3/34 (8.8%)

Abbreviations: MWA, microwave ablation; RFA: radiofrequency ablation.

[a]Short term reflects ≤ 5 year follow-up.

[b]Mean and range of follow-up and summary statistics of successful treatment not described for pheochromocytoma versus paraganglioma cohorts.[47]

[c]Successful treatment defined as complete necrosis at follow-up imaging after a single ablation session.

[d]Successful treatment defined as resolution of biochemical abnormality.

[e]Mean and range of follow-up and summary statistics of successful treatment not described for RFA versus cryoablation cohorts.[46]

[f]One tumor treated twice.

[9]Excludes one patient with 8.2 cm tumor treated with cryoablation for tumor debulking rather than curative intent.

intravenous phentolamine, enabling completion of the MWA treatment and with no subsequent clinical sequlae.[45] Of those patients in the series published by Wolf et al who were treated with percutaneous MWA ($n = 4$ tumors), no local tumor progression was identified over a mean follow-up period of 14.5 months (mean tumor size, 5.1 cm).[39] Similarly, Wang et al treated five patients with adrenal metastases using MWA (mean tumor size, 3.5 cm) and observed no evidence of local tumor progression at a median of 19.2 months.[49]

2.8.2 Adrenocortical Carcinoma and Adrenocortical Carcinoma Metastases

Experience treating locally recurrent and metastatic adrenocortical carcinoma has been described by Wood et al, who employed percutaneous RFA to treat 15 tumors in eight patients. All patients had unresectable tumors or were poor candidates for surgery.[33] RFA in this cohort had minimal morbidity and was particularly effective for tumors ≤ 5 cm in diameter, of which 8 of 12 (67%) were observed to be successfully treated, with no local tumor progression over the follow-up period (mean 10.3 months). One patient developed a delayed abscess after RFA of a 9 cm tumor, which was treated successfully with antibiotics and catheter drainage; no instances of hypertensive crisis were reported in this series.[33] Results by Li et al suggest similar challenges in treating large (> 5 cm) adrenocortical carcinomas with percutaneous ablation. One patient of this series underwent MWA for a 6.1 cm primary left adrenocortical carcinoma, with residual tumor detected on 1-month follow-up CT, successfully treated with repeat ablation.[45]

2.8.3 Pheochromocytoma Metastases

Metastases from adrenal pheochromocytoma have been successfully treated with percutaneous RFA, which is of practical value given the difficulties encountered with management of surgically unresectable metastatic disease and in the setting of metastasis-related symptoms.[9,47] Two published reports have employed percutaneous RFA for metastatic adrenal pheochromocytoma. Venkatesan et al summarized the treatment of seven hepatic and osseous metastases from pheochromocytoma in six patients (mean tumor size 3.4 cm, range 2.2–6 cm).[9] All patients were evaluated for surgical resection but were not surgical candidates because of disease at other sites or rapidly growing disease and refusal to undergo surgery.[9] α- and β-adrenergic and catecholamine synthesis inhibition was achieved with preprocedural administration of phenoxybenzamine, atenolol, and α-methyl-paratyrosine, respectively, and intraprocedural anesthesia monitoring was used in all cases. Successful ablation was achieved in six of seven metastases over a mean 12.3-month follow-up period (range, 2.5–28), with no intra- or postprocedural episodes of hypertensive crisis observed. Blood samples were obtained before, after, and during specific intervals within the RFA sessions (e.g., during needle electrode insertion into the tumor, during the initial application of the RFA current, and during probe repositioning in the tumor). Interestingly, elevations in plasma catecholamine levels were observed during RFA procedural maneuvers compared to baseline and postablation values, which corresponded temporally with elevations in dynamic mean arterial pressure and heart rate.[9] Dynamic mean arterial pressure elevations occurring as rapidly as 1 mm Hg/s were observed with application of RFA current, all of which responded to prompt administration of intravenous antihypertensives, cessation of the RFA current, or both.[9] McBride et al described experience treating a total of seven hepatic and diaphragmatic metastases from pheochromocytoma in three patients within a larger cohort of 47 pheochromocytoma and paraganglioma metastases treated with RFA, cryoablation, and ethanol ablation.[47] Mean tumor size in the patients with metastatic pheochromocytoma was 1.9 cm, with a range of 1.4 to 3.5 cm. Follow-up, although not described explicitly for those patients with metastatic pheochromocytoma, was available in 27 of all treated patients in their study, with successful treatment reported in 15 of 27 patients (52%). Major complications were reported in two ablation sessions. These included one case of hypertensive lability after RFA, although it was not specified as to whether this was attributed to a patient with pheochromocytoma or paraganglioma. In addition, one periprocedural death after RFA of metastatic pheochromocytoma to the diaphragmatic crus resulted from complications of colonic and duodenal perforation observed after ablation.[47] Although the majority of metastatic pheochromocytoma tumors treated with RFA and reported in these two studies achieved successful local control, the application of RFA for pheochromocytomas should be considered an area for further study, and larger studies with long-term follow-up are needed. Careful preprocedure screening, intra- and postprocedural monitoring, and awareness of hemodynamic risk mitigation are also critical to reducing complications. These warrant the involvement of experienced and informed operators and multidisciplinary teams.[9]

Pearls ■

- Percutaneous thermal ablative therapies, including RFA, MWA, and cryoablation have been successfully used in the treatment of adrenal malignancy, including adrenal metastases, locally recurrent and metastatic adrenocortical carcinoma, and metastatic pheochromocytoma.
- The interventional oncologist must be mindful of the risk of intraprocedural hypertensive crisis during adrenal tumor ablation. A significantly higher rate of intraprocedural hypertension has been described in patients undergoing adrenal tumor ablation compared to nonadrenal abdominal tumors.
- Vigilance concerning the risk of hypertensive crisis is particularly essential during pheochromocytoma ablation. Attention to pre-, intra-, and postablation medical management is critical, including preablation endocrine and anesthesia consultation, consideration for intraprocedural general anesthesia, and postablation monitoring of hemodynamics.
- Specific intraprocedural technical maneuvers can greatly influence the likelihood of successful ablation of adrenal malignancy, including decubitus, prone, or transhepatic patient positioning, and hydrodissection for protection of vulnerable regional anatomy.
- Communication with the anesthesiologist is critical during ablation of pheochromocytoma, along with attention to procedural maneuvers that may represent a higher risk for hypertensive crisis (needle manipulation, repositioning, or removal).

2.9 Conclusions

Current data concerning the treatment of adrenal malignancy with percutaneous image-guided thermal ablation of adrenal tumors with RFA, MWA, and cryoablation suggest these therapies may lead to acceptable short-term outcomes and a low rate of complications. With appropriate periprocedural management, these therapies can be employed to treat certain adrenal metastases, locally recurrent and metastatic adrenocortical carcinoma, and metastatic adrenal pheochromocytoma. Ongoing management controversies include the comparative utility of these thermal ablation modalities in the treatment of adrenal malignancy, although some modality-specific advantages, including larger ablation zones associated with MWA and ice ball visualization with cryoablation, have been observed for adrenal malignancy ablation, as has been seen in other organs.[41] Further study is warranted to confirm the long-term efficacy of percutaneous ablation for adrenal malignancy, its relative efficacy compared to standard-of-care curative and palliative oncological therapies, and its impact on overall survival.

References

[1] Boland GW, Blake MA, Hahn PF, Mayo-Smith WW. Incidental adrenal lesions: principles, techniques, and algorithms for imaging characterization. Radiology 2008; 249(3): 756–775

[2] Kloos RT, Gross MD, Francis IR, Korobkin M, Shapiro B. Incidentally discovered adrenal masses. Endocr Rev 1995; 16 (4): 460–484

[3] Low G, Dhliwayo H, Lomas DJ. Adrenal neoplasms. Clin Radiol 2012; 67(10): 988–1000

[4] Ethier MD, Beland MD, Mayo-Smith W. Image-guided ablation of adrenal tumors. Tech Vasc Interv Radiol 2013; 16(4): 262–268

[5] Golden SH, Robinson KA, Saldanha I, Anton B, Ladenson PW. Clinical review: Prevalence and incidence of endocrine and metabolic disorders in the United States: a comprehensive review. J Clin Endocrinol Metab 2009; 94 (6): 1853–1878

[6] Libè R, Fratticci A, Bertherat J. Adrenocortical cancer: pathophysiology and clinical management. Endocr Relat Cancer 2007; 14(1): 13–28

[7] Lenders JW, Eisenhofer G, Mannelli M, Pacak K. Phaeochromocytoma. Lancet 2005; 366(9486): 665–675

[8] Reisch N, Peczkowska M, Januszewicz A, Neumann HP. Pheochromocytoma: presentation, diagnosis and treatment. J Hypertens 2006; 24(12): 2331–2339

[9] Venkatesan AM, Locklin J, Lai EW et al. Radiofrequency ablation of metastatic pheochromocytoma. J Vasc Interv Radiol 2009; 20(11): 1483–1490

[10] Paul CA, Virgo KS, Wade TP, Audisio RA, Johnson FE. Adrenalectomy for isolated adrenal metastases from non-adrenal cancer. Int J Oncol 2000; 17(1): 181–187

[11] Lo CY, van Heerden JA, Soreide JA et al. Adrenalectomy for metastatic disease to the adrenal glands. Br J Surg 1996; 83 (4): 528–531

[12] Kim SH, Brennan MF, Russo P, Burt ME, Coit DG. The role of surgery in the treatment of clinically isolated adrenal metastasis. Cancer 1998; 82(2): 389–394

[13] Xiao YY, Tian JL, Li JK, Yang L, Zhang JS. CT-guided percutaneous chemical ablation of adrenal neoplasms. Am J Roentgenol 2008; 190(1): 105–110

[14] Venkatesan AM, Locklin J, Dupuy DE, Wood BJ. Percutaneous ablation of adrenal tumors. Tech Vasc Interv Radiol 2010; 13 (2): 89–99

[15] Uppot RN, Gervais DA. Imaging-guided adrenal tumor ablation. Am J Roentgenol 2013; 200(6): 1226–1233

[16] Sudheendra D, Wood B. Thermal ablation of the adrenal gland. In: Mauro M, Murphy K, Thomson K, Venbrux A, Zollikofer C, eds. Image-Guided Interventions. Amsterdam, Netherlands: Elsevier; 2008:1606–1612

[17] Tuncali K, vanSonnenbe , rg E, Shankar S, Mort , ele KJ, Cibas ES, Silverman SG. Evaluation of patients referred for percutaneous ablation of renal tumors: importance of a preprocedural diagnosis. Am J Roentgenol 2004; 183(3): 575–582

[18] Olson JA, Wells SA. The pituitary and adrenal glands. In: Sabiston DC, ed. Textbook of Surgery: The Biological Basis of Modern Surgical Practice. Montreal, QC: WB Saunders; 1997:684–687

[19] Chini EN, Brown MJ, Farrell MA, Charbonea , u JW. Hypertensive crisis in a patient undergoing percutaneous radiofrequency ablation of an adrenal mass under general anesthesia. Anesth Analg 2004; 99(6): 1867–1869

[20] Atwell TD, Wass CT, Charboneau JW, Callstrom MR, Farrell MA, Sengupta S. Malignant hypertension during cryoablation of an adrenal gland tumor. J Vasc Interv Radiol 2006; 17 (3): 573–575

[21] Onik G, Onik C, Medary I et al. Life-threatening hypertensive crises in two patients undergoing hepatic radiofrequency ablation. Am J Roentgenol 2003; 181(2): 495–497

[22] Mamlouk MD, vanSonnenberg E, Stringfellow G, Smith D, Wendt A. Radiofrequency ablation and biopsy of metastatic pheochromocytoma: emphasizing safety issues and dangers. J Vasc Interv Radiol 2009; 20(5): 670–673

[23] Rhim H, Goldberg SN, Dodd GD, III et al. Essential techniques for successful radio-frequency thermal ablation of malignant hepatic tumors. Radiographics 2001; 21(Spec No): S17–S35, discussion S36–S39

[24] Shah DR, Green S, Elliot A, McGahan JP, Khatri VP. Current oncologic applications of radiofrequency ablation therapies. World J Gastrointest Oncol 2013; 5(4): 71–80

[25] Saldanha DF, Khiatani VL, Carrillo TC et al. Current tumor ablation technologies: basic science and device review. Semin Intervent Radiol 2010; 27(3): 247–254

[26] Simon CJ, Dupuy DE, Mayo-Smith WW. Microwave ablation: principles and applications. Radiographics 2005; 25 Suppl 1: S69–S83

[27] Martin RC, Scoggins CR, McMasters KM. Safety and efficacy of microwave ablation of hepatic tumors: a prospective review of a 5-year experience. Ann Surg Oncol 2010; 17(1): 171–178

[28] Wright AS, Sampson LA, Warner TF, Mahvi DM, Lee FT, Jr. Radiofrequency versus microwave ablation in a hepatic porcine model. Radiology 2005; 236(1): 132–139

[29] Zhang L, Wang N, Shen Q, Cheng W, Qian GJ. Therapeutic efficacy of percutaneous radiofrequency ablation versus microwave ablation for hepatocellular carcinoma. PLoS ONE 2013; 8(10): e76119

[30] Alexander ES, Dupuy DE. Lung cancer ablation: technologies and techniques. Semin Intervent Radiol 2013; 30(2): 141–150

[31] Ahmed M, Brace CL, Lee FT, Jr, Goldberg SN. Principles of and advances in percutaneous ablation. Radiology 2011; 258(2): 351–369

[32] Kujala N, Beland M. Principles of cryoablation. In: Mueller P, Adam A, eds. Interventional Oncology: A Practical Guide for the Interventional Oncologist. New York, NY: Springer; 2012:39–49

[33] Wood BJ, Abraham J, Hvizda JL, Alexander HR, Fojo T. Radiofrequency ablation of adrenal tumors and adrenocortical carcinoma metastases. Cancer 2003; 97(3): 554–560

[34] Mayo-Smith WW, Dupuy DE. Adrenal neoplasms: CT-guided radiofrequency ablation—preliminary results. Radiology 2004; 231(1): 225–230

[35] Yamakado K, Takaki H, Yamada T et al. Incidence and cause of hypertension during adrenal radiofrequency ablation. Cardiovasc Intervent Radiol 2012; 35(6): 1422–1427

[36] Fransson BA, Keegan RD, Ragle CA, Haldorson GJ, Greene SA. Hemodynamic changes during laparoscopic radiofrequency ablation of normal adrenal tissue in dogs. Vet Surg 2009; 38 (4): 490–497

[37] Mendiratta-Lala M, Brennan DD, Brook OR et al. Efficacy of radiofrequency ablation in the treatment of small functional adrenal neoplasms. Radiology 2011; 258(1): 308–316

[38] Liu SY, Ng EK, Lee PS et al. Radiofrequency ablation for benign aldosterone-producing adenoma: a scarless technique to an old disease. Ann Surg 2010; 252(6): 1058–1064

[39] Wolf FJ, Dupuy DE, Machan JT, Mayo-Smith WW. Adrenal neoplasms: Effectiveness and safety of CT-guided ablation of 23 tumors in 22 patients. Eur J Radiol 2012; 81(8): 1717–1723

[40] Venkatesan AM, Wood BJ, Gervais DA. Percutaneous ablation in the kidney. Radiology 2011; 261(2): 375–391

[41] Pua BB, Solomon SB. Ablative therapies in adrenal tumors: primary and metastatic. J Surg Oncol 2012; 106(5): 626–631

[42] Zagoria RJ. Imaging-guided radiofrequency ablation of renal masses. Radiographics 2004; 24 Suppl 1: S59–S71

[43] Levinson AW, Su LM, Agarwal D et al. Long-term oncological and overall outcomes of percutaneous radio frequency ablation in high risk surgical patients with a solitary small renal mass. J Urol 2008; 180(2): 499–504, discussion 504

[44] Weingärtner K, Gerharz EW, Bittinger A, Rosai J, Leppek R, Riedmiller H. Isolated clinical syndrome of primary aldosteronism in a patient with adrenocortical carcinoma. Case report and review of the literature. Urol Int 1995; 55(4): 232–235

[45] Li X, Fan W, Zhang L et al. CT-guided percutaneous microwave ablation of adrenal malignant carcinoma: preliminary results. Cancer 2011; 117(22): 5182–5188

[46] Welch BT, Callstrom MR, Carpenter PC et al. A single-institution experience in image-guided thermal ablation of adrenal gland metastases. J Vasc Interv Radiol 2014; 25 (4): 593–598

[47] McBride JF, Atwell TD, Charboneau WJ, Young WF, Jr, Wass TC, Callstrom MR. Minimally invasive treatment of metastatic pheochromocytoma and paraganglioma: efficacy and safety of radiofrequency ablation and cryoablation therapy. J Vasc Interv Radiol 2011; 22(9): 1263–1270

[48] Carrafiello G, Laganà D, Recaldini C et al. Imaging-guided percutaneous radiofrequency ablation of adrenal metastases: preliminary results at a single institution with a single device. Cardiovasc Intervent Radiol 2008; 31(4): 762–767

[49] Wang Y, Liang P, Yu X, Cheng Z, Yu J, Dong J. Ultrasound-guided percutaneous microwave ablation of adrenal metastasis: preliminary results. Int J Hyperthermia 2009; 25(6): 455–461

[50] Arima K, Yamakado K, Suzuki R et al. Image-guided radiofrequency ablation for adrenocortical adenoma with Cushing syndrome: outcomes after mean follow-up of 33 months. Urology 2007; 70(3): 407–411

Chapter 3

Ablation of Lung Cancer, Pulmonary Metastatic Disease, and Chest Wall Malignancy

3

3 Ablation of Lung Cancer, Pulmonary Metastatic Disease, and Chest Wall Malignancy

Charles McGraw, Scott Genshaft, Fereidoun Abtin, Antonio Gutierrez, and Robert Suh

3.1 Introduction

The role of thermal ablation in the treatment of thoracic malignancies has been growing for more than a decade. It has become an established treatment alternative to surgical resection in patients with both primary lung cancer and metastatic disease, as well as in patients with locally recurrent tumor following treatment. Emerging indications include treatment of primary and secondary tumors of the pleura and chest wall, as well as palliative ablation for painful soft tissue and bone lesions.

For early-stage, non–small cell lung cancer (NSCLC) (stage I/II), surgical resection or lobectomy remains the treatment of choice.[1] However, many patients are deemed medically inoperable for lobectomy or refuse surgery. Studies have shown that patients who receive some form of therapy for early-stage lung cancer demonstrate better outcomes than those who do not receive any form of therapy.[2] Therefore, a sizeable proportion of medically inoperable, early-stage lung cancer can benefit from less invasive therapies, such as percutaneous thermal ablation.

Approximately 20% of patients with lung metastases and resected primary soft tissue tumors have a limited number of metastases isolated to the lung and are potential candidates for surgical resection or metastasectomy.[3] Although surgical metastasectomy may result in improved disease-free survival in properly selected patients, multiple surgical resections may diminish pulmonary capacity.[4] Therefore, lung-sparing techniques, including percutaneous thermal ablation, are an attractive option in those candidates with limited metastatic disease or limited recurrent or residual disease following prior surgical resection, chemotherapy, or radiotherapy.

Management of malignancies of the chest wall and pleura is a promising new and not fully evaluated indication for thoracic tumor ablation. A growing body of data supports the efficacy of thermal ablation in treating soft tissue lesions,[5] and application to these tissues in the thorax is a natural extension. Although the published data specifically addressing the application of thermal ablation to pleural and chest wall disease are

limited, our institutional experience has yielded promising results in the treatment of thymoma, mesothelioma, and metastatic disease, including, but not limited to, chondrosarcoma.

3.2 Principles of Thermal Ablation

3.2.1 Radiofrequency Ablation

Radiofrequency ablation (RFA) is based on a thermal energy delivery system that causes agitation of ionic dipolar molecules, resulting in frictional heating of the surrounding tissues and fluids. The primary challenge in the application of RF energy to tumors in the lung is the disparity of tissue characteristics between normally aerated lung and tumor. The lung acts as an insulator, due to its naturally high impedance, which can limit the extension of an ablation zone to include a margin, compromising the likelihood of local treatment success. This insulation by the normal lung has the positive effect of increasing the central temperature of a solid mass that has been directly punctured by the ablation needle, the so-called oven-effect.[6]

Pleural and chest wall tumors tend to have characteristics similar to those of adjacent tissue; therefore the ablation zone tends to be more predictable. The potential traversal of nerves and the possibility of nerve injury (e.g., phrenic nerve, brachial plexus), related either to electrode placement or to ablation, are important considerations in treatment planning and delivery.[7] On a practical level, heat-based ablations, particularly RFA, can result in significant intraprocedural discomfort, which may require increased conscious sedation, and, possibly, general anesthesia. Additionally, some patients may experience postablative pain secondary to tissue charring, and, occasionally, neuropathic pain from nerve ablation.[8,9]

3.2.2 Microwave Ablation

Microwave ablation (MWA) is performed by microwave energy (900–2,450 MHz) inducing dipole excitation, which in turn causes the water molecules to spin, transferring some of their kinetic energy and creating friction, resulting in heat generation and tissue hyperthermia.[10] The microwave antenna emits electromagnetic radiation into tissue without the necessity of an electrical current; thus carbonization and gas pockets around the antenna do not interfere as much with energy deposition, resulting in higher intratumoral temperatures and more robust ablations as compared to RFA.[11]

3.2.3 Percutaneous Cryotherapy

In contradistinction to the heat-based ablative techniques, percutaneous cryotherapy (PCT) uses dissipation of extreme cold temperatures as its mode of cell death. This results in a zone of cooling below freezing and ice ball formation, which is often visible on computed tomography (CT).

On a practical note, cryoablation systems allow for application of a "stick" mode, which decreases the probe temperature to −10°C, forming a small ice ball and allowing for probe immobilization with respect to adjacent tumor or tissue. This can be used after satisfactory placement of a probe to facilitate additional probe placement, or to move the targeted tumor in lung parenchyma away from critical structures during cryoablation.

3.2.4 Special Equipment

Radiofrequency Ablation

Currently, commercially available RFA electrodes are either single-needle or multitined, with a gradual increasing trend toward use of single-needle electrodes. The zone of ablation may be increased for each probe by overlapping treatment regions for a single electrode, using programmed tine expansion, using multiple electrodes with a switch box generator, or diffusing hypertonic saline through specially designed electrodes into the tumor. Generally speaking, multiple electrodes should not be spaced farther than 2 cm apart in order to allow for complete coalescence of overlapping zones of ablation.

Dispersive, large surface area grounding pads are required and need to be carefully applied over the patient's body, avoiding underlying bone prominences, and excess hair should be removed prior to pad placement to facilitate skin adhesion and ensure firm contact.

Microwave Ablation

Microwave generators allow single or multiple antennas to be activated simultaneously. Higher intratumoral temperatures are achieved as a result of an improved convection profile in comparison to RFA, resulting in larger ablation volumes with shorter ablation times with less heat sink phenomenon. No dispersive or grounding pads are required, and the absence of electrical stimulation, as with RFA, confers less pain as a result of nerve irritation, of particular importance when treating juxtapleural and chest wall lesions, which can often be quite painful during RFA as a result of intercostal nerve stimulation.

Percutaneous Cryoablation

There are two commercially available PCA systems that offer cryoprobes in sizes ranging from 1.2 to 3.8 mm in diameter. In theory, both systems achieve ice of similar dimension that is based on cryoprobe diameter; however, in our practice, the 2.4 mm probes are preferred to achieve adequate lethal ice.

PCA offers many advantages over the other thermal ablative techniques: the lack of electrical current allows for safe use in patients with implantable cardiac devices, the level of pain during and after ablation is decreased in comparison to RFA and MWA (of particular importance when addressing juxtapleural and pleural/chest wall tumors), and hypodense ice is easily visualized when ablating within soft tissues. Furthermore, some suggest that PCT is favored when addressing juxtapleural and paramediastinal lung lesions and pleural and chest wall lesions because it preserves tissue collagenous architecture.[12]

An issue inherent to cryoablation is the relatively large-caliber probes (usually at least 2.4 mm or 13 G) compared to the 17 G heat-based probes, which can make skewering small tumors within the relatively more compliant lung difficult or impossible. This can be overcome by placement of at least two probes at the periphery of a lesion, the so-called chopstick approach, with commercially available generators able to accommodate up to 20 probes.

Within the lung, the authors use a triple-freeze technique (3-min freeze–3-min passive thaw–7-min freeze–3-min passive thaw–7-min freeze) with intermittent short 3-min passive thaw cycles after freeze cycles causing the airspaces to fill with pulmonary fluid and hemorrhage, significantly increasing thermal conductivity and allowing for extension of the ablation zone (▶ Fig. 3.1). In the chest wall and pleura, we typically employ a double-freeze technique with a longer, 8-minute

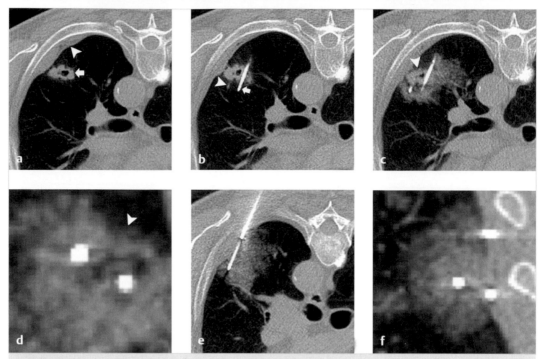

Fig. 3.1 Percutaneous cryotherapy (PCT) with parenchymal hemorrhage extending the ablation zone. **(a)** With the patient in a prone position, axial images in lung windows demonstrate a cavitary nodule *(arrow)* in the left lower lobe representing metastatic renal cell carcinoma. Note the prior 1% lidocaine administration within the extrapleural space *(arrowhead)* prior to probe placement. **(b)** Preablation images demonstrate the placement of two probes; one with the superomedial *(arrow)* and the other partially visualized in the inferolateral *(arrowhead)* portions of the nodule. **(c)** Axial images through the superior portion of the nodule demonstrate a lack of hemorrhage surrounding the superolateral *(arrowhead)* aspect of the nodule. **(d)** This lack of hemorrhage encompassing the nodule *(arrowhead)* is confirmed on a coronal view. **(e, f)** An additional probe is placed within the superolateral aspect of the nodule with subsequent cryoablation, which demonstrates hemorrhage and therefore the likely ablation margin encompassing the nodule on **(e)** axial and **(f)** coronal views. Note: the ice ball representing the ablation margin is not well visualized on these images.

passive thaw cycle, unless the anticipated ablative margin extends into the adjacent pulmonary parenchyma.

3.3 Indications

Proper patient selection is highly dependent on the anticipated goal to be achieved. Although no strict criteria for patient selection exists, emerging goals for percutaneous thermal ablation in the lung, chest wall, and pleura thus far have been established to include (1) potential for cure in early stage (stage I) NSCLCs that are medically inoperable or if the patient refuses surgery; (2) prolongation of survival in those with limited recurrent or metastatic disease to the lung and chest wall/pleura; (3) cytoreduction of large tumors to potentially alter the susceptibility of viable tumor tissue

to chemotherapy or radiotherapy; (4) palliation of symptoms, particularly pain in peripheral tumors invading the pleural and chest wall[13]; and (5) ablation of tumors adjacent to vital structures to limit or slow invasion.

3.4 Contraindications

Thoracic ablative procedures have few absolute and relative contraindications, which are similar to those of image-guided biopsy of the lung. Absolute contraindications include acute pneumonia, severe pulmonary arterial hypertension (> 40 mm Hg), and uncorrectable coagulopathy. Relative contraindications include poor lung function (forced expiratory volume in the first second of expiration [FEV_1] < 1 L), prior pneumonectomy, or single-functioning lung, because the potential complications of pulmonary hemorrhage, pneumothorax, or hemothorax with poor or limited respiratory reserve may cause respiratory failure. Pacemakers and pacemaker wires, which can conduct electrical current from radiofrequency and, to a lesser degree, microwave energies along the pacemaker wires can result in application of thermal energy in unintended remote locations. Additionally, a pacemaker may malfunction during RFA. Patients with pacemakers can still receive RFA provided the pacemaker is turned off prior to the procedure.[14]

3.5 Preprocedure Workup

Preprocedural evaluation of a patient typically includes a patient history, with focus on cardiopulmonary status, pulmonary infection, bleeding diatheses, and medications. Platelet count and coagulation profile are essential. Pulmonary function tests should be reviewed to check for adequacy of oxygenation, pulmonary reserve, flow-volume spirometry, and fitness for sedation and lung reduction, particularly in those patients with lung disease or prior resection.

The presence of a pacemaker or automatic implantable cardioverter defibrillator (AICD), especially in a patient with constant dependence, should increase consideration of PCT and MWA, rather than RFA, which can cause device malfunction. Alternatively, if RFA is the preferred ablative technique, and the patient has limited dependence on a cardiac pacer, a deactivated pacemaker with transvenous or temporary external cardiac pacing is an acceptable strategy.

A thorough medication history should be obtained with attention to anticoagulant and antiplatelet medications, which should be stopped or tapered prior to the anticipated procedure. Conversion to subcutaneous or low molecular weight heparin can be considered for those patients on oral anticoagulants, which can be stopped at least 24 hours prior to the procedure.

Histopathologic diagnosis of the lesion(s) should be obtained before the ablation. Biopsy can be performed prior to the ablation as a separate session or immediately prior to the ablation as a concurrent session. At our institution, we prefer to perform the percutaneous biopsy approximately 1 week prior to the ablation to allow for perilesional hemorrhage to resolve, to confirm the final pathology, and for clear tumor margins to be apparent at the time of the ablation. Furthermore, longer procedure times, or a delayed or postponed ablation procedure related to biopsy complications, may result when biopsy occurs prior to ablation as a concurrent session.

There is no standardized agreement on the pre- or postprocedural administration of antibiotics. At our institution, we typically do not give antibiotics for most chest ablations.

Ideally, a preprocedure chest CT scan should be performed within 4 weeks of the anticipated procedure to assess (1) tumor size and number; (2) lesion shape and location in relation to vessels, bronchi, and other vital structures; (3) the presence of comorbid lung disease, including advanced bullous disease, radiation injury, or infection; and (4) a safe percutaneous access route.

PCT of the chest is typically performed under conscious sedation, although general anesthesia is at times warranted during ablations that require a higher degree of monitoring. No matter the choice of anesthesia employed during thermal ablation of the chest, it must be efficient at both controlling pain and maximizing the reproducibility of the target tumor position to facilitate accurate probe placement. Additionally, there is an increased risk of pneumothorax from positive pressure ventilation with general anesthesia.[15] For these reasons, most experienced operators prefer conscious sedation in nearly all percutaneous thermal ablations of the thorax.

On occasion, general anesthesia is preferred, including in cases with increased risk of bleeding, in patients with tenuous respiratory status, or to allow for selective intubation of a bronchus to improve positioning of the contralateral-targeted pulmonary lesion in relation to vital structures. The most common indication for the escalation of sedation level to general anesthesia is when using RFA for treatment of chest wall and pleural lesions, a procedure that is often quite painful.[9]

3.6 Selection Criteria

Studies have repeatedly identified certain lesion characteristics for which ablation can be expected to achieve a complete result of total tumor kill without recurrence (▶ Table 3.1 and ▶ Fig. 3.2). These include size, location, number of lesions, and adjacent structures.

3.6.1 Size

Lesions < 3 to 3.5 cm[13,16] are more likely to be fully treated than larger lesions. Multiple RFAs and

Table 3.1 Comparison between various factors that influence the choice of ablative modality from less favorable (+) to more favorable (+ + +)

Comparative technologies			
Parameter(s)	Radiofrequency	Microwave	Cryoablation
< 3 cm	+ + +	+ + +	+ + +
> 3 cm	+ (up to 3)[a]	+ + + (up to 3)[a]	+ + (up to 20)[a]
≤ 1.5 cm pleura	+ (pain)	+ (air leak)	+ + +
Chest wall and pleura	+	+ +	+ + +
Mediastinum	+	+	+ +
Sinks (heat/cold)	+	+ + +	+ +
Pacer and AICD	+	+ +	+ + +
Coagulopathy	+ + +	+ + +	+
Maneuverability	(+)	(+)	+

Abbreviation: AICD, automatic implantable cardioverter defibrillator.
[a]The number of simultaneous applicators for each respective therapeutic modality.

cryoprobes are used for lesions > 2 cm. MWA is preferred for larger lesions, with its ability to treat up to 3.5 cm (▶ Fig. 3.3) and possibly larger lesions.

3.6.2 Location

For completely intraparenchymal lesions, any of the three percutaneous ablative therapies can be used. For juxtapleural, pleural, and chest wall lesions, cryoablation is preferred to the heat-based ablative therapies due to less patient discomfort and fewer complications.[17]

3.6.3 Number of Lesions

For metastatic disease, there are ideally fewer than six pulmonary lesions, which is loosely based on metastasectomy data showing decreased survival with an increasing number of resections.[18]

3.6.4 Adjacent Structures

Ablation adjacent to a pulmonary artery or vein measuring > 3 mm,[19,20] or large bronchus,[21] using RFA or PCT, may result in incomplete ablation margins due to heat sink or cold sink, respectively. MWA reduces, but does not completely negate, this heat sink phenomenon[10] (▶ Fig. 3.4).

PCT is preferred for lesions adjacent to the hilum and vital mediastinal structures, such as the aorta, heart, esophagus, and trachea, due to the preservation of the tissues' collagenous architecture and

visualization of ice (▶ Fig. 3.5). In some situations, the ability to "stick" the cryoprobe to the tumor allows the targeted tissue to be torqued away from adjacent structures.

Similarly, cryoablation is preferred for pleural and chest wall lesions because it results in less pain and tissue injury as compared to RFA and MWA, respectively.

3.7 Technique

3.7.1 Choice of Imaging Modality

CT is typically the modality of choice for image-guided placement of ablation probes within and around tumors within the lung, pleura, and chest wall. CT offers excellent tumor conspicuity, particularly when located within the lung. Current systems have the ability to quickly acquire volumetric data and render multiplanar reformations to accurately portray tumor–probe relationships. Although traditional CT imaging is limited by its lack of real-time guidance, CT fluoroscopy allows for real-time, or near real-time, visualization of probe placement.

3.7.2 Anatomy and Approaches

There are techniques that are common to any ablative technique in the lung. If possible, preferential positioning on the CT table should allow the applicator to be introduced along a line that represents

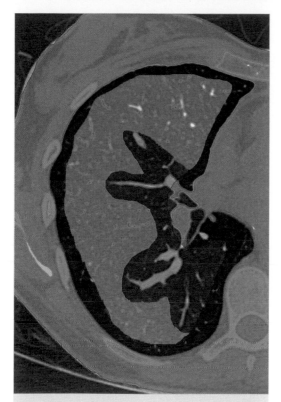

Fig. 3.2 Thermal energy preference map based on the authors' experience (yellow, radiofrequency ablation; red, microwave ablation; blue, cryoablation). All modalities can be used for lesions < 3 cm; however, microwave is preferred for lesions > 3 cm as well those lesions that are adjacent to vessels or bronchi > 3 mm in diameter. Cryoablation is the preferred modality in the peripheral lung, close to the pleura, chest wall, hilum, mediastinum, or vital structures.

the shortest distance from the skin to the target tumor. Exceptions to this technique include juxtapleural nodules, which typically require a long intrapulmonary needle path tangential to the pleura, which maximizes targeting of the tumor with the active tip and prevents bronchopleural fistula formed by backward ablation across the visceral pleura along the probe shaft (▶ Fig. 3.6 and ▶ Fig. 3.7). Likewise, hilar lesions are best approached by an abronchovascular route along the axial radiations from the hilum.

When all factors are equal, a posterior approach with the patient in the prone position is preferred to a supine approach, given that the posterior ribs are subject to less respiratory motion. The ablation path should ideally pass over the superior aspect

of the rib to avoid injury to the subcostal neurovascular bundle.

Percutaneous thermal ablation of chest wall and pleural malignancy demands technical considerations distinct from those of lung tumors. Although heat and cold ablative therapies have been used in the soft tissue, our clinical experience is strictly confined to PCT.

In general, recurrent tumor in the pleura tends to be elongated. When possible, cryoprobes are placed in the lesions along the tumor's long axis, allowing the oblong geometry of the ensuing ice ball to provide maximum coverage of the targeted tumor. With cryoprobes placed along the long axis, repeat freeze–thaw cycles can be performed at multiple stations from deep to superficial along the long axis of the targeted tumor, obviating the need for additional cryoprobe use. Our unpublished data from recurrent mesothelioma treatment supports effective local control when a 7 mm margin is achieved; the adequacy of this guideline as it pertains to other malignancies of the pleura will require further study.

3.7.3 Technical Aspects

Once the patient is comfortably positioned on the CT table, an initial preprocedural CT scan is performed, and a site of skin entry is marked using a radiopaque marker. Local anesthesia is achieved with 1% lidocaine solution using a 19-gauge or smaller coaxial system to the parietal pleura, where a generous amount (at least 5–10 mL) of 1% lidocaine, or longer-acting 0.5% bupivacaine, is administered to achieve pleural anesthesia (▶ Fig. 3.8). The applicator is then positioned into or adjacent to the lesion using an extrapleural tandem needle technique or, on occasion, through an insulated coaxial cannula. It is important that the patient be instructed to maintain a similar size breath hold (typically suspended at the end of inspiration) during all intermittent CT scans and incremental advancements of the applicators in the chest wall and lung toward the lesion. This is especially critical for lesions in the lung bases, along the diaphragm, where lung movement with respect to the chest wall is greatest.

An understanding of the imaging appearance of the ablation zone is imperative. Immediately following RFA or MWA in the lung, focal ground-glass opacity is seen on CT and corresponds to the coagulation necrosis, congestion, inflammation, and pulmonary hemorrhage involving the tumor and adjacent lung. Because it does not solely

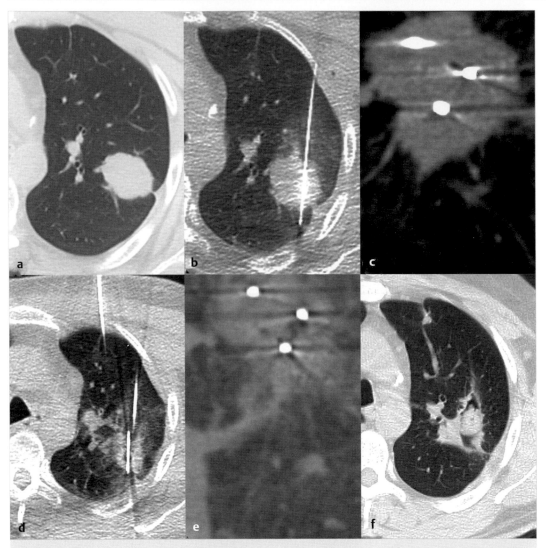

Fig. 3.3 Microwave ablation of a large colorectal metastasis. **(a)** Axial image in lung windows demonstrates a 3.5 cm left upper lobe colorectal metastasis. **(b)** An axial preablation image demonstrates one of three antennas in the superior aspect of the nodule. **(c)** A coronal preablation image demonstrates positioning of the antennas approximately 2 cm apart and 1 cm from the mass's margin. **(d, e)** Axial and coronal ablation images demonstrate tumor desiccation with tumor volume loss and ground glass surrounding the mass. **(f)** A follow-up CT at 2 months demonstrates interval cavitation and decrease in size of the ablation site.

correspond to coagulation necrosis, the ground-glass opacity should ideally extend 5 to 10 mm beyond the tumor margin to achieve complete tumor necrosis (▶ Fig. 3.9). Similarly, due to nonlethal temperature of the outer isotherms, the hypodense ice ball from PCT within the purposely induced perilesional parenchymal hemorrhage or the chest wall soft tissues should extend 5 to 10 mm beyond the approximate tumor margin (▶ Fig. 3.10).

At the completion of lung heat-based ablation (RFA and MWA), many operators perform tract cauterization of the lung parenchyma with lower-power application while withdrawing the applicator from the lung, but ensuring that the generator is shut off prior to the exposed tip reaching the extrathoracic soft tissues. Theoretically, this may lower the probability of parenchymal hemorrhage, tumor tract seeding, and pneumothorax.[22]

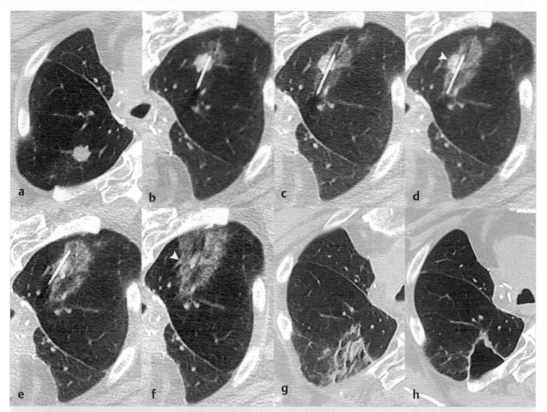

Fig. 3.4 Microwave ablation requiring repositioning due to heat sink effect. **(a)** Axial images in lung windows demonstrate a colorectal metastasis in the right lower lobe. **(b)** Ablation images with the patient in the prone position demonstrate the antenna appropriately positioned within the nodule. Axial images during 5 minutes **(c)** and 10 minutes **(d)** at 90 W demonstrate surrounding ground glass, which spares the medial aspect of the nodule *(arrowhead)*. **(e)** Given the inadequate ablation margin medially, the antenna is repositioned to the medial aspect of the nodule. **(f)** An additional 5 minutes at 90 W demonstrates an adequate ablation margin medially *(arrowhead)*. Postablation images demonstrate ablation zone hemorrhage and inflammation **(g)** at 1 month with subsequent cavitation **(h)** at 2 months.

3.7.4 Advanced Techniques

Several techniques can be used to increase the distance of the applicator from vital structures to minimize collateral tissue damage. Fixating the probe with ice within or immediately adjacent to targeted tissue during cryoablation allows enough security to torque the probe, mobilizing the ablation zone away from adjacent structures. This technique is particularly useful to move the zone of ablation away from nerves (e.g., phrenic) and critical structures (e.g., esophagus). A second technique is the induction of an iatrogenic pneumothorax or pneumoperitoneum in order to air-insulate the targeted tumor and injury-prone structures (► Fig. 3.11). Finally, when using cryoablation in the chest wall, a sterile glove filled with

warm water placed on the skin or an infusion of a mixture of sterile water and lidocaine into the subcutaneous tissues may present frostbite of the overlying skin.[23]

3.8 Complications

The most frequent complications—pneumothorax, pleural effusion, and hemothorax—are shared in all three types of lung ablation to varying degrees (► Table 3.2). Although pneumothorax remains the most common complication, occurring in approximately 15 to 40% of percutaneous lung ablations, depending on the thermal energy used, only approximately 10 to 15% of pneumothoraces require manual aspiration or chest tube placement (► Fig. 3.12).[23,24,25,26,27,28] A gradual pleural

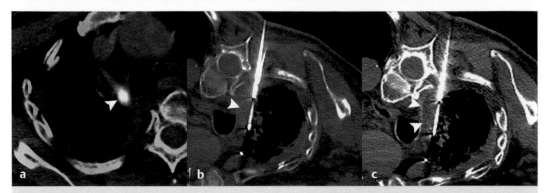

Fig. 3.5 Percutaneous cryotherapy (PCT) of a paratracheal mesothelioma recurrence. **(a)** An axial fused positron emission tomography computed tomographic image demonstrates a hypermetabolic focus *(arrowhead)* in the right paratracheal region, representing recurrent mesothelioma. **(b)** With the patient in a prone position, a single cryoprobe was positioned within the ill-defined soft tissue fullness *(arrowhead)* of the right paratracheal region. **(c)** An ice ball *(arrowheads)* following PCT encompasses the soft tissue mass but preserves integrity of adjacent trachea, partly due to the cold sink effect.

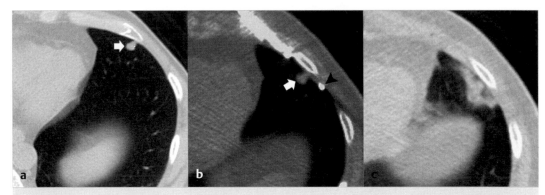

Fig. 3.6 Tangential approach for a juxtapleural osteosarcoma metastasis using radiofrequency ablation (RFA). **(a)** Axial computed tomographic image in lung windows demonstrates an irregular nodule *(arrow)* abutting the pleura in the left upper lobe. **(b)** Ablation image demonstrates RFA probe placement adjacent to the nodule *(arrowhead, probe tip; arrow, nodule),* tangential to the pleura to ensure adequate ablation of the juxtapleural component of metastasis. **(c)** Postablation images demonstrate adequate coverage of the nodule with ground glass.

effusion is a relatively common sequela of percutaneous ablation, occurring in approximately 15 to 20% of patients. Few (4%) require intervention for symptom relief. A rapidly accumulating pleural effusion detected by CT or radiography during the immediate postprocedural period should warrant expedited clinical evaluation to exclude a potentially lethal hemothorax and to prompt immediate intervention, such as embolization or ligation of the bleeding vessel, if required.

Unique to RFA and less commonly MWA, is postablation syndrome (PAS), likely related to the release of inflammatory cytokines at the site of ablation into the systemic circulation. This occurs in roughly 40% of patients undergoing RFA and an infrequent 2% of MWA patients.[23,26,28] The symptoms include low-grade fever, chills, malaise, myalgia, anorexia, and nausea, and they typically ensue within the first 24 to 48 hours and last up to 7 to 14 days. Treatment is largely symptomatic and involves antipyretics, pain control, and antitussives, as needed.[29]

Less common complications include infection, bronchopleural fistula, pulmonary hemorrhage,

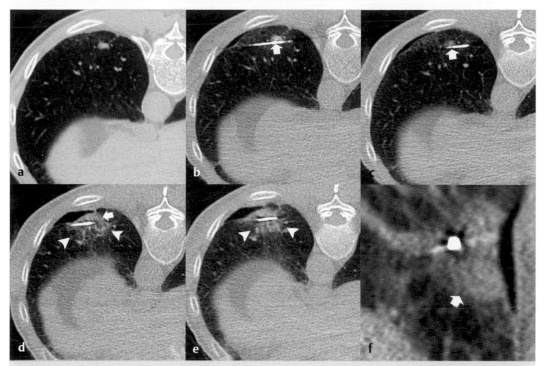

Fig. 3.7 Tangential approach for microwave ablation (MWA) of a biopsy-proven NSCLC in the juxtapleural left lower lobe. **(a)** Axial computed tomographic image in lung windows with the patient in the prone position demonstrates a juxtapleural spiculated nodule in the left lower lobe. **(b, c)** Consecutive axial images demonstrate placement of the antenna adjacent to the tumor *(arrow)*, but with the tumor intervening between the probe and the pleura to prevent ablation injury to the pleura. Note is made of a trace pneumothorax related to probe placement. **(d, e)** Consecutive axial images demonstrate adequate ablation margins *(arrowheads)* with ground glass and airspace consolidation encompassing the tumor *(arrow)* with associated volume loss of the adjacent lung. **(f)** A coronal image confirms the ablation margin, consisting of airspace consolidation *(arrow)* and surrounding ground glass, encompassing the tumor.

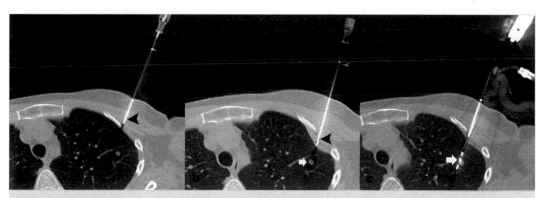

Fig. 3.8 Pleural anesthesia prior to percutaneous thermal ablation. **(a)** Axial computed tomography (CT) demonstrates a 19-gauge coaxial needle *(arrowhead)* with the tip terminating in extrapleural soft tissues. **(b)** Postanesthesia, a 19-gauge coaxial needle *(arrowhead)* has been advanced into the extrapleural space with a convex collection of 10 mL of 1% lidocaine in the extrapleural space. The targeted lung lesion *(arrow)* is along the path of the needle. **(c)** Intraprocedural CT images demonstrate subsequent microwave ablation antenna placement *(arrow)* within the pulmonary tumor.

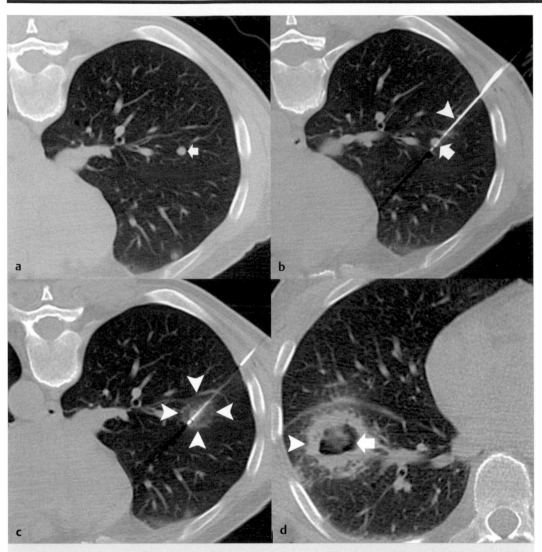

Fig. 3.9 Imaging end point with radiofrequency ablation (RFA). **(a)** Preablation computed tomographic (CT) image in lung window demonstrates a right lower lobe pericentimeter biopsy-proven non–small cell lung cancer *(arrow)*. **(b)** With the patient in a prone position, a single radiofrequency electrode *(arrowhead)* was inserted into the nodule *(arrow)*. **(c)** Ablation images demonstrate adequate coverage of the tumor with ground glass *(arrowheads)*. **(d)** In an axial CT image 1 week later the zone of ablation shows interval cavitation *(arrow)* with surrounding consolidation *(arrowhead)*.

neural injury, tumor seeding, and air embolism. Bronchopleural fistula is of particular concern with aggressive ablation, especially MWA, of peripheral pulmonary, pleural, and chest wall lesions, resulting in a communication between the peripheral airway or lung and the pleural space.[30] It requires prolonged catheter drainage and, possibly, escalating adjunctive treatments, including autologous pleural blood patch or sealant placement or surgical wedge resection[31,32,33](▸ Fig. 3.13).

3.9 Postprocedural Management and Follow-up Evaluation

3.9.1 Postprocedural Management

Following the ablation procedure, patients recover in the posttreatment care unit with the punctured lung dependent. With an anterior lung puncture,

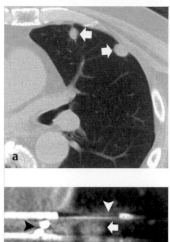
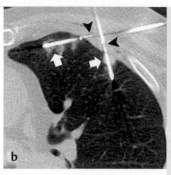
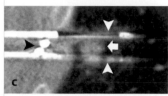
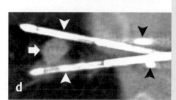
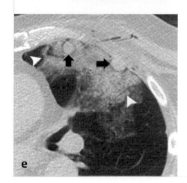
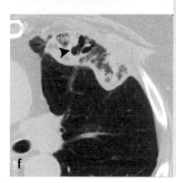

Fig. 3.10 Percutaneous cryotherapy (PCT) of two colorectal metastases in the left upper lobe using two cryoprobes for each lesion. **(a)** Preprocedure computed tomographic (CT) image demonstrates two juxtapleural nodules *(arrows)* in the left upper lobe, an ideal case for using PCT. **(b)** Axial images demonstrate two probes *(black arrowheads)* adjacent to or within each nodule (white arrows). **(c)** Sagittal and **(d)** coronal images confirm two probes *(white arrowheads)* adjacent to or slightly within each nodule *(arrow)*. Smaller lesions can be difficult to skewer when using the large-caliber cryoprobes and in this case required two cryoprobes each for adequate ablation margins. The respective crossing cryoprobes *(black arrowheads)* are noted in each image. **(e)** Immediate postablation images demonstrate extensive perilesional hemorrhage *(white arrowheads)* encompassing the margins of the targeted nodule (black arrows). **(f)** Follow-up CT approximately 3 weeks later demonstrates hemorrhage resolution with an ablation zone showing central cavitation *(arrowhead)*.

the patient is placed in ipsilateral decubitus position to decrease the risk of delayed pneumothorax and to reduce bleeding into the central airway, while vital signs and oxygenation are frequently monitored. For lung ablations, chest radiographs are generally obtained at 2 and 4 hours postprocedure to check for complications, such as pneumothorax; however, they may be acquired less frequently, if at all, in certain situations in which the lung parenchyma was not traversed, such as in chest wall ablations. On occasion, if the patient is symptomatic, follow-up chest radiographs at 24 and/or 48 hours following the ablation can assess for interval pleural effusion, airspace consolidations, or delayed or progressive pneumothorax.

3.9.2 Follow-up Evaluation

Following discharge, periodic imaging is required to identify any complications, confirm expected postablation appearances, exclude local tumor progression, and screen for disease progression at other intra- and extrathoracic sites. Although there is no proven standardized imaging modality or protocol within the literature, many feel that CT with interval positron emission tomographic (PET)-CT can be helpful in determining the efficacy of the ablation[34,35] (► Fig. 3.14).

Given that the common pathological end point of ablation, regardless of thermal energy used, is coagulation necrosis, many of the imaging findings are strikingly similar across the modalities. Although the descriptions of the timing of radiographic findings are beyond the scope of this chapter, in general, the size of the zone of ablation may be larger compared to the preablation tumor for the first 3 to 6 months (2 months in PCT), but should generally be smaller after 6 months (► Fig. 3.15 and ► Fig. 3.16).[34,36,37]

3.10 Outcomes

Much of the data on percutaneous thermal ablation in the lung has been generated for RFA.

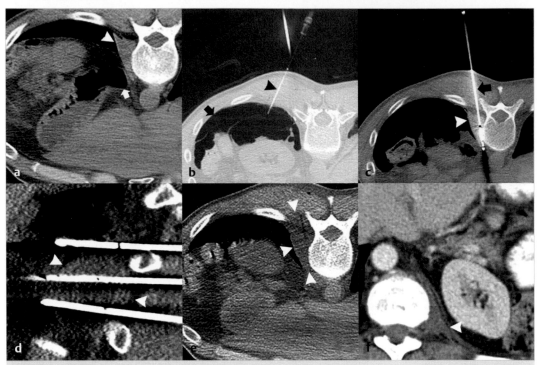

Fig. 3.11 Malignant thymoma recurrence along the left paraspinal space requiring intentional pneumoretroperitoneum prior to percutaneous cryotherapy. **(a)** Axial computed tomographic (CT) image in soft tissue windows with the patient in a prone position demonstrates a soft tissue mass *(arrowhead)* along the left paraspinal region, representing malignant thymoma recurrence. The relatively decompressed stomach *(arrow)* abuts the soft tissue mass. **(b)** A 19-gauge coaxial needle *(arrowhead)* was introduced into the retroperitoneum with subsequent injection of room air to cause a large retropneumoperitoneum *(arrow)*. **(c)** A preablation CT image demonstrates one of three cryoprobes *(black arrow)* is positioned within the mass *(white arrowhead)*. The stomach has been displaced from the expected ablation margin. **(d)** The three cryoprobe positions in relation to the mass *(arrowheads)* are confirmed on a sagittal reformatted CT. **(e)** A postablation CT demonstrates the hypodense ice ball *(arrowheads)* encompassing the previously seen mass with extension of the ice ball into the left neural foramen. **(f)** Follow-up CT performed 3 months later demonstrates interval decrease in size and increased hypodensity of the left paraspinal tumor *(arrowhead)*, likely representing scar tissue.

Compounding the limited outcome data for thermal ablation in the lung is the heterogeneity of the patient population, lesions treated, and criteria for treatment.

3.10.1 Radiofrequency Ablation

Survival following thermal ablation is dependent on many factors. For patients with NSCLC, survival is strongly correlated with clinical tumor stage, such that potential cure can be achieved in stage 1A and 1B NSCLC. Better survival is associated with smaller baseline tumor size, which theoretically allows for achieving complete necrosis. Simon and colleagues reported that the median survival for medically inoperable stage 1 NSCLC was 29 months with 1-, 2-, 3-, 4-, and 5-year survival rates

of 78%, 57%, 36%, 27%, and 27%, respectively.[25] Reemphasizing the importance of tumor size was the fact that local tumor progression rates over time were significantly lower in patients with smaller index lesions (≤ 3 vs. > 3 cm, $p < 0.002$) with median time to progression of ≤ 3 cm being 45 months and > 3 cm being 12 months. Similar survival rates were found by Lencioni and colleagues in a prospective, intention-to-treat, multicenter clinical trial for inoperable NSCLC with RFA.[38] The 1- and 2-year survival rates for inoperable NSCLC were 70% and 48%, respectively, and the 2-year survival for stage I NSCLC was 75%. In a retrospective review in 50 patients undergoing RFA for inoperable stage I NSCLC, Hiraki and colleagues found the 1-, 2-, 3-, 4-, and 5-year overall survivals to be 94%, 86%, 74%, 67%, and 61%,

Table 3.2 Complication percentages associated with radiofrequency ablation (RFA), microwave ablation (MWA), and percutaneous cryotherapy (PCT)

Summary pulmonary RFA[54]		MWA[26]	PCT[23]
Complications	%		
Pneumothorax	42.7	39	12
Minor	28.3	27	11
Chest tube	14.4	12	1.4
Pleural effusions	14.8	21	14
Pain	14.1	2	
Pyrexia	4.4	2	42
Hemoptysis	4.3	6	62
Pneumonia	1.5		
Abscesses	0.4	3	
Bronchopleural fistula	0.4		
Subcutaneous emphysema	0.2		5
Burn/skin injury		3	5
Acute respiratory distress/ hospital admission		2/15	
Procedure-related death	0.2		1

resepctively.[39] Interestingly, tumor size had no prognostic significance. Additionally, there was no significant survival difference ($p = 0.057$) between overall survival of stage Ia and stage Ib patients.

Given the poor outcomes of surgical resection, chemotherapy and radiation therapy in unresectable recurrent NSCLC, a retrospective review on the outcomes of RFA in 44 patients and 51 tumor targets was performed by Kodoma and colleagues.[40] The 1-, 3-, and 5-year overall survival rates were 97.7%, 72.9%, and 55.7%, respectively. There were 5 of 41 patients with recurrences over the 5 years, 3 of which were successfully retreated with RFA. The 1-, 3-, and 5-year secondary local tumor progression rates were 5.4%.

RFA as an adjunctive role with chemotherapy in stage III and IV NSCLC performed superiorly to chemotherapy alone with overall survival of 42 months versus 29 months, respectively ($p = 0.03$).[41] Combination therapy of mostly RFA with external-beam radiation therapy and brachytherapy in medically inoperable stage I and II NSCLC in 41 patients by Grieco et al found overall survival rates of 86.8% at 1 year, 70.4% at 2 years, and 57.1% at 3 years, which was felt to represent improved

survival compared to either treatment modality alone.[42]

A number of factors have been found to influence survival and local control in patients undergoing RFA in the setting of pulmonary metastatic disease, including tumor size ≤ 3 cm, absence of extrapulmonary metastases at the time of ablation,[43] single metastasis, normal carcinoembryonic antigen (CEA) prior to therapy in colorectal metastases, prolonged disease-free interval between primary therapy and development of first metastases, and initial complete response to ablation.[44, 45] Local control is affected by smaller tumor size (≤ 1.5–3.5 cm) and lack of a subtending bronchus > 2 mm.[46,47]

> ### Pearls
>
> - Thermal ablation is an effective treatment alternative in select patients with primary or secondary lung or chest wall malignancies.
> - The choice of RFA, MWA, or PCT depends on operator comfort as well as patient and tumor characteristics, including, but not limited to, tumor size and location.
> - Thermal ablation in the lung and chest wall can be safely performed as an outpatient procedure with up to 4 hours of postprocedural observation.
> - Complications are relatively similar across the various thermal energies, although pneumothorax tends to be the most common, which occasionally requires chest tube insertion.
> - The survival outcomes of thermal ablation in the lung across the various energy modalities approach those of surgical resection and radiation therapy.
> - PCT is the preferred modality of treatment for chest wall and pleural lesions because it is less painful than RFA and MWA.
> - The data regarding chest wall and pleural malignancies are limited, but in our experience has a significant role in local control and palliation for recurrent mesothelioma, thymoma, and metastatic disease.

In inoperable patients with colorectal pulmonary metastatic disease, Chua and colleagues found that the median progression-free survival was 11 months (95% confidence interval 9–14), and the median overall survival was 51 months. The 3- and 5-year survival rates were 60% and 45%, respectively,[43] which compares well with the

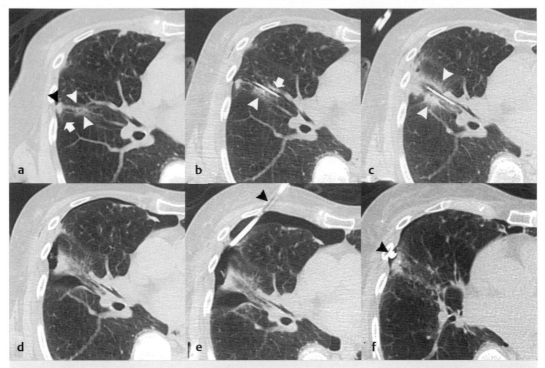

Fig. 3.12 Postablation pneumothorax complicating microwave ablation of a biopsy-proven non–small cell lung cancer. **(a)** Preablation axial CT image in lung windows demonstrates a semisolid lesion with ill-defined borders in the right middle lobe *(white arrowheads)*, which is adjacent to the right major fissure *(white arrow)*. Note is made of postbiopsy changes lateral to the tumor (black arrowhead) related to a biopsy performed approximately 3 weeks earlier. **(b)** The antenna is positioned adjacent to the lesion *(arrowhead)* without crossing the adjacent major fissure. The antenna intervenes between the large pulmonary vessel *(arrow)*, a potential cause of heat sink, and the lesion. **(c)** Ablation image demonstrates coverage of the tumor margin with ground glass and airspace consolidation *(arrowheads)*. **(d)** On the CT image following antenna removal, a small pneumothorax was present, which slowly increased on a subsequent CT scan performed 5 minutes later (image not shown), confirming an air leak. **(e)** A 12F chest tube *(arrowhead)* was placed into the pleural space. **(f)** The small to moderate pneumothorax *(arrowhead)* was aspirated with a trace residual pneumothorax. The chest tube side holes approximate the presumed region of air leak. The patient was discharged home later that day with a Heimlich valve connected to the chest tube. The chest tube was removed 3 days later once the air leak had resolved.

surgical metastasectomy rate. Nakamura and colleagues reported that complete tumor ablation of sarcoma pulmonary metastases was a significant factor for prognosis, with the 1- and 3-year survival rates of 88.9% and 59.2% with complete ablation versus 29.6% and 0% with incomplete tumor ablation.[48] Furthermore, Simon and colleagues reported 1-, 2-, 3-, 4-, and 5-year survival rates for colorectal metastases as 87%, 78%, 57%, 57%, and 57%, respectively.[25]

As with NSCLC, there is likely an adjunctive role of RFA with chemotherapy in the setting of pulmonary metastatic disease. Inoue and colleagues demonstrated a significant difference in survival between those patients with colorectal metastases receiving chemotherapy and RFA and in those receiving chemotherapy alone at 88% and 33%, respectively, at 3 years.[44] Chua and colleagues found that the use of adjunct systemic chemotherapy was an independent predictor for overall survival in patients undergoing RFA for unresectable colorectal pulmonary metastases.[47]

3.10.2 Microwave Ablation

Unlike RFA, outcome data are limited regarding MWA therapy for lung cancer or pulmonary metastatic disease, although results would be expected

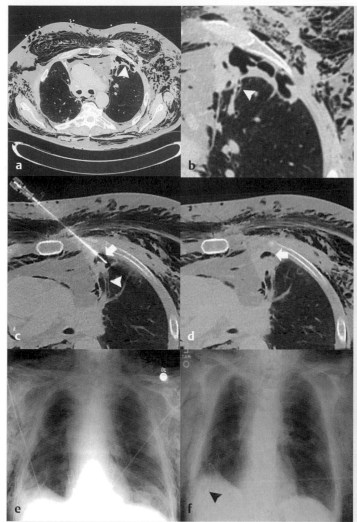

Fig. 3.13 Novel technique for percutaneous treatment of percutaneous cryotherapy (PCT)-related bronchomediastinal fistula. **(a)** Axial computed tomographic (CT) images were obtained 3 months following PCT of left upper lobe colorectal metastases and demonstrate extensive subcutaneous emphysema and mediastinum without a pneumothorax. The cavitary ablation site *(arrowhead)* communicates with the chest wall and mediastinum (not shown). **(b)** A magnified view demonstrates a bronchus *(arrowhead)* supplying the cavitary ablation site and the likely culprit for the persistent air leak. **(c)** A 19-gauge coaxial needle *(arrowhead)* was advanced into the cavitary ablation site *(arrow)* and offending bronchus. **(d)** Surgical sealant was administered through the outer cannula of the coaxial needle filling the cavitary site *(arrow)*. **(e)** In comparison of portable chest X-ray prior to procedure to **(f)** 1 day after the procedure, there is significant reduction in the subcutaneous emphysema and pneumomediastinum, consistent with a successfully treated postablation persistent air leak. Note is made of a mediastinal drain *(arrowhead)* on **(f)** follow-up chest X-ray that was placed during surgical sealant administration for immediate decompression of pneumomediastinum.

to be at least as good for MWA because ablation zones trend toward being more robust, with less thermal sink effect. Wolf et al reported their results on mixed pulmonary tumors and found 1-, 2-, and 3-year overall survivals of 65%, 55%, and 45%, respectively. Unlike RFA, the overall survivals were not affected by index lesions > 3 cm in size; however, there was a statistically significant decrease in local control for those tumors > 3 cm in size.[26]

In a group of mixed pulmonary malignancies, Lu and colleagues found clinical efficacy and comparable survival rates for NSCLC and pulmonary metastatic disease, respectively, to prior studies with MWA and RFA. Most notably though there was no significant difference in local progression between tumors < 3 cm and tumors 3 to 4 cm;

however, there was increased local progression for those tumors > 4 cm.[49]

Risk factors for local tumor progression in primary and metastatic pulmonary lesions following MWA include the following: tumor diameter (> 1.55 cm), tumor shape (irregular, vs. round or oval), low applied energy (< 26.7 J/mm³), and pleural adhesion. Notably, adjacency to vessels > 3 mm in diameter had no significant correlation with local tumor progression.[50]

3.10.3 Cryoablation

Like MWA, there are limited outcome data for PCT in pulmonary malignancies. Compared with RFA and sublobar resection in medically inoperable stage I NSCLC, PCT had similar outcomes with 3-

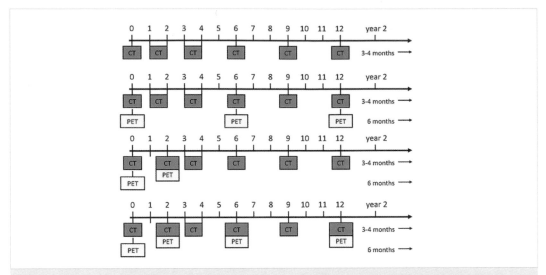

Fig. 3.14 Follow-up imaging algorithm from our institution. Timetables for follow-up may have several different appearances using computed tomography alone or in combination with positron emission tomography.

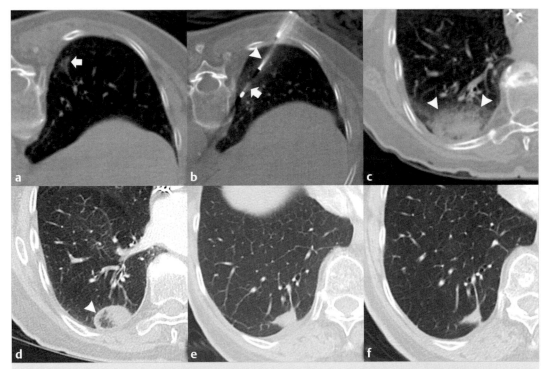

Fig. 3.15 Imaging changes following percutaneous cryotherapy (PCT) of a biopsy-proven non–small cell lung cancer. **(a)** Preablation computed tomographic (CT) image in lung windows with the patient in the prone position demonstrates an irregular semisolid lesion *(arrow)* in the right lower lobe. **(b)** A procedural CT scan demonstrates the cryoprobe *(arrowhead)* within the lesion *(arrow)*. **(c)** A postprocedure CT image with the patient in the supine position demonstrates extensive hemorrhage and airspace consolidation *(arrowheads)* in the region of the previously seen tumor. **(d)** An axial CT image in lung windows performed 5 weeks following the procedure demonstrates a more discrete, consolidative appearance to the ablation site *(arrowheads)*. **(e)** Follow-up CT images at approximately 5 and **(f)** nearly 9 months shows the expected findings of continued involution of the cryoablation zone.

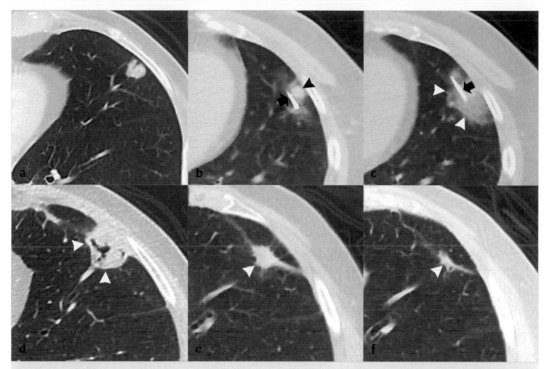

Fig. 3.16 Imaging changes following radiofrequency ablation (RFA) of a biopsy-proven non–small cell lung cancer. **(a)** An irregular, juxtapleural tumor is seen on axial computed tomographic (CT) image in lung windows. **(b)** An RFA single-tined needle *(arrow)* is placed adjacent to the tumor *(arrowhead)*. **(c)** Following subsequent ablation, there is ground glass and airspace consolidation *(arrowheads)* surrounding a tangentially viewed RFA probe *(arrow)*. **(d)** On a 1-month follow-up CT image, the zone of ablation *(arrowheads)* is more defined with central cavitation. **(e)** At 3-month follow-up CT, the zone of ablation *(arrowhead)* has decreased in size. **(f)** Follow-up CT over 5 years from RFA shows the zone of ablation retracting to a thin, linear scar *(arrowhead)* without evidence of recurrence.

year overall survival rates of 77% versus 87.1% with sublobar resection and 87.5% with RFA ($p > 0.05$). There was little difference in the cancer-specific survival with PCT versus the other two treatment options.[51]

In a retrospective review of 71 consecutive patients with mixed pulmonary tumors, but mostly metastatic disease, Yashiro et al found that 1-, 2-, and 3-year local progression-free rates were 80.4%, 69%, and 67.7%, respectively. Presence of a vessel ≥ 3 mm no more than 3 mm from the edge of the tumor was associated with local progression.[52]

Yamauchi et al found that, in 160 medically inoperable stage I NSCLCs treated with PCT, the 2- and 3-year overall survival was 88% and 88%, respectively. The mean disease-free 2- and 3-year survival was 78% and 67%, respectively. Importantly, there was no decrease in pulmonary function tests, similar to RFA, as would be seen with surgical resection or radiation therapy.[53]

References

[1] Spira A, Ettinger DS. Multidisciplinary management of lung cancer. N Engl J Med 2004; 350(4): 379–392

[2] McGarry RC, Song G, des Rosiers P, Timmerman R. Observation-only management of early stage, medically inoperable lung cancer: poor outcome. Chest 2002; 121(4): 1155–1158

[3] Burt MMN, Ginsberg RJ. Surgical treatment of lung carcinoma. In: Baue AE, ed. Glenn's Thoracic and Cardiovascular Surgery. 6th ed. Stamford, CT: Appleton & Lange; 1996:421–443

[4] Welter S, Cheufou D, Ketscher C, Darwiche K, Maletzki F, Stamatis G. Risk factors for impaired lung function after pulmonary metastasectomy: a prospective observational study of 117 cases. Eur J Cardiothorac Surg 2012; 42(2): e22–e27

[5] Littrup PJ, Bang HJ, Currier BP et al. Soft-tissue cryoablation in diffuse locations: feasibility and intermediate term outcomes. J Vasc Interv Radiol 2013; 24(12): 1817–1825

[6] Goldberg SN, Gazelle GS, Compton CC, McLoud TC. Radiofrequency tissue ablation in the rabbit lung: efficacy and complications. Acad Radiol 1995; 2(9): 776–784

[7] Hiraki T, Gobara H, Mimura H et al. Brachial nerve injury caused by percutaneous radiofrequency ablation of apical lung cancer: a report of four cases. J Vasc Interv Radiol 2010; 21(7): 1129–1133

[8] Gadaleta C, Mattioli V, Colucci G et al. Radiofrequency ablation of 40 lung neoplasms: preliminary results. Am J Roentgenol 2004; 183(2): 361–368

[9] VanSonnenberg E, Shankar S, Morrison PR et al. Radiofrequency ablation of thoracic lesions: part 2, initial clinical experience—technical and multidisciplinary considerations in 30 patients. Am J Roentgenol 2005; 184(2): 381–390

[10] Simon CJ, Dupuy DE, Mayo-Smith WW. Microwave ablation: principles and applications. Radiographics 2005; 25 Suppl 1: S69–S83

[11] Wright AS, Lee FT, Jr, Mahvi DM. Hepatic microwave ablation with multiple antennae results in synergistically larger zones of coagulation necrosis. Ann Surg Oncol 2003; 10(3): 275–283

[12] Maiwand MO, Homasson JP. Cryotherapy for tracheobronchial disorders. Clin Chest Med 1995; 16(3): 427–443

[13] Lee JM, Jin GY, Goldberg SN et al. Percutaneous radiofrequency ablation for inoperable non-small cell lung cancer and metastases: preliminary report. Radiology 2004; 230 (1): 125–134

[14] Skonieczki BD, Wells C, Wasser EJ, Dupuy DE. Radiofrequency and microwave tumor ablation in patients with implanted cardiac devices: is it safe? Eur J Radiol 201 1; 79(3): 343–346

[15] Rose SC. Radiofrequency ablation of pulmonary malignancies. Semin Respir Crit Care Med 2008; 29(4): 361–383

[16] Akeboshi M, Yamakado K, Nakatsuka A et al. Percutaneous radiofrequency ablation of lung neoplasms: initial therapeutic response. J Vasc Interv Radiol 2004; 15(5): 463–470

[17] Abtin FWC, Golshan A, Suh R. CT guided percutaneous cryoablation of thoracic tumors: technical feasibility, early efficacy and imaging of 27 treated tumors. Paper presented at: Scientific session 8, #713, 2nd World Congress of Thoracic Imaging and Diagnosis in Chest Disease; May 30–June 2, 2009; Valencia, Spain

[18] Murthy SC, Kim K, Rice TW et al. Can we predict long-term survival after pulmonary metastasectomy for renal cell carcinoma? Ann Thorac Surg 2005; 79(3): 996–1003

[19] Steinke K, Haghighi KS, Wulf S, Morris DL. Effect of vessel diameter on the creation of ovine lung radiofrequency lesions in vivo: preliminary results. J Surg Res 2005; 124(1): 85–91

[20] Hinshaw JL, Lee FT, Jr. Cryoablation for liver cancer. Tech Vasc Interv Radiol 2007; 10(1): 47–57

[21] Oshima F, Yamakado K, Akeboshi M et al. Lung radiofrequency ablation with and without bronchial occlusion: experimental study in porcine lungs. J Vasc Interv Radiol 2004; 15(12): 1451–1456

[22] Yamakado K, Akeboshi M, Nakatsuka A et al. Tumor seeding following lung radiofrequency ablation: a case report. Cardiovasc Intervent Radiol 2005; 28(4): 530–532

[23] Wang H, Littrup PJ, Duan Y, Zhang Y, Feng H, Nie Z. Thoracic masses treated with percutaneous cryotherapy: initial experience with more than 200 procedures. Radiology 2005; 235 (1): 289–298

[24] Rose SC, Thistlethwaite PA, Sewell PE, Vance RB. Lung cancer and radiofrequency ablation. J Vasc Interv Radiol 2006; 17 (6): 927–951, quiz 951

[25] Simon CJ, Dupuy DE, DiPetrillo TA et al. Pulmonary radiofrequency ablation: long-term safety and efficacy in 153 patients. Radiology 2007; 243(1): 268–275

[26] Wolf FJ, Grand DJ, Machan JT, Dipetrillo TA, Mayo-Smith WW, Dupuy DE. Microwave ablation of lung malignancies: effectiveness, CT findings, and safety in 50 patients. Radiology 2008; 247(3): 871–879

[27] Dorsey ER, Jarjoura D, Rutecki GW. The influence of controllable lifestyle and sex on the specialty choices of graduating U.S. medical students, 1996–2003. Acad Med 2005; 80(9): 791–796

[28] Wasser EJ, Dupuy DE. Microwave ablation in the treatment of primary lung tumors. Semin Respir Crit Care Med 2008; 29(4): 384–394

[29] Zhu JC, Yan TD, Morris DL. A systematic review of radiofrequency ablation for lung tumors. Ann Surg Oncol 2008; 15 (6): 1765–1774

[30] Sakurai J, Hiraki T, Mukai T et al. Intractable pneumothorax due to bronchopleural fistula after radiofrequency ablation of lung tumors. J Vasc Interv Radiol 2007; 18(1 Pt 1): 141–145

[31] Wagner JM, Hinshaw JL, Lubner MG et al. CT-guided lung biopsies: pleural blood patching reduces the rate of chest tube placement for postbiopsy pneumothorax. Am J Roentgenol 2011; 197(4): 783–788

[32] Shackcloth MJ, Poullis M, Jackson M, Soorae A, Page RD. Intrapleural instillation of autologous blood in the treatment of prolonged air leak after lobectomy: a prospective randomized controlled trial. Ann Thorac Surg 2006; 82(3): 1052–1056

[33] Droghetti A, Schiavini A, Muriana P et al. Autologous blood patch in persistent air leaks after pulmonary resection. J Thorac Cardiovasc Surg 2006; 132(3): 556–559

[34] Abtin FG, Eradat J, Gutierrez AJ, Lee C, Fishbein MC, Suh RD. Radiofrequency ablation of lung tumors: imaging features of the postablation zone. Radiographics 2012; 32(4): 947–969

[35] Beland MD, Wasser EJ, Mayo-Smith WW, Dupuy DE. Primary non-small cell lung cancer: review of frequency, location, and time of recurrence after radiofrequency ablation. Radiology 2010; 254(1): 301–307

[36] Vogl TJ, Naguib NN, Gruber-Rouh T, Koitka K, Lehnert T, Nour-Eldin NE. Microwave ablation therapy: clinical utility in treatment of pulmonary metastases. Radiology 2011; 261 (2): 643–651

[37] Ito N, Nakatsuka S, Inoue M et al. Computed tomographic appearance of lung tumors treated with percutaneous cryoablation. J Vasc Interv Radiol 2012; 23(8): 1043–1052

[38] Lencioni R, Crocetti L, Cioni R et al. Response to radiofrequency ablation of pulmonary tumours: a prospective, intention-to-treat, multicentre clinical trial (the RAPTURE study). Lancet Oncol 2008; 9(7): 621–628

[39] Hiraki T, Gobara H, Mimura H, Matsui Y, Toyooka S, Kanazawa S. Percutaneous radiofrequency ablation of clinical stage I non-small cell lung cancer. J Thorac Cardiovasc Surg 2011; 142(1): 24–30

[40] Kodama H, Yamakado K, Takaki H et al. Lung radiofrequency ablation for the treatment of unresectable recurrent non-small-cell lung cancer after surgical intervention. Cardiovasc Intervent Radiol 2012; 35(3): 563–569

[41] Lee H, Jin GY, Han YM et al. Comparison of survival rate in primary non-small-cell lung cancer among elderly patients treated with radiofrequency ablation, surgery, or chemotherapy. Cardiovasc Intervent Radiol 2012; 35(2): 343–350

[42] Grieco CA, Simon CJ, Mayo-Smith WW, DiPetrillo TA, Ready NE, Dupuy DE. Percutaneous image-guided thermal ablation and radiation therapy: outcomes of combined treatment for 41 patients with inoperable stage I/II non-small-cell lung cancer. J Vasc Interv Radiol 2006; 17(7): 1117–1124

[43] Chua TC, Sarkar A, Saxena A, Glenn D, Zhao J, Morris DL. Long-term outcome of image-guided percutaneous radiofrequency ablation of lung metastases: an open-labeled prospective trial of 148 patients. Ann Oncol 2010; 21(10): 2017–2022

[44] Inoue Y, Miki C, Hiro J et al. Improved survival using multimodality therapy in patients with lung metastases from colorectal cancer: a preliminary study. Oncol Rep 2005; 14(6): 1571–1576

[45] Yamakado K, Inoue Y, Takao M et al. Long-term results of radiofrequency ablation in colorectal lung metastases: single center experience. Oncol Rep 2009; 22(4): 885–891

[46] Sakurai J, Hiraki T, Mimura H et al. Radiofrequency ablation of small lung metastases by a single application of a 2-cm expandable electrode: determination of favorable responders. J Vasc Interv Radiol 2010; 21(2): 231–236

[47] Chua TC, Thornbury K, Saxena A et al. Radiofrequency ablation as an adjunct to systemic chemotherapy for colorectal pulmonary metastases. Cancer 2010; 116(9): 2106–2114

[48] Nakamura T, Matsumine A, Yamakado K et al. Lung radiofrequency ablation in patients with pulmonary metastases from musculoskeletal sarcomas [corrected].[corrected] Cancer 2009; 115(16): 3774–3781

[49] Lu Q, Cao W, Huang L et al. CT-guided percutaneous microwave ablation of pulmonary malignancies: Results in 69 cases. World J Surg Oncol 2012; 10: 80

[50] Vogl TJ, Worst TS, Naguib NN, Ackermann H, Gruber-Rouh T, Nour-Eldin NE. Factors influencing local tumor control in patients with neoplastic pulmonary nodules treated with microwave ablation: a risk-factor analysis. Am J Roentgenol 2013; 200(3): 665–672

[51] Zemlyak A, Moore WH, Bilfinger TV. Comparison of survival after sublobar resections and ablative therapies for stage I non-small cell lung cancer. J Am Coll Surg 2010; 211(1): 68–72

[52] Yashiro H, Nakatsuka S, Inoue M et al. Factors affecting local progression after percutaneous cryoablation of lung tumors. J Vasc Interv Radiol 2013; 24(6): 813–821

[53] Yamauchi Y, Izumi Y, Hashimoto K et al. Percutaneous cryoablation for the treatment of medically inoperable stage I non-small cell lung cancer. PLoS ONE 2012; 7(3): e33223

[54] Chan VO, McDermott S, Malone DE, Dodd JD. Percutaneous radiofrequency ablation of lung tumors: evaluation of the literature using evidence-based techniques. J Thorac Imaging 2011; 26(1): 18–26

Chapter 4

Hepatocellular Carcinoma: Ablation

4

4 Hepatocellular Carcinoma: Ablation

Riccardo Lencioni

4.1 Introduction

Hepatocellular carcinoma (HCC) is currently the second leading cause of cancer-related death worldwide.[1] Unlike most solid cancers, future incidence and mortality rates for HCC were projected to largely increase in several regions around the world over the next decade.[2,3]

HCC is increasingly diagnosed at an early, asymptomatic stage owing to surveillance of high-risk patients.[4] Patients with early-stage HCC require careful therapeutic management. Given the complexity of the disease, multidisciplinary assessment of tumor stage, liver function, and physical status is required for proper therapeutic planning. Patients with early-stage HCC should be considered for any of the available curative therapies, including surgical resection, liver transplantation, and image-guided ablation.[5,6,7]

Image-guided ablation is recommended for patients with early-stage HCC when surgical options are precluded.[5,6,7] Although tumor ablation procedures can be performed at laparoscopy or surgery, most procedures aimed at treating HCC are performed with a percutaneous approach. Hence several authors refer to these procedures as percutaneous therapies. Over the past 25 years, several methods for focal tumor destruction have been developed and clinically tested.[8] Although radiofrequency ablation (RFA) has been the most popular technique, several alternate technologies, including thermal and nonthermal methods, have recently attracted attention because they appear to be able to overcome some specific limitations of RFA.[9,10,11]

4.2 Indications and Contraindications

A multidisciplinary team must perform a careful clinical, laboratory, and imaging assessment of each individual patient to evaluate the patient's eligibility for image-guided ablation. Laboratory tests should include a full evaluation of the patient's coagulation status. A prothrombin time ratio > 50% and a platelet count > 50,000/µL are required to keep the risk of bleeding at an acceptably low level. The tumor staging protocol should include triple-phase computed tomography (CT) or magnetic resonance imaging (MRI) of the liver as well as imaging examinations to rule out extra-hepatic disease, as appropriate.

To be considered for image-guided ablation, patients should have either a single tumor smaller than 5 cm or as many as three nodules smaller than 3 cm each, no evidence of vascular invasion or extrahepatic spread, an Eastern Cooperative Oncology Group (ECOG) performance status test of 0 or 1, and liver cirrhosis in Child–Pugh class A or B.[5,6,7] Pretreatment imaging must carefully define the location of each lesion with respect to surrounding structures. Lesions located along the surface of the liver can be considered for thermal ablation, although their treatment requires adequate expertise and may be associated with a higher risk of complications. Thermal ablation of superficial lesions that are adjacent to any part of the gastrointestinal tract must be avoided because of the risk of thermal injury of the gastric or bowel wall. The colon appears to be at greater risk than the stomach or small bowel for thermally mediated perforation. Gastric complications are rare, likely owing to the relatively greater wall thickness of the stomach or the rarity of surgical adhesions along the gastrohepatic ligament. Thermal ablation of lesions adjacent to the gallbladder or to the hepatic hilum is at risk of thermal injury of the biliary tract. In experienced hands, thermal ablation of tumors located in the vicinity of the gallbladder was shown to be feasible, although associated in most cases with self-limited iatrogenic cholecystitis. In contrast, thermal ablation of lesions adjacent to hepatic vessels is possible because flowing blood usually protects the vascular wall from thermal injury. In these cases, however, there may be an increased risk of incomplete treatment of the neoplastic tissue close to the vessel because of the heat loss by convection.

Further studies are needed to establish whether novel technologies will expand the clinical role of image-guided ablation with respect to thermal ablation—RFA and microwave ablation (MWA). In particular, promising data have been reported on the safety and efficacy of nonthermal technologies, such as irreversible electroporation (IRE), in treating tumors in proximity to vital structures. It has to be pointed out, however, that the oldest and cheapest ablation technique, percutaneous ethanol injection (PEI), remains a viable option for small HCC tumors unsuitable for thermal ablation.

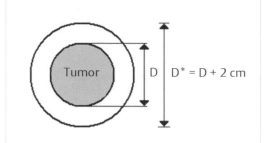

Fig. 4.1 Schematic model of a thermal ablation. The target diameter of the ablation zone (D*) must be ideally 2 cm larger than the diameter of the tumor that undergoes treatment (D).

4.3 Technique

RFA is currently established as the standard ablative modality.[12,13] However, several alternate energy-based methods for focal tissue destruction have recently become available. These novel ablation technologies destroy a tumor either through thermal (heat or cold) or nonthermal mechanisms. Whatever the ablative modality, the ablation of appropriate margins beyond the visible borders of the tumor is necessary to achieve therapeutic results similar to those achieved with surgery. Ideally, a 360°, 0.5 to 1 cm thick ablative margin should be produced all around the target tumor. This cuff would ensure that the peripheral portion of the lesion as well as any microscopic invasions located in its close proximity have been eradicated (▶ Fig. 4.1).

RFA systems function in the 375 to 500 KHz range. Most devices currently used are monopolar in that there is a single active electrode, with current dissipated at one or more return grounding pads. Bipolar devices have two active electrode applicators, usually placed in close proximity to achieve contiguous coagulation between the two electrodes, or on a single electrode. Several electrode types are available for clinical RFA, including internally cooled electrodes and multitined expandable electrodes with or without perfusion.[12,13]

MWA systems function at 915 MHz or 2.45 GHz frequencies. These wavelengths have specific physical properties with regard to tissue permeability and antenna design. Microwaves can generate very high temperatures in very short time periods, potentially leading to improved treatment efficiency and larger ablation zones, with less susceptibility to heat sink effects. Multiple microwave antennas can be powered simultaneously to take advantage of thermal synergy when placed in close proximity or widely spaced to ablate several tumors simultaneously.

The term *cryoablation* should be exclusively used for all methods of destroying tissue by the application of low temperature freezing, or alternating freezing and thawing or slight heating. Rapid tissue freezing and thawing produce the greatest cytotoxic effects by disrupting cellular membranes and inducing cell death. A distinct advantage of cryoablation is the ability to monitor the ice-ball formation during the procedure.

IRE includes those technologies and devices that cause cell death through the repeated application of short-duration high-voltage electrical pulses that create irreversible injuries to cellular membranes. Although there may be some hyperthermic ablative changes with higher power applications, the mechanism of cell death with IRE is thought to be predominantly nonthermal. Hence, issues associated with perfusion-mediated tissue cooling are not relevant for this technology. IRE is administered under general anesthesia with administration of a neuromuscular blocking agent to prevent undesirable muscle contraction, and by using cardiac gating to synchronize pulse delivery with the absolute refractory period to prevent cardiac arrhythmias.

Other energy-based ablation technologies include laser ablation and high-intensity focused ultrasound. These technologies have been adopted by a few centers worldwide for the treatment of malignant liver tumors.

4.4 Imaging

Targeting of the lesion can be performed with ultrasound, CT, or MRI (▶ Fig. 4.2). The guidance system is chosen largely on the basis of operator preference and local availability of dedicated equipment, such as CT fluoroscopy or open MRI systems. Real-time ultrasound/CT (or ultrasound/MRI) fusion imaging systems may improve the ability to guide and monitor liver tumor ablation procedures. During the procedure, important aspects to be monitored include how well the tumor is being covered and whether any adjacent normal structures are being affected at the same time. Although the transient hyperechoic zone that is seen at ultrasound within and surrounding a tumor during and immediately after RFA can be used as a rough guide to the extent of tumor

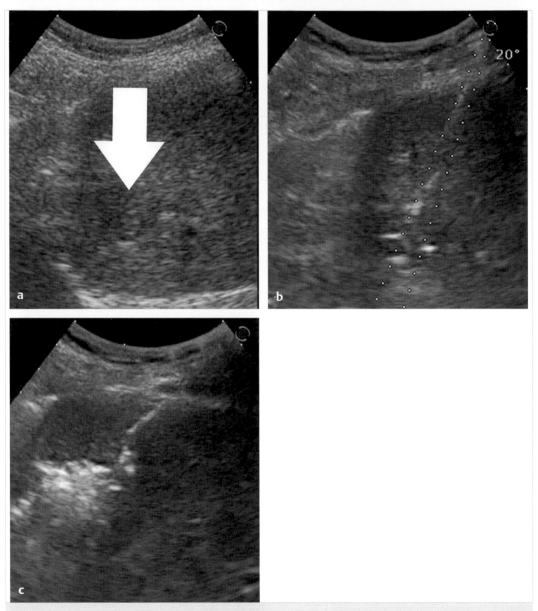

Fig. 4.2 Ultrasound-guided radiofrequency ablation (RFA) of a small hepatocellular carcinoma. **(a)** The tumor is localized via intercostal ultrasound scanning *(arrow)*. **(b)** A multitined expandable needle for RFA is advanced and precisely deployed within the lesion. **(c)** At the end of the procedure, a large hyperechoic cloud covering the tumors is seen on ultrasound.

destruction, MRI is currently the only imaging modality with validated techniques for real-time temperature monitoring.

Contrast-enhanced imaging performed at the end of the procedure may allow an initial evaluation of treatment effects. However, 1-month CT or MRI examinations are recognized as the standard to assess treatment outcome. CT and MRI show successful ablation as a nonenhancing area with or without a peripheral enhancing rim (▶ Fig. 4.3). The enhancing rim that may be observed along the periphery of the ablation zone appears as a relatively concentric, symmetric, and uniform process in an area with smooth inner margins. This is a

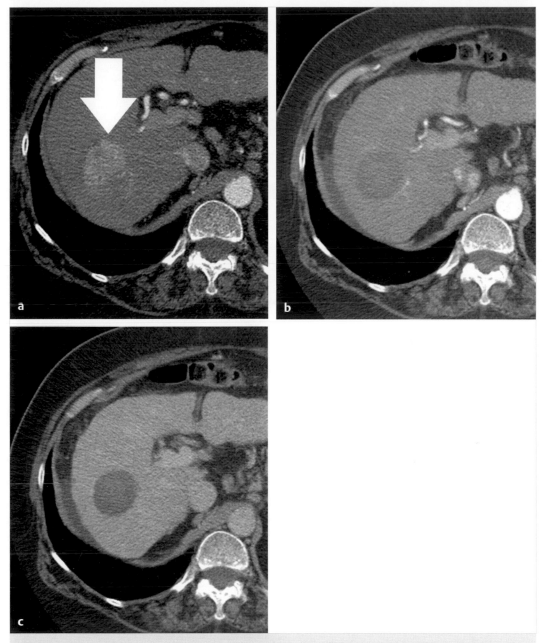

Fig. 4.3 Complete response of hepatocellular carcinoma (HCC) after radiofrequency ablation. **(a)** Pretreatment computed tomography (CT) shows hypervascular HCC with typical arterial phase enhancement *(arrow)*. **(b)** CT obtained 1 month after treatment shows nonenhancing areas in both the arterial and **(c)** the portal venous phase replacing the tumor and consistent with complete ablation.

transient finding that represents a benign physiological response to thermal injury (initially, reactive hyperemia; subsequently, fibrosis and giant cell reaction). Benign periablational enhancement needs to be differentiated from irregular peripheral enhancement due to residual tumor that occurs at the treatment margin. In contrast to benign periablational enhancement, residual unablated tumor often grows in scattered, nodular, or eccentric patterns. Later follow-up imaging studies should be aimed at detecting the recurrence of the treated lesion (i.e., local tumor progression), the development of new hepatic lesions, or the emergence of extrahepatic disease.

4.5 Complications

Several multicenter surveys have reported acceptable morbidity and mortality rates for RFA of liver tumors. The mortality rate ranged from 0.1 to 0.5%, the major complication rate ranged from 2.2 to 3.1%, and the minor complication rate ranged from 5 to 8.9%.[14] The most common causes of death were sepsis, hepatic failure, colon perforation, and portal vein thrombosis, while the most common complications were intraperitoneal bleeding, hepatic abscess, bile duct injury, hepatic decompensation, and grounding pad burns.[15,16,17] Minor complications and side effects were usually transient and self-limiting. An uncommon late complication of RF ablation can be tumor seeding along the needle track. In patients with HCC, tumor seeding occurred in 8 (0.5%) of 1,610 cases in a multicenter survey.[15] Lesions with subcapsular location and an invasive tumoral pattern, as shown by a poor differentiation degree, seem to be at higher risk for such a complication.[18] Although these data indicate that RFA is a relatively safe procedure, a careful assessment of the risks and benefits associated with the treatment has to be made in each individual patient by a multidisciplinary team.

4.6 Clinical Data and Outcomes

The use of RFA for local ablation of early-stage HCC is supported by a large amount of data and robust clinical evidence. Five randomized, controlled trials (RCTs) have compared RFA versus PEI for the treatment of early-stage HCC. These investigations consistently showed that RFA has a higher anticancer effect than PEI, leading to a better local control of the disease[19,20,21,22,23] (▶ Table 4.1). The assessment of the impact of RFA on survival has been more controversial. Although a survival benefit was identified in the three RCTs performed in Asia, the two European RCTs failed to show statistically significant differences in overall survival between patients who received RFA and those treated with PEI, despite the trend favoring RFA (▶ Table 4.1). In patients with early-stage HCC treated with percutaneous ablation, long-term survival is often the result of different sequential interventions, given that about than 80% of the patients will develop recurrent intrahepatic HCC

nodules within 5 years of the initial treatment and will received additional therapies.[24] Nevertheless, three independent meta-analyses including all RCTs have confirmed that treatment with RFA offers a survival benefit as compared with PEI, particularly for tumors larger than 2 cm, thus establishing RFA as the standard percutaneous technique.[25,26,27] For studies that reported major complications, however, the incidence in RFA-treated patients was 4.1% (95% confidence interval [CI], 1.8–6.4%), compared to 2.7% (95% CI, 0.4–5.1%) observed in PEI-treated patients.[28] This difference was not statistically significant; nevertheless, this safety profile should be taken into consideration as part of the overall risk/benefit profile in each case.

Recent reports on long-term outcomes of RFA-treated patients have shown that, in patients with Child–Pugh class A and early-stage HCC, 5-year survival rates are as high as 51 to 64% and may reach 76% in patients who meet the Barcelona Clinic Liver Cancer (BCLC) criteria for surgical resection[24,29,30,31] (▶ Table 4.2). Caution, however, is needed when interpreting and generalizing these results, in particular in light of studies that suggest a nonnegligible rate of incomplete histopathological response after RFA. In fact, the ability of RFA to achieve complete tumor eradication appears to be dependent on tumor size and location. In particular, histological studies performed in liver specimens of patients who underwent RFA as a bridge treatment to transplantation showed that the presence of large (≥ 3 mm) abutting vessels result in a drop of the rate of complete tumor necrosis to < 50% because of the heat loss due to perfusion-mediated tissue cooling within the area to be ablated.[32]

Several attempts have been made to increase the effect of RFA in HCC treatment. Because heat efficiency is the difference between the amount of heat produced and the amount of heat lost, most investigators devote their attention to strategies that aim primarily at minimizing heat loss due to perfusion-mediated tissue cooling. Given that HCC is mostly nourished by the hepatic artery, a combination of RFA and balloon catheter occlusion of the tumor arterial supply or prior transarterial chemoembolization (TACE) has been used to increase heat efficiency.[33,34,35,36] The combination of TACE and RFA did not show significant clinical benefit when applied to the treatment of small (< 3 cm) HCC.[37] However, such an approach did show significant advantages, in terms of both local tumor control and survival, when used in intermediate-sized

Table 4.1 Randomized, controlled trials comparing radiofrequency ablation versus percutaneous ethanol injection for the treatment of early-stage hepatocellular carcinoma

Reference	Initial CR	Treatment failure[a]	Overall survival		
			1 y	3 y	*P*
Lencioni et al[19]					
RFA (*n* = 52)	91%	8%	88	81	NS
PEI (*n* = 50)	82%	34%	96	73	
Lin et al[20]					
RFA (*n* = 52)	96%	17%	82	74	0.014
PEI (*n* = 52)	88%	45%	61	50	
Shiina et al[21]					
RFA (*n* = 118)	100%	2%	90	80	0.02
PEI (*n* = 114)	100%	11%	82	63	
Lin et al[22]					
RFA (*n* = 62)	97%	16%	88	74	0.031
PEI (*n* = 62)	89%	42%	96	51	
Brunello et al[23]					
RFA (*n* = 70)	96%	34%	88	59	NS
PEI (*n* = 69)	66%	64%	96	57	

Abbreviations: CR, complete response; NS, not significant; PEI, percutaneous ethanol injection; RFA, radiofrequency ablation.
[a] Includes initial treatment failure (incomplete response) and late treatment failure (local recurrence).

(3–5 cm) HCC[38,39] as well as in recurrent HCC after prior hepatectomy.[40]

The largest RCT conducted so far included 189 patients with HCC < 7 cm.[41] Patients were randomly assigned to receive TACE combined with RFA (TACE-RFA; *n* = 94) or RFA alone (*n* = 95). The 1-, 3-, and 4-year overall survivals for the TACE-RFA group and the RFA group were 92.6%, 66.6%, and 61.8% and 85.3%, 59%, and 45.0%, respectively. The corresponding recurrence-free survivals were 79.4%, 60.6%, and 54.8% and 66.7%, 44.2%, and 38.9%, respectively. Patients in the TACE-RFA group had better overall survival and recurrence-free survival than patients in the RFA group (hazard ratio [HR], 0.525; 95% CI, 0.335–0.822; *P* = 0.002; HR, 0.575; 95% CI, 0.374–0.897; *P* = 0.009, respectively). On logistic regression analyses, treatment allocation, tumor size, and tumor number were significant prognostic factors for overall survival, whereas treatment allocation and tumor number were significant prognostic factors for recurrence-free survival.

Although TACE followed by RFA has been the most popular combination, alternate strategies have been investigated. In particular, drug-eluting bead (DEB)-TACE has been performed after RFA, rather than before, following a different rationale.[42] In a standard RFA, one can take advantage of only those temperatures that are sufficient by themselves to induce coagulative necrosis (> 50–55°C). However, there are large zones of sublethal heating created during RF application in tissues surrounding the electrode, that are not being used to achieve sustained treatment effect. Experimental studies in animal tumor models have shown that lowering the temperature threshold at which cell death occurs by combining sublethal temperature with cell exposure to chemotherapeutic agents increases tumor necrosis, apparently occurring in tissues heated to 45 to 50°C. It has been hypothesized that the administration of DEB to tumors incompletely killed by RFA could increase the anticancer effect, as a result of both the delivery of highly concentrated doxorubicin

Table 4.2 Studies reporting 5-year survival of patients with early-stage hepatocellular carcinoma who received radiofrequency ablation as first-line nonsurgical treatment

Reference	Patients no.	Overall survival 1 year	3 year	5 year
Lencioni et al[24]				
Child-Pugh A	144	100	76	51
Child-Pugh B	43	89	46	31
Tateishi et al[29]				
Child-Pugh A	221	96	83	63
Child-Pugh B-C[a]	98	90	65	31
Choi et al[30]				
Child–Pugh A	359	NA	78	64
Child–Pugh B	160	NA	49	38
N'Kontchou et al[31]				
BCLC resectable[b]	67	NA	82	76
BCLC unresectable	168	NA	49	27

Abbreviation: BCLC, Barcelona Clinic Liver Cancer.
[a]Only 4 of 98 patients had Child-Pugh C cirrhosis.
[b]BCLC criteria for resection include single tumor, normal bilirubin level (< 1.5 mg/dL), and absence of significant portal hypertension.

into a relatively small volume of residual viable neoplastic tissue and the reduced cell resistance to the drug caused by the exposure to sublethal heating.

In a pilot clinical study, DEB-TACE was performed within 24 hours of RFA to take advantage of the reactive hyperemia induced by RF application to facilitate delivery of the microspheres to the tumor-bearing area. In fact, marked periablational hypervascularity was observed at the time of the angiographic study. DEB administration resulted in a substantial increase in tissue destruction, leading to confirmed complete response (CR) of the target lesion in 12 (60%) of 20 patients bearing large tumors refractory to standard RF treatment[42] (► Fig. 4.4). DEB-enhanced RFA was well tolerated, with no major complications associated with the technique. Nevertheless, after this initial evaluation of efficacy and safety, further clinical investigation is warranted to prove the clinical benefit of this approach.

Pearls

- Indication to use image-guided ablation should be discussed by a multidisciplinary team after careful assessment of tumor stage, liver function, and performance status.
- Accurate pretreatment planning, including selection of the ablation technology, imaging guidance, and approach, is key to success.
- Ablation protocols are usually based on the ablation size charts provided by the manufacturer. However, the actual ablation zone may vary in clinical setting, depending on tissue vascularization, tissue conductivity, local interactions, and settings of the system, among other factors.
- Tumors are generally assumed to be spherical. If the difference between the longest axis and the shortest axis of a tumor is 1 cm or greater, appropriate changes to the ablation strategy may be warranted in view of the ellipsoidal shape of the target.
- Imaging aspects that are particularly important include tumor size, shape, and location within the organ relative to blood vessels as well as to critical structures that might be at risk for injury.
- Changes in the actual position of the electrodes with respect to planned position can potentially lead to incomplete ablation or thermal injury of structures located in the vicinity of the target tumor: appropriate changes to the ablation protocol may be warranted based on the actual position of the electrodes.
- Posttreatment response assessment and follow-up protocols are fundamental components of the treatment strategy.

Is RFA still the best technique for tumor ablation? Several novel alternatives are currently being tested clinically. MWA, in particular, is emerging as a valuable alternative to RFA and seems to have potential to improve the rate of complete ablation achieved with RFA in multiple tumors or in tumors that are > 2 to 3 cm as well as tumors in a perivascular location.[43,44] A review of the literature on the use of MWA for hepatic tumors included published studies in the English language with at least 30 patients per study.[43] The authors concluded that MWA may be optimal when larger necrosis zones and/or ablation of multiple lesions are the objective. The data reviewed supported the

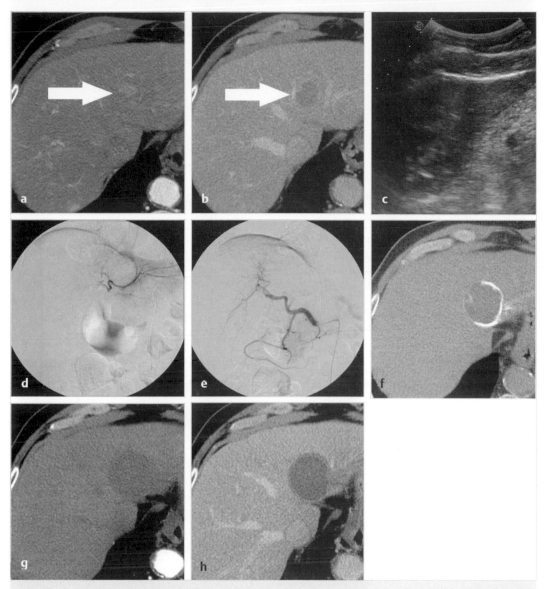

Fig. 4.4 Hepatocellular carcinoma (HCC) treated with a combination of radiofrequency ablation (RFA) and drug-eluting bead transarterial chemoembolization (DEB-TACE). **(a, b)** Pretreatment computed tomography (CT) shows hypervascular HCC located in close proximity to the heart *(arrows)*. **(c)** RFA is carried out under ultrasound guidance by using a multitined expandable electrode. **(d, e)** Treatment is completed with intra-arterial injection of 2 mL of 100 to 300 µm DEB uploaded with 50 mg of doxorubicin. **(f)** CT obtained immediately after the procedure confirms accumulation of the injected material along the periphery of the ablation zone. **(g, h)** Follow-up CT scans show a complete response.

potential advantage noted for ablation of HCC lesions > 3 cm, but did not support treatment of HCC lesions < 3 cm.[43] In a recent multi-institutional study including 450 patients treated with 473 MWA procedures in four leading U.S. institutions (139 HCC, 198 colorectal cancer (CRC) liver metastases, 61 neuroendocrine liver metastases, and 75 other), complete ablation was confirmed for 839 of 865 tumors (97%) on follow-up cross-sectional imaging, and the local recurrence rate was 6%.[44] In another large series including 100 patients, a matched comparison of MWA and RFA was performed.[45] The two groups were evaluated for ablation success, ablation recurrence, and ablation time, all of which were significantly improved in the MWA group. Ablation and operative times were significantly shortened in the MWA group, primarily related to the ability to do simultaneous ablations with multiple probes. The authors concluded that MWA of hepatic tumors is a safe and effective method for treating unresectable hepatic tumors, with a low rate of local recurrence.

IRE shows promise for the treatment of small tumors located in the vicinity of bile ducts and blood vessels.[46,47,48] In the first clinical study published on the use of IRE in liver tumor treatment, factors analyzed included patient and tumor characteristics, treatment-related complications, and local recurrence-free survival for ablated lesions. The series included 44 patients.[46] Tumor histologies included CRC metastasis ($n = 20$), HCC ($n = 14$), and others ($n = 10$). Initial success was achieved in 46 (100%) treatments. Five patients had nine adverse events, with all complications resolving within 30 days. There was a trend toward higher recurrence rates for tumors > 4 cm (HR 3.236, 95% CI: 0.585–17.891; $P = 0.178$). A recent systematic review of safety and efficacy of IRE concluded that, in cases where other techniques are unsuitable, IRE is a promising modality for the ablation of tumors near bile ducts and blood vessels.[48]

More data are needed to define the potential for other energy-based ablation technologies, such as cryoablation, in the specific field of liver tumor treatment. A recent safety study on 42 patients with HCC reported 13 (39.4%) complications out of 33 cryoablation procedures versus 8 (26.7%) complications out of 30 RFA procedures, including 2 (6.1%) severe/fatal complications for cryoablation procedures versus 1 (3.3%) for RFA. The authors concluded that no significant difference was seen in the overall safety of cryoablation and RFA in the treatment of HCC in patients with cirrhosis.[49]

Advances in ablation systems and devices are highly warranted. However, progress in imaging guidance and monitoring is also key to success. To be able to compete with surgical resection, image-guided ablation needs to be able to offer more accurate prediction of the outcome in each individual patient. Variability in outcomes needs to be minimized via careful treatment planning (► Fig. 4.5). Also, the outcome of the ablation procedure needs to be carefully documented by providing sound evidence that an "A0" treatment has been achieved.

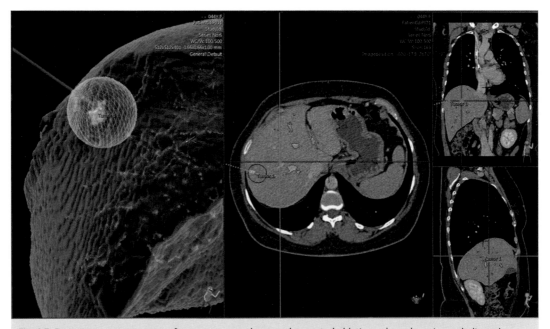

Fig. 4.5 Pretreatment assessment of target tumor volume and expected ablation volume by using a dedicated workstation (Maxio, Perfint Healthcare) enables accurate planning of the procedure.

References

[1] International Agency for Research on Cancer. World Health Organization. GLOBOCAN 2012: estimated cancer incidence, mortality, and prevalence worldwide in 2012. http://globocan.iarc.fr. Accessed May 20, 2014

[2] Olsen AH, Parkin DM, Sasieni P. Cancer mortality in the United Kingdom: projections to the year 2025. Br J Cancer 2008; 99(9): 1549–1554

[3] Davis GL, Alter MJ, El-Serag H, Poynard T, Jennings LW. Aging of hepatitis C virus (HCV)-infected persons in the United States: a multiple cohort model of HCV prevalence and disease progression. Gastroenterology 2010; 138(2): 513–521, 521.e1–521.e6

[4] Fong ZV, Tanabe KK. The clinical management of hepatocellular carcinoma in the United States, Europe, and Asia: a comprehensive and evidence-based comparison and review. Cancer 2014; 120(18): 2824–2838

[5] Bruix J, Sherman M American Association for the Study of Liver Diseases. Management of hepatocellular carcinoma: an update. Hepatology 2011; 53(3): 1020–1022

[6] European Association for the Study of the Liver. European Organisation for Research and Treatment of Cancer. EASL-EORTC clinical practice guidelines: management of hepatocellular carcinoma. J Hepatol 2012; 56(4): 908–943

[7] Verslype C, Rosmorduc O, Rougier P ESMO Guidelines Working Group. Hepatocellular carcinoma: ESMO-ESDO Clinical Practice Guidelines for diagnosis, treatment and follow-up. Ann Oncol 2012; 23 Suppl 7: vii41–vii48

[8] Lencioni R, Crocetti L. Local-regional treatment of hepatocellular carcinoma. Radiology 2012; 262(1): 43–58

[9] Erinjeri JP, Clark TWI. Cryoablation: mechanism of action and devices. J Vasc Interv Radiol 2010; 21(8) Suppl: S187–S191

[10] Lubner MG, Brace CL, Ziemlewicz TJ, Hinshaw JL, Lee FT, Jr. Microwave ablation of hepatic malignancy. Semin Intervent Radiol 2013; 30(1): 56–66

[11] Lu DS, Kee ST, Lee EW. Irreversible electroporation: ready for prime time? Tech Vasc Interv Radiol 2013; 16(4): 277–286

[12] Gervais DA, Goldberg SN, Brown DB, Soulen MC, Millward SF, Rajan DK. Society of Interventional Radiology position statement on percutaneous radiofrequency ablation for the treatment of liver tumors. J Vasc Interv Radiol 2009; 20(7) Suppl: S342–S347

[13] Crocetti L, de Baere T, Lencioni R. Quality improvement guidelines for radiofrequency ablation of liver tumours. Cardiovasc Intervent Radiol 2010; 33(1): 11–17

[14] Rhim H. Complications of radiofrequency ablation in hepatocellular carcinoma. Abdom Imaging 2005; 30(4): 409–418

[15] Livraghi T, Solbiati L, Meloni MF, Gazelle GS, Halpern EF, Goldberg SN. Treatment of focal liver tumors with percutaneous radio-frequency ablation: complications encountered in a multicenter study. Radiology 2003; 226(2): 441–451

[16] de Baère T, Risse O, Kuoch V et al. Adverse events during radiofrequency treatment of 582 hepatic tumors. Am J Roentgenol 2003; 181(3): 695–700

[17] Bleicher RJ, Allegra DP, Nora DT, Wood TF, Foshag LJ, Bilchik AJ. Radiofrequency ablation in 447 complex unresectable liver tumors: lessons learned. Ann Surg Oncol 2003; 10(1): 52–58

[18] Llovet JM, Vilana R, Brú C et al. Barcelona Clínic Liver Cancer (BCLC) Group. Increased risk of tumor seeding after percutaneous radiofrequency ablation for single hepatocellular carcinoma. Hepatology 2001; 33(5): 1124–1129

[19] Lencioni RA, Allgaier HP, Cioni D et al. Small hepatocellular carcinoma in cirrhosis: randomized comparison of radiofrequency thermal ablation versus percutaneous ethanol injection. Radiology 2003; 228(1): 235–240

[20] Lin SM, Lin CJ, Lin CC, Hsu CW, Chen YC. Radiofrequency ablation improves prognosis compared with ethanol injection for hepatocellular carcinoma < or =4 cm. Gastroenterology 2004; 127(6): 1714–1723

[21] Shiina S, Teratani T, Obi S et al. A randomized controlled trial of radiofrequency ablation with ethanol injection for small hepatocellular carcinoma. Gastroenterology 2005; 129(1): 122–130

[22] Lin SM, Lin CJ, Lin CC, Hsu CW, Chen YC. Randomised controlled trial comparing percutaneous radiofrequency thermal ablation, percutaneous ethanol injection, and percutaneous acetic acid injection to treat hepatocellular carcinoma of 3 cm or less. Gut 2005; 54(8): 1151–1156

[23] Brunello F, Veltri A, Carucci P et al. Radiofrequency ablation versus ethanol injection for early hepatocellular carcinoma: A randomized controlled trial. Scand J Gastroenterol 2008; 43(6): 727–735

[24] Lencioni R, Cioni D, Crocetti L et al. Early-stage hepatocellular carcinoma in patients with cirrhosis: long-term results of percutaneous image-guided radiofrequency ablation. Radiology 2005; 234(3): 961–967

[25] Orlando A, Leandro G, Olivo M, Andriulli A, Cottone M. Radiofrequency thermal ablation vs. percutaneous ethanol injection for small hepatocellular carcinoma in cirrhosis: meta-analysis of randomized controlled trials. Am J Gastroenterol 2009; 104(2): 514–524

[26] Cho YK, Kim JK, Kim MY, Rhim H, Han JK. Systematic review of randomized trials for hepatocellular carcinoma treated with percutaneous ablation therapies. Hepatology 2009; 49(2): 453–459

[27] Germani G, Pleguezuelo M, Gurusamy K, Meyer T, Isgrò G, Burroughs AK. Clinical outcomes of radiofrequency ablation, percutaneous alcohol and acetic acid injection for hepatocellular carcinoma: a meta-analysis. J Hepatol 2010; 52(3): 380–388

[28] Bouza C, López-Cuadrado T, Alcázar R, Saz-Parkinson Z, Amate JM. Meta-analysis of percutaneous radiofrequency ablation versus ethanol injection in hepatocellular carcinoma. BMC Gastroenterol 2009; 9: 31

[29] Tateishi R, Shiina S, Teratani T et al. Percutaneous radiofrequency ablation for hepatocellular carcinoma. An analysis of 1000 cases. Cancer 2005; 103(6): 1201–1209

[30] Choi D, Lim HK, Rhim H et al. Percutaneous radiofrequency ablation for early-stage hepatocellular carcinoma as a first-line treatment: long-term results and prognostic factors in a large single-institution series. Eur Radiol 2007; 17(3): 684–692

[31] N'Kontchou G, Mahamoudi A, Aout M et al. Radiofrequency ablation of hepatocellular carcinoma: long-term results and prognostic factors in 235 Western patients with cirrhosis. Hepatology 2009; 50(5): 1475–1483

[32] Lu DS, Yu NC, Raman SS et al. Radiofrequency ablation of hepatocellular carcinoma: treatment success as defined by histologic examination of the explanted liver. Radiology 2005; 234(3): 954–960

[33] Rossi S, Garbagnati F, Lencioni R et al. Percutaneous radiofrequency thermal ablation of nonresectable hepatocellular carcinoma after occlusion of tumor blood supply. Radiology 2000; 217(1): 119–126

[34] Veltri A, Moretto P, Doriguzzi A, Pagano E, Carrara G, Gandini G. Radiofrequency thermal ablation (RFA) after transarterial chemoembolization (TACE) as a combined therapy for unresectable non-early hepatocellular carcinoma (HCC). Eur Radiol 2006; 16(3): 661–669

[35] Helmberger T, Dogan S, Straub G et al. Liver resection or combined chemoembolization and radiofrequency ablation improve survival in patients with hepatocellular carcinoma. Digestion 2007; 75(2–3): 104–112

[36] Yamasaki T, Kurokawa F, Shirahashi H, Kusano N, Hironaka K, Okita K. Percutaneous radiofrequency ablation therapy for patients with hepatocellular carcinoma during occlusion of hepatic blood flow. Comparison with standard percutaneous radiofrequency ablation therapy. Cancer 2002; 95(11): 2353–2360

[37] Shibata T, Isoda H, Hirokawa Y, Arizono S, Shimada K, Togashi K. Small hepatocellular carcinoma: is radiofrequency ablation combined with transcatheter arterial chemoembolization more effective than radiofrequency ablation alone for treatment? Radiology 2009; 252(3): 905–913

[38] Morimoto M, Numata K, Kondou M, Nozaki A, Morita S, Tanaka K. Midterm outcomes in patients with intermediate-sized hepatocellular carcinoma: a randomized controlled trial for determining the efficacy of radiofrequency ablation combined with transcatheter arterial chemoembolization. Cancer 2010; 116(23): 5452–5460

[39] Kim JH, Won HJ, Shin YM et al. Medium-sized (3.1–5.0 cm) hepatocellular carcinoma: transarterial chemoembolization plus radiofrequency ablation versus radiofrequency ablation alone. Ann Surg Oncol 2011; 18(6): 1624–1629

[40] Takaki H, Yamakado K, Sakurai H et al. Radiofrequency ablation combined with chemoembolization: treatment of recurrent hepatocellular carcinomas after hepatectomy. Am J Roentgenol 2011; 197(2): 488–494

[41] Peng ZW, Zhang YJ, Chen MS et al. Radiofrequency ablation with or without transcatheter arterial chemoembolization in the treatment of hepatocellular carcinoma: a prospective randomized trial. J Clin Oncol 2013; 31(4): 426–432

[42] Lencioni R, Crocetti L, Petruzzi P et al. Doxorubicin-eluting bead-enhanced radiofrequency ablation of hepatocellular carcinoma: a pilot clinical study. J Hepatol 2008; 49(2): 217–222

[43] Boutros C, Somasundar P, Garrean S, Saied A, Espat NJ. Microwave coagulation therapy for hepatic tumors: review of the literature and critical analysis. Surg Oncol 2010; 19(1): e22–e32

[44] Groeschl RT, Pilgrim CH, Hanna EM et al. Microwave ablation for hepatic malignancies: a multiinstitutional analysis. Ann Surg 2014; 259(6): 1195–1200

[45] Martin RC, Scoggins CR, McMasters KM. Safety and efficacy of microwave ablation of hepatic tumors: a prospective review of a 5-year experience. Ann Surg Oncol 2010; 17(1): 171–178

[46] Cannon R, Ellis S, Hayes D, Narayanan G, Martin RC, II. Safety and early efficacy of irreversible electroporation for hepatic tumors in proximity to vital structures. J Surg Oncol 2013; 107(5): 544–549

[47] Silk MT, Wimmer T, Lee KS et al. Percutaneous ablation of peribiliary tumors with irreversible electroporation. J Vasc Interv Radiol 2014; 25(1): 112–118

[48] Scheffer HJ, Nielsen K, de Jong MC et al. Irreversible electroporation for nonthermal tumor ablation in the clinical setting: a systematic review of safety and efficacy. J Vasc Interv Radiol 2014; 25(7): 997–1011, quiz 1011[Epub ahead of print]

[49] Dunne RM, Shyn PB, Sung JC et al. Percutaneous treatment of hepatocellular carcinoma in patients with cirrhosis: a comparison of the safety of cryoablation and radiofrequency ablation. Eur J Radiol 2014; 83(4): 632–638

Chapter 5

Hepatocellular Carcinoma: Chemoembolization

5

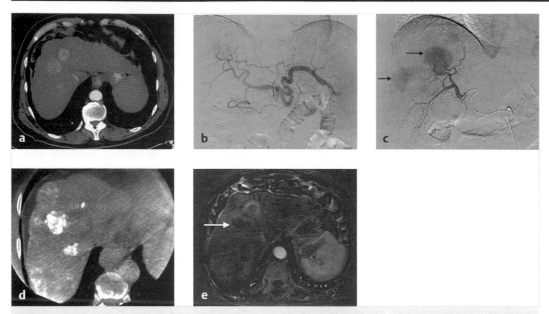

Fig. 5.1 A 60-year-old man with Child–Pugh A cirrhosis secondary to chronic hepatitis C. **(a)** Baseline contrast-enhanced computed tomography (CT) demonstrates multiple arterial enhancing tumors, predominantly in the right lobe. Due to the presence of bilobar hepatocellular carcinoma (HCC) and portal hypertension, he is not a candidate for surgical resection. **(b)** Catheterization and digital subtraction angiography (DSA) of the celiac trunk was performed with a 5 French Simmons-1 catheter (AngioDynamics), demonstrating conventional hepatic arterial anatomy. **(c)** Selective catheterization and DSA of the right hepatic artery with a 2.8 French microcatheter shows multiple hypervascular tumors *(arrows)*. Chemoembolization was performed in a lobar fashion due to multifocal HCC, using doxorubicin mixed with ethiodized oil, followed by infusion of 300 to 500 μm particles. **(d)** Noncontrast CT obtained immediately after chemoembolization shows ethiodized oil staining of multiple tumors in the right hepatic lobe. **(e)** Follow-up contrast-enhanced magnetic resonance imaging demonstrates a lack of enhancement of the tumors *(white arrow)*, consistent with the treatment response.

phase in order to assess the number, location, and size of the hypervascular tumors.

Chemotherapy and embolic combinations vary considerably. The lack of standardization is in part due to the paucity of available randomized literature comparing different treatment specifics.[11] As a result, no single chemoembolic platform is the standard. Therefore, the most common formulation used in the United States will be discussed. Oil-based chemoembolization has been traditionally done. Multiple agents can be combined, such as cisplatin, mitomycin-C, and doxorubicin; however, the limited availability of some of these agents has resulted in many centers now using a single agent. This consists of mixing 50 to 100 mg doxorubicin with 10 to 20 mL ethiodized oil (Guebert, Indiana). Although no survival benefit exists for systemic doxorubicin in the setting of HCC, localized intra-arterial delivery allowing high intratumoral and low systemic concentrations of the drug can result in significant tumor response

and prolonged survival. The oil acts as an emulsifying agent and a lipophilic carrier in order to allow localized drug delivery without rapid washout. Infusion is performed under live fluoroscopic guidance to prevent reflux of chemotherapy and assess for arterial stasis. When infusing, complete stasis should be avoided because it will prevent future repeat treatments if necessary. After infusion of chemotherapy, follow-up embolization is performed. Gelatin slurry (Pfizer), embospheres (Merit), and PVA (Boston Scientific) are the most commonly used embolic agents. Again, complete stasis should be avoided in order to allow for repeat treatments. Furthermore, it has been shown that achieving stasis does not result in better response or better patient outcomes.[12]

Embolization with DEB has gained popularity over traditional oil-based chemoembolization. Due to the prolonged binding properties of DEBs with doxorubicin, the drug is slowly released into the tumor, reaching higher local concentration and

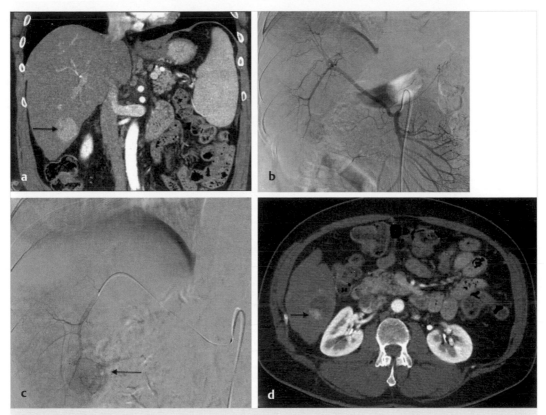

Fig. 5.2 A 50-year-old man with Child–Pugh B cirrhosis secondary to chronic hepatitis C. **(a)** Coronal contrast-enhanced computed tomography (CT) shows a 3.1 cm tumor *(arrow)* in the right hepatic lobe, segment V. Because he was within the Milan criteria, chemoembolization was performed for the purposes of bridging to liver transplantation. **(b)** Catheterization and digital subtraction angiography (DSA) of the superior mesenteric artery were performed with a 5 French Simmons-1 catheter, demonstrating a replaced right hepatic artery. **(c)** Selective catheterization and DSA of the segment V branch of the right hepatic artery with a 2.8 French microcatheter shows a single hypervascular tumor *(arrow)*. Chemoembolization was performed using doxorubicin drug-eluting beads. **(d)** Follow-up axial contrast-enhanced CT shows near complete necrosis with a small nodular area of residual enhancement *(arrow)*, consistent with a partial response. The patient underwent a second round of chemoembolization, with eventual complete response on follow-up imaging.

decreased systemic concentration when compared to oil-based chemoembolization. This may allow for decreased side effects and improved tolerance in some patients.[13] The most common formulation is to combine 50 to 150 mg doxorubicin with 100 to 300 μm particles (LC Beads, Biocompatibles, Inc.).[14] A 50 to 75 mg doxorubicin vial is reconstituted with 2 mL of sterile water. The saline from the LC bead vial is removed. The reconstituted doxorubicin solution is directly added to the bead vial, and then 60 minutes are needed to allow the drug to bind to the beads. The total mixture is diluted with nonionic iodinated contrast (20–30 mL). Infusion should be done using intermittent fluoroscopy, with a slow injection rate. After delivery of the beads, postembolization angiography is performed. Similar to oil-based chemoembolization, arterial stasis should be avoided in order to allow for future repeated treatments.

5.6 Postprocedure Management and Follow-up Evaluation

Patients are often admitted for overnight observation and pain and nausea control. Patients should receive adequate intravenous hydration until they are taking a normal amount of oral fluids. Pain can be treated with narcotics (e.g., oral oxycodone, intravenous morphine, or dilaudid). Acetaminophen should be avoided given the risk of liver dysfunction. Nausea can be controlled with 5-HT3 antagonists (palonosetron, ondansetron) and metoclopramide. Antibiotics are often continued, especially if the patient has biliary incompetence. This usually includes a third-generation cephalosporin and metronidazole. Discharge medications include medications for pain, nausea, and constipation related to opioid use.

A noncontrast CT scan following oil-based chemoembolization can help identify ethiodized oil distribution and potentially guide the need for future treatments (▶ Fig. 5.1). Follow-up should include an outpatient Interventional Radiology (IR) clinic visit, imaging (multiphase CT or MRI), and laboratory evaluation (complete blood count, comprehensive metabolic panel, and nonmaternal alpha-fetoprotein if it was positive at baseline) at 1 month. If a second round of treatment is already planned (e.g., chemoembolization to the contralateral lobe), then imaging at 1 month can be deferred. Toxicity is assessed at follow-up and is categorized using Common Terminology Criteria for Adverse Events (CTCAE), version 4. Repeat chemoembolization should be considered if follow-up imaging demonstrates persistent enhancement of tumors (i.e., incomplete necrosis), assuming toxicity was tolerable from previous chemoembolization (▶ Fig. 5.2). Subsequent rounds of chemoembolization require a repeat thorough investigation to determine arterial supply to the tumors. An incomplete response can be due to feeding vessels arising from extrahepatic origins. For example, tumors in the hepatic dome may be supplied by the right inferior phrenic artery (▶ Fig. 5.3). Tumors in segment IV may be supplied by the right internal mammary artery. If complete response is achieved, surveillance imaging is performed every 3 months to assess for recurrent or new tumor.

The decision to discontinue chemoembolization therapy is controversial. If toxicity is intolerable to the patient or if persistent enhancement or tumor progression occurs despite multiple rounds of chemoembolization, then alternative treatment options should be pursued.

5.7 Side Effects and Complications

Postembolization syndrome is the most common side effect of chemoembolization. This is a constellation of symptoms, including low-grade fever, abdominal pain, nausea, vomiting, and ileus. It often occurs up to 48 to 72 hours following chemoembolization and can last up to 1 week.[1] It should be treated symptomatically because it is generally transient.

Serious complications from chemoembolization are fortunately uncommon in well-selected patients. Liver failure occurs infrequently, at a reported rate of 1 to 3%. Risk factors include compromised liver function (Child–Pugh class C), portal vein thrombosis, and large amounts of hepatic tissue treated. Unfortunately, there is no definitive therapy for liver failure in this setting other than liver transplantation. Treatment is supportive in nature. The use of superselective chemoembolization rather than lobar treatment in decompensated cirrhotics (Child–Pugh class C), decreases the risk of hepatotoxicity.[15]

Bilomas occur in a small percentage of patients following chemoembolization, with the vast majority of bilomas detected on follow-up imaging being asymptomatic (▶ Fig. 5.4). Asymptomatic bilomas should not be actively treated, but they may be a relative contraindication for future liver-directed therapy. If bilomas are symptomatic, percutaneous drainage may be necessary. Abscess is a rare complication of hepatic chemoembolization. Biliary obstruction or a prior biliary procedure has been shown to represent an increased risk for post-chemoembolization abscess.[16] Given the trend in the literature demonstrating a higher risk of abscess in patients with bilioenteric anastomosis or biliary instrumentation, more aggressive prophylactic antibiotic regimens should be administered for 7 to 10 days after treatment. Some also advocate a bowel prep and initiating antibiotics up to 7 days before the procedure to decrease the risk of abscess.[17]

5.8 Clinical Data and Outcomes

A summary of noteworthy clinical trials is listed in ▶ Table 5.1. Results of two prospective randomized, clinical trials have shown a survival benefit for use of chemoembolization versus supportive care in patients with unresectable HCC. In a randomized prospective trial, Llovet et al compared survival between chemoembolization, bland embolization, and best supportive care in 112 patients.[5] The majority of patients in this study had hepatitis C virus–induced liver disease, and many patients had multifocal tumors and/or clinically symptomatic ascites. Chemoembolization

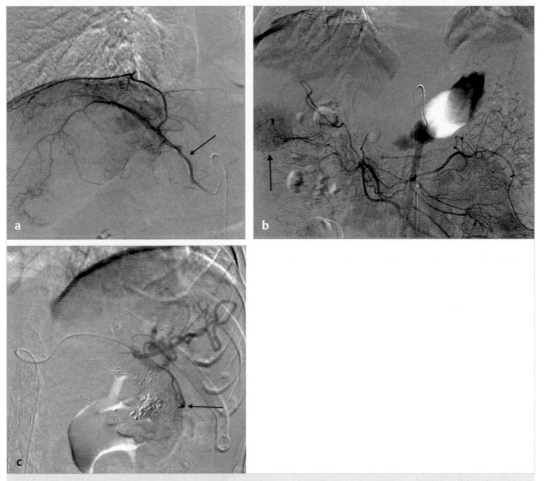

Fig. 5.3 Collateral supply to hepatocellular carcinoma. **(a)** Hypervascular tumors in the right hepatic dome are fed by the right inferior phrenic artery *(arrow)*. **(b)** Tumor *(arrow)* in the right hepatic lobe is supplied by jejunal branches off the superior mesenteric artery. **(c)** After receiving multiple rounds of treatment, residual tumor *(arrow)* in segment III of the left hepatic lobe is supplied by a branch of the splenic artery.

was performed using doxorubicin mixed with ethiodized oil, followed by embolization with gelatin fragments. Survival probabilities at 1 year and 2 years were 75% and 50% for embolization, 82% and 63% for chemoembolization, and 63% and 27% for control (chemoembolization vs. control $p = 0.009$). Similarly, Lo et al compared chemoembolization with best supportive care in 80 patients, predominantly with hepatitis B virus induced cirrhosis. Chemoembolization was performed using cisplatin mixed with ethiodized oil, followed by embolization with gelatin fragments. Chemoembolization resulted in a superior tumor response on imaging compared to supportive care, and survival was significantly better in the chemoembolization group (1 year, 57%; 2 years, 31%; 3 years,

26%) than in the control group (1 year, 32%; 2 years, 11%; 3 years, 3%; $P = 0.002$).[5] Although death from liver failure was more frequent in patients who received chemoembolization, the liver function of the survivors was not significantly different between the two groups.

A Cochrane review reported on an evaluation of nine clinical trials to determine survival advantage of chemoembolization over supportive care.[18] The authors' analysis concluded "there is not sufficient evidence to support or refute chemoembolization or bland embolization for patients with unresectable HCC." However, there are several drawbacks to the Cochrane review. First, numerous trials were excluded in the analysis because a placebo or best supportive care arm was not included. Since

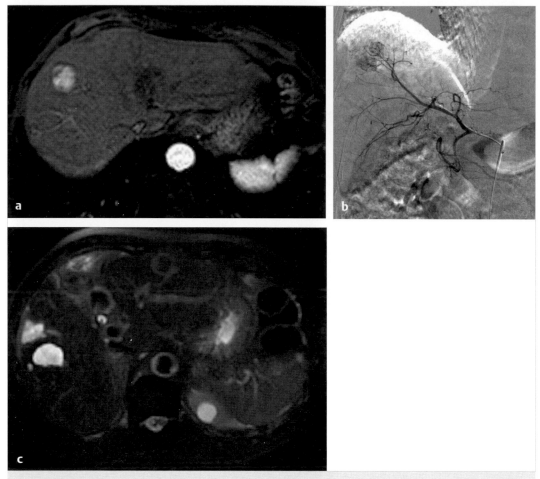

Fig. 5.4 Complication after chemoembolization. **(a)** A single hepatocellular carcinoma (HCC) is present in segment VIII of the liver. **(b)** HCC in the right hepatic lobe is fed by multiple small branches of the right hepatic artery. **(c)** After undergoing chemoembolization, multiple fluid collections develop in the right hepatic lobe, consistent with bilomas.

chemoembolization has now become the standard of care, performing trials with placebo arms is not feasible. Second, the nine included studies were published prior to 2002. Since then, technique and patient selection have evolved considerably, which has improved outcomes in terms of tumor response, and hence survival and complications. Using more commonly accepted inclusion criteria and recent techniques of selective chemoembolization, a prospective study of 99 patients undergoing chemoembolization demonstrated a median survival of 3.1 years with 1- and 2-year survivals of 90% and 75%, respectively.[19] Other meta-analyses have also demonstrated a survival benefit with chemoembolization.[20]

The largest series of chemoembolization assessed survival in 8,510 patients with HCC. A chemotherapeutic agent, ethiodized oil, and gelatin sponge were used in the study's protocol. A median survival of 34 months was reported, with 1-, 3-, 5-, and 7-year survival reported at 82%, 47%, 26%, and 16%, respectively. Multiple factors were associated with shorter survival: degree of liver dysfunction, elevated alpha-fetoprotein level, tumor size, number of tumors, and degree of portal vein invasion.[21]

The first major prospective randomized, controlled trial of DEB compared the safety and efficacy of doxorubicin DEB-chemoembolization versus oil-based chemoembolization. The trial

Table 5.1 Clinical trials of chemoembolization

Author	N	Patients	Technique	Response	Survival	TTP
Llovet et al[5]	112	Child–Pugh A or B Okuda I or II	TACE vs. bland embolization vs. supportive care		1 y: 82% vs. 75% vs. 63% 2 y: 63% vs. 50% vs. 27%	
Lo et al[4]	80	All stages	TACE vs. supportive care	Objective response: 39% vs. 6%	1 y: 57% vs. 32% 2 y: 31% vs. 11% 3 y: 26% vs. 3%	
Takayasu et al[21]	8510	All stages	Conventional TACE		1 y: 82% 3 y: 47% 5 y: 26% 7 y: 16%	
Lammer et al[13]	201	BCLC A/B	Conventional TACE vs. DEB-TACE	Objective response: 52% vs. 44%		
Malagari et al[19]	84	Child–Pugh A or B	DEB-TACE vs. bland embolization	Complete response: 27% vs. 14% Partial response: 46% vs. 42%	1 y: 85% vs. 76%	42 vs. 36 mo
Lencioni et al[27]	307	BCLC B	DEB-TACE vs. sorafenib + DEB-TACE			166 vs. 169 d
Ikeda et al[26]	99	Child–Pugh A or B; ECOG 0–2	Conventional TACE	Complete response: 42% Partial response: 31% Stable disease: 18% Disease progression: 7%	1 y: 90% 2 y: 75%	7.8 mo

Abbreviations: BCLC, Barcelona Clinic Liver Cancer; d, days; DEB, drug-eluting bead; ECOG, Eastern Cooperative Oncology Groupmo, months; TACE, transcatheter arterial chemoembolization; y, years.

included 212 patients with unresectable HCC, ECOG performance status of 0 or 1, preserved liver function (Child–Pugh class A or B), and absence of vascular invasion. The study failed to meet its primary end point of statistically significant imaging superiority in the DEB-chemoembolization group. However, patients with advanced disease (Child–Pugh class B, ECOG 1, bilobar or recurrent disease) in the DEB-chemoembolization group demonstrated higher rates of objective tumor response on imaging, lower rates of acute hepatotoxicity, and lower rates of doxorubicin-related toxicity compared to patients in the oil-based chemoembolization group.[13] Since this trial, the technique of DEB-chemoembolization has evolved, with the use of smaller particles (100–300 µm) showing promising results with improved response and decreased toxicity.[22,23]

Several studies have assessed the potential for improved local tumor response when combining chemoembolization with radiofrequency ablation (RFA).[7] In a prospective randomized trial, RFA was compared to RFA in addition to chemoembolization for tumors ≤ 7 cm. The recurrence-free survivals at 1, 3, and 4 years for chemoembolization + RFA versus RFA alone were 79.4%, 60.6%, and 54.8% and 66.7%, 44.2%, and 38.9%, respectively. Meta-analyses of combination therapies have shown that there is no significant survival benefit for combination treatment of small tumors (< 3 cm). However, benefit may exist for intermediate-sized tumors (3–5 cm).[7,24]

Since the approval of sorafenib for HCC in 2008, there has been great interest in combining systemic and locoregional therapies. The combination of sorafenib and chemoembolization was proved to be safe in a prospective phase 2 trial.[25] However, a comparison of DEB-chemoembolization versus DEB-chemoembolization in combination with sorafenib did not show improved survival or significant improvement in time to progression (169 vs. 166 days).[27]

Chemoembolization practices will continue to evolve as ongoing research helps optimize technique and patient selection.

Pearls

- Chemoembolization is the most commonly performed procedure for patients with unresectable HCC.
- Appropriate candidates for chemoembolization include the following: ineligible for curative treatment, adequate hepatic function (Child–Pugh class A or B), acceptable functional performance status, absence of portal vein thrombosis, absence of extrahepatic metastases.
- Chemoembolization can also be used in conjunction with other therapies or as a bridge to transplant.
- Chemoembolization should include a complete diagnostic arteriogram of the superior mesenteric artery (SMA) and celiac circulation to evaluate hepatic arterial variants. Superselective catheterization and treatment should be performed if possible in order to maximize tumor deposition of chemotherapeutic agents and minimize hepatic toxicity.
- Several different chemoembolic techniques have been employed with varying degrees of success. The lack of adequate comparative studies makes recommendation of an absolute strategy challenging.
- Postembolization syndrome should be expected to varying degrees in most patients and should not be confused for evidence of complication. Patients should be managed postprocedure by an interventional radiologist familiar with expected symptoms and complications.
- DEB chemoembolization may have improved toxicity compared to oil-based chemoembolization, but significant differences in tumor response rates or survival have not yet been proved.

References

[1] El-Serag HB, Marrero JA, Rudolph L, Reddy KR. Diagnosis and treatment of hepatocellular carcinoma. Gastroenterology 2008; 134(6): 1752–1763

[2] Brown DB, Gould JE, Gervais DA et al. Society of Interventional Radiology Technology Assessment Committee and the International Working Group on Image-Guided Tumor Ablation. Transcatheter therapy for hepatic malignancy: standardization of terminology and reporting criteria. J Vasc Interv Radiol 2009; 20(7) Suppl: S425–S434

[3] Yamada R, Sato M, Kawabata M, Nakatsuka H, Nakamura K, Takashima S. Hepatic artery embolization in 120 patients with unresectable hepatoma. Radiology 1983; 148(2): 397–401

[4] Lo C-M, Ngan H, Tso W-K et al. Randomized controlled trial of transarterial lipiodol chemoembolization for unresectable hepatocellular carcinoma. Hepatology 2002; 35(5): 1164–1171

[5] Llovet JM, Real MI, Montaña X et al. Barcelona Liver Cancer Group. Arterial embolisation or chemoembolisation versus symptomatic treatment in patients with unresectable hepatocellular carcinoma: a randomised controlled trial. Lancet 2002; 359(9319): 1734–1739

[6] Hong K, Khwaja A, Liapi E, Torbenson MS, Georgiades CS, Geschwind JF. New intra-arterial drug delivery system for the treatment of liver cancer: preclinical assessment in a rabbit model of liver cancer. Clin Cancer Res 2006; 12(8): 2563–2567

[7] Morimoto M, Numata K, Kondou M, Nozaki A, Morita S, Tanaka K. Midterm outcomes in patients with intermediate-sized hepatocellular carcinoma: a randomized controlled trial for determining the efficacy of radiofrequency ablation combined with transcatheter arterial chemoembolization. Cancer 2010; 116(23): 5452–5460

[8] Benson AB, III, Abrams TA, Ben-Josef E et al. NCCN clinical practice guidelines in oncology: hepatobiliary cancers. J Natl Compr Canc Netw 2009; 7(4): 350–391

[9] Luo J, Guo RP, Lai EC et al. Transarterial chemoembolization for unresectable hepatocellular carcinoma with portal vein tumor thrombosis: a prospective comparative study. Ann Surg Oncol 2011; 18(2): 413–420

[10] Tognolini A, Louie J, Hwang G, Hofmann L, Sze D, Kothary N. C-arm computed tomography for hepatic interventions: a practical guide. J Vasc Interv Radiol 2010; 21(12): 1817–1823

[11] Llovet JM, Di Bisceglie AM, Bruix J et al. Panel of Experts in HCC-Design Clinical Trials. Design and endpoints of clinical trials in hepatocellular carcinoma. J Natl Cancer Inst 2008; 100(10): 698–711

[12] Jin B, Wang D, Lewandowski RJ et al. Chemoembolization endpoints: effect on survival among patients with hepatocellular carcinoma. Am J Roentgenol 2011; 196(4): 919–928

[13] Lammer J, Malagari K, Vogl T et al. PRECISION V Investigators. Prospective randomized study of doxorubicin-eluting-bead embolization in the treatment of hepatocellular carcinoma: results of the PRECISION V study. Cardiovasc Intervent Radiol 2010; 33(1): 41–52

[14] Lencioni R, de Baere T, Burrel M et al. Transcatheter treatment of hepatocellular carcinoma with Doxorubicin-loaded DC Bead (DEBDOX): technical recommendations. Cardiovasc Intervent Radiol 2012; 35(5): 980–985

[15] Kothary N, Weintraub JL, Susman J, Rundback JH. Transarterial chemoembolization for primary hepatocellular carcinoma in patients at high risk. J Vasc Interv Radiol 2007; 18(12): 1517–1526, quiz 1527

[16] Johnson GE, Ingraham CR, Nair AV, Padia SA. Hepatic abscess complicating transarterial chemoembolization in a patient with liver metastases. Semin Intervent Radiol 2011; 28(2): 193–197

[17] Patel S, Tuite CM, Mondschein JI, Soulen MC. Effectiveness of an aggressive antibiotic regimen for chemoembolization in patients with previous biliary intervention. J Vasc Interv Radiol 2006; 17(12): 1931–1934

[18] Oliveri RS, Wetterslev J, Gluud C. Transarterial (chemo)embolisation for unresectable hepatocellular carcinoma. Cochrane Database Syst Rev 2011; 3(3): CD004787

[19] Malagari K, Pomoni M, Kelekis A et al. Prospective randomized comparison of chemoembolization with doxorubicin-eluting beads and bland embolization with BeadBlock for hepatocellular carcinoma. Cardiovasc Intervent Radiol 2010; 33(3): 541–551

[20] Llovet JM, Bruix J. Systematic review of randomized trials for unresectable hepatocellular carcinoma: Chemoembolization improves survival. Hepatology 2003; 37(2): 429–442

[21] Takayasu K, Arii S, Ikai I et al. Liver Cancer Study Group of Japan. Prospective cohort study of transarterial chemoembolization for unresectable hepatocellular carcinoma in 8510 patients. Gastroenterology 2006; 131(2): 461–469

[22] Padia SA, Shivaram G, Bastawrous S et al. Safety and efficacy of drug-eluting bead chemoembolization for hepatocellular carcinoma: comparison of small-versus medium-size particles. J Vasc Interv Radiol 2013; 24(3): 301–306

[23] Kalva SP, Pectasides M, Liu R et al. Safety and effectiveness of chemoembolization with drug-eluting beads for advanced-stage hepatocellular carcinoma. Cardiovasc Intervent Radiol 2014; 37(2): 381–387

[24] Wang W, Shi J, Xie W-F. Transarterial chemoembolization in combination with percutaneous ablation therapy in unresectable hepatocellular carcinoma: a meta-analysis. Liver Int 2010; 30(5): 741–749

[25] Pawlik TM, Reyes DK, Cosgrove D, Kamel IR, Bhagat N, Geschwind JF. Phase II trial of sorafenib combined with concurrent transarterial chemoembolization with drug-eluting beads for hepatocellular carcinoma. J Clin Oncol 2011; 29 (30): 3960–3967

[26] Lencioni R, Zou J, Leberre M, Meinhardt G. Sorafenib (SOR) or placebo (PL) in combination with transarterial chemoembolization (TACE) for intermediate-stage hepatocellular carcinoma (SPACE). J Clin Oncol 2010; 28(15) Suppl: 178

[27] Ikeda M, Arai Y, Park SJ et al. Japan Interventional Radiology in Oncology Study Group (JIVROSG). Korea Interventional Radiology in Oncology Study Group (KIVROSG). Prospective study of transcatheter arterial chemoembolization for unresectable hepatocellular carcinoma: an Asian cooperative study between Japan and Korea. J Vasc Interv Radiol 2013; 24(4): 490–500

Chapter 6

Hepatocellular Carcinoma: Radioembolization

6 Hepatocellular Carcinoma: Radioembolization

Avnesh S. Thakor, Arash Eftekhari, Edward Wolfgang Lee, Darren Klass, and David Liu

6.1 Introduction

6.1.1 Hepatocellular Carcinoma Overview

Hepatocellular carcinoma (HCC) is the sixth most common cancer in the world and the third leading cause of cancer mortality worldwide. Although HCC occurs more commonly in regions with a higher incidence of hepatitis, such as in Asia Pacific and Southern Europe, the National Cancer Institute (NCI) and the American Cancer Society (ACS) report the age-standardized incidence rate of HCC at 2.1 per 100,000 population in North America. Both the incidence and mortality rate related to HCC in the United States continue to rise with an estimated 30,640 new cases of HCC diagnosed in 2013 and 21,670 new deaths related to HCC.[1]

Risk factors for the development of HCC include viral hepatitis, alcohol abuse, nonalcoholic steatohepatitis (NASH), intake of aflatoxin-contaminated food, diabetes, obesity, and certain hereditary conditions, such as hemochromatosis. The main viruses associated with the development of HCC are the hepatitis B virus (HBV) and hepatitis C virus (HCV); indeed, 50% of HCC cases worldwide are associated with HBV infection, with a further 25% associated with HCV.[2] The end stage of chronic inflammation in the liver, as best characterized by chronic viral infections, is hepatic cirrhosis. This is characterized by a decrease in hepatocyte proliferation and an increase in parenchymal fibrosis, which ultimately results in compromised hepatic function. In the progression of chronic inflammation to fibrosis, there is an upregulation of mitogenic pathways due to increased levels of cytokines (i.e., tumor growth factor, TGF-β1) and reactive oxygen species (ROS) released from damaged liver parenchymal cells, which lead to the propagation of monoclonal populations.[3] These clonal nests of hepatocytes contain telomerase erosions and chromosome aberrations, which limit the proliferative, and hence regenerative, capacity of the liver.[4,5] The altered gene expression in these dysplastic hepatocytes predisposes them to becoming premalignant, and, over time, developing into HCC. Because HBV and HCV can also cause HCC independent of cirrhosis, other pathogenic mechanisms have also been postulated, including the integration of HBV DNA into the host genome (where it can cause gene deletions, rearrangements, and chromosome instability) and the synthesis of several oncogenic proteins by HCV.[6]

6.2 Radiobiology, Mechanisms of Action and General Approach

6.2.1 Basic Principles

Selective internal radiation therapy (SIRT), also known as radioembolization and/or radiomicrosphere therapy in its current commercial form, uses yttrium-90 (^{90}Y) as a form of brachytherapy whereby microspheres loaded with ^{90}Y are permanently implanted in the target tumor vascular bed within the liver via intra-arterial administration. SIRT aims to selectively deliver radiation to liver tumors while limiting the dose delivered to normal liver parenchyma through the exploitation of the phenomenon of neovascularization of hepatic primary tumors originating exclusively via the hepatic arterial supply. This process allows for the deposition of ^{90}Y microspheres to preferentially implant within liver tumors in a 3 to 20:1 ratio, as compared to the normal liver parenchyma.[7] Although conventional external beam whole liver radiotherapy treatment is not well tolerated, radiotherapy to smaller portions of the liver is well tolerated without significant complications, provided a sufficient amount of normal liver parenchyma is spared.[8] Treatment with ^{90}Y can be currently delivered either as a resin (SIR-Spheres, Sirtex Medical Inc., Sydney, Australia) or as a glass microsphere (TheraSphere, BTG Ltd, Ottawa, Canada). As ^{90}Y decays, it emits high-energy β-radiation (0.97 mEv), which travels a mean of 2.5 mm from the physical microsphere. A single microparticle does not significantly contribute to the overall response to treatment; it is the collective effect of multiple microparticles that creates a cumulative isodose cloud of lethal radiation exposure (via crossfire) in the range of 100 to 1,000 gray (Gy) for a limited time (^{90}Y decays to zirconium-90 [^{90}Z] with a half-life of 64.2 h)[9] (▶ Fig. 6.1). The microparticle size used for SIRT is on average 20 to 60 μm, which is small enough for the particles to enter the tumor vascular network, but large enough to prevent arteriovenous shunting (in most situations).[10]

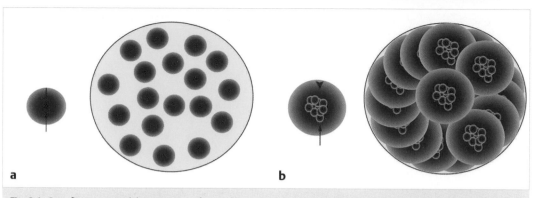

Fig. 6.1 Crossfire concept. **(a)** Deposition of a single microsphere *(arrow)* within tumor tissue results in a radiation kill zone of approximately 2.5 mm, which in turn leads to inadequate whole tumor volume irradiation. **(b)** It takes several microclusters *(arrowhead)* of spheres *(arrow)* with a combined gray of "X" to kill the tumor tissue. These microclusters also have to overlap sufficiently to achieve crossfire between the microclusters.

6.2.2 Mechanism of Action of Selective Internal Radiation Therapy

SIRT's mechanism of action is fundamentally different from that of chemoembolization; in fact, the term *radio embolization* is a misnomer because no significant effect or response has been demonstrated by the physical particle itself, even when angiographic embolization of nonradioactive microspheres has been performed.[11] Chemoembolization relies on the occlusion of vessels of the tumor, thereby creating stasis and hence maximum exposure of the chemotherapeutic agent to the ischemic environment created within the tumor. In contrast, blood flow and oxygen are essential for SIRT to allow ROS generation via the ionization of water molecules from the emitted β-radiation. This, in turn, results in damage to DNA and activation of apoptosis via an increase in the ratio of BAX:BCL-2 gene expression.[12] Furthermore, cancer cells are more susceptible to oxidative stress due to their relatively low concentration of superoxide dismutase (SOD) and their increased production of superoxide ($^{\bullet}O_2^-$) from their higher aerobic metabolism.[13] SOD is an antioxidant that quenches $^{\bullet}O_2^-$ before it can react with hydroxyl radicals (OH$^{\bullet}$) to produce hydrogen peroxide (H_2O_2). Direct double-strand DNA breaks also account for a significant proportion of cellular death. As such, the resin and glass microspheres used for SIRT are small enough to have little or no embolic effect on the medium- to small-sized hepatic arteries, thereby maintaining adequate tissue oxygenation.[11]

6.3 Indications for Radioembolization

6.3.1 Staging Systems Used in Chronic Liver Disease

The severity of any underlying chronic liver disease can be assessed using two scoring systems, independent of whether or not the patient has HCC.

The Child–Pugh score is used to assess both the prognosis of underlying chronic liver disease (i.e., cirrhosis) and the necessity of treatment of liver transplantation (▶ Table 6.1). Based on the patient's serum bilirubin, serum albumin, and international normalized ratio (INR), and the clinical presence of ascites or hepatic encephalopathy, patients are scored from 5 to 15 points based on a linear regression model. Depending on the score, patients are then placed in a class A to C, which reflects their likely mortality over the next year. Class A = 5–6 points with a 100% 1-year survival, class B = 7 to 9 points with an 81% 1-year survival, and class C = 10 to 15 points with a 45% 1-year survival.

The second scoring system used to assess the severity of chronic liver disease is the Model for End-Stage Liver Disease (MELD) score, which is based on the following equation:

Table 6.1 Childs–Pugh score

Variable	1 point	2 points	3 points
Total bilirubin, μmol/L (mg/dL)	< 34 (< 2)	34–50 (2–3)	> 50 (> 3)
Serum albumin, g/dL	> 3.5	2.8–3.5	< 2.8
International normalized ratio	< 1.70	1.71–2.30	> 2.30
Ascites	None	Mild	Moderate to severe
Hepatic encephalopathy	None	Grade I–II	Grade III–IV

Table 6.2 Model for end-stage liver disease (MELD) score

MELD score	Mortality (%)
> 40	71.3
30–39	52.6
20–29	19.6
10–19	6
< 9	1.9

Equation 6.1

$$MELD = 3.78(Ln\ bilirubin[mg/dL]) + 11.2(Ln\ INR) + 9.57(Ln\ creatinine[mg/dL]) + 6.43$$

This system was initially used to predict the 3-month mortality following a transjugular intrahepatic portosystemic shunt (TIPS) procedure but was also found to be useful for prioritizing recipients of a liver transplant. In hospitalized patients, the 3-month mortality is based on a patient's MELD score (▶ Table 6.2).

6.4 The Barcelona Clinic Liver Cancer Staging System for HCC

There are several staging systems used to stratify patients with HCC to guide appropriate primary therapeutic treatment and adjuvant therapy, to estimate survival prognosis, and to exchange information without ambiguity.[14] Because patients with HCC often have underlying cirrhosis, the severity of the underlying liver disease, the patient's functional status, and the extent of the HCC neoplasm require consideration. The most widely accepted model is the Barcelona Clinic Liver Cancer (BCLC) staging system, which has been shown to be best for guiding treatment in early-stage disease, especially in identifying when there is potential benefit from curative therapies. The

BCLC classification was formed from several cohort studies and randomized clinical trials conducted by the Barcelona group; the classification uses variables related to tumor stage, liver functional status, physical status, and cancer-related symptoms and links the stage of the disease to a specific treatment strategy via an algorithm (▶ Fig. 6.2).[4]

6.5 Treatment Selection for Patients with HCC

The treatment selection for HCC depends on the tumor size, morphology (e.g., portal vein thrombus), and location, as well as the presence of comorbidities (including the extent of the underlying hepatic reserve) and the presence or absence of extrahepatic disease. Historically, intermediate-stage patients (stage B) have been offered conventional Lipiodol-based (Guerbet, Paris, France) chemoembolization. In this population therapeutic intent is balanced between the preservation of hepatic function (against the background of cirrhosis) and the progression of tumor, because both factors ultimately contribute to overall survival. By conventional BCLC criteria, patients with advanced disease (stage C, which includes a myriad of clinical conditions, including portal vein invasion, lower performance status, and extrahepatic metastatic disease) who are considered to have no locoregional option may be relegated to a palliative therapeutic option using sorafenib (Nexavar, Bayer Pharmaceuticals). Finally, in patients with end-stage disease (stage D, Bayer Pharmaceuticals, Leverkusen, Germany), only palliative treatment is offered because the terminal stages of liver decompensation and tumor progression preclude any meaningful benefit.[15,16]

As more advanced techniques and targeted therapies develop, their evaluation with respect to advanced disease states, quality of life, side-effect/toxicity profile, and depth of response warrants

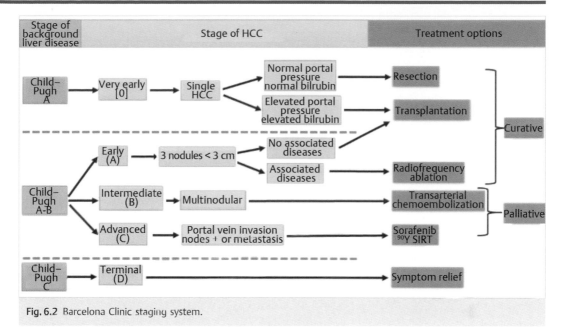

Fig. 6.2 Barcelona Clinic staging system.

further consideration. Specifically, the role of radioembolization or SIRT within the context of these factors has resulted in hybridization of the BCLC staging system, leading to the incorporation of this less toxic and potentially more effective locoregional therapy within the treatment algorithm. From the BCLC classification, patients with HCC who are candidates for transarterial chemoembolization (TACE) include stage A patients with nonablatable and nonresectable disease, and stage B patients with either unilobar disease or those with a limited number of nodules (1–5). In these patients, the main reason for considering SIRT over TACE includes a better treatment-related quality of life (i.e., less postembolization syndrome and no inpatient stay following treatment) and increased depth of radiographic response; however, no clear survival advantage has been demonstrated in this population.[17] The advantages of SIRT become clearer in the following specific situations (that also include subcategories of BCLC C patients): (1) poor candidates for TACE—stage B patients with bilobar disease or those with multiple tumors (>5), (2) cases where TACE has previously failed; (3) cases where TACE is contraindicated (e.g. those with portal vein thrombosis), (4) elderly populations, (5) poor Eastern Cooperative Oncology Group (ECOG) performance status (≤2), and (6) patients who are under consideration for downstaging to surgical resection or transplantation (► Table 6.3).

6.6 General Approach to Selective Internal Radiation Therapy

SIRT can be offered to patients with either segmental, unilobar, or bilobar disease. However, prior to SIRT administration, considerations include the following: hepatic reserve, tumor morphology, and potential for nontargeted embolization (due to deposition in nonhepatic mesenteric vessels or intrahepatic/tumoral arterioportal shunts). Practically, these factors are assessed during clinical consultation, review of imaging, and mesenteric angiography with technetium-99 m macroaggregated serum albumin (^{99m}Tc-MAA) administration. The mapping procedure allows for selective embolization techniques, which can eliminate nontarget mesenteric vessels and/or optimize administration through the consolidation of intrahepatic vessels under the principle of redistribution.

6.7 Contraindications to Radioembolization

6.7.1 Lung Shunt

In all cases of HCC, due to the complex process of angiogenesis and the ongoing autonecrosis/remodeling occurring within tumor microvasculature, functional arteriovenous shunts develop,

Table 6.3 Summary of the efficacy outcomes in key studies using SIRT/radioembolization in hepatocellular carcinoma (▶ Table 6.5)

Lead Author/Year	n	Treatment	Cohort	Median survival (months), | p-value				
				Whole cohort	BCLC stage A	BCLC stage B	BCLC stage B/C	BCLC stage C
Comparative studies								
Gramenzi 2014[69]	63	SIR-Spheres	BCLC A/B/C	13.2 mo		22.1 mo		6.0 mo
	74	Sorafenib	BCLC A/B/C	14.4 mo | 0.96		20.4 mo | 0.88		8.4 mo | 0.88
Moreno-Luna 2013[70]	61	TheraSphere	BCLC A/B/C	15 mo	23.9 mo	16.8 mo		8.4 mo
	55	cTACE	BCLC A/B/C	14.4 mo | 0.47	18.6 mo | 0.40	13 mo | 0.16		10.1 mo | 0.47
Iñarrairaegui 2012[71]	6	SIR-Spheres > radical therapy	UNOS T3 uncensored	Not reached | nr				
	15	SIR-Spheres	UNOS T3	22 mo				
Salem 2011[17]	123	TheraSphere	BCLC A/B/C	20.5 mo	27.3 mo	17.2 mo		22.1 mo
	122	cTACE	BCLC A/B/C	17.4 mo | 0.23	45.4 mo | 0.74	17.5 mo | 0.42		9.3 mo | 0.04
Lance 2011[72]	38	SIR-Spheres	NR	8.0 mo				
	35	cTACE	NR	10.3 mo | 0.33				
Kooby 2010[73]	27	SIR-Spheres	Okuda I–III	6 mo				
	44	cTACE	Okuda I–III	6 mo | 0.74				

Table 6.3 continued

Lead Author/Year	n	Treatment	Cohort	Median survival (months),	p-value
Carr 2010[74]	99	TheraSphere	NR	11.5 mo	<0.05
	691	cTACE	NR	8.5 mo	
D'Avola 2009[75]	35	SIR-Spheres	First-line	16 mo	<0.001
	43	Std Tx or BSC	First-line	8 mo	
Lewandowski 2009[76]	43	TheraSphere	UNOS T3	35.7 mo	0.18
	43	cTACE	Censored	18.7 mo	
	43	TheraSphere	UNOS T3	41.6 mo	0.008
	43	cTACE	Uncensored	19.2 mo	
Woodall 2007[77]	20	90Y glass m/s	No PVT	13.9 mo	0.01
	15	90Y glass m/s	BCLC C + PVT	2.7 mo	
	17	Screen failures	= PVT	5.2 mo	
Goin 2005[21]	34	TheraSphere	Okuda I/II	12.4 mo	NR
	38	cTACE	Okuda I/II	11.3 mo	

Noncomparative studies

Lead Author/Year	n	Treatment	Cohort	Median survival (months),	p-value
Chow 2014[78]	29	SIR-Spheres + sorafenib	BCLC B/C	20.3 mo	8.6 mo

Table 6.3 continued

Lead Author/Year	n	Treatment	Cohort	Median survival (months),	p-value			
Khor 2014[79]	103	SIR-Spheres	BCLC A/B/C			23.8 mo	11.8 mo
Mazzaferro 2013[80]	52	TheraSphere	BCLC B/C	15 mo		18 mo	13 mo
Sangro 2011[23]	325	SIR-Spheres	BCLC A/B/C	12.8 mo	24.4 mo	16.9 mo	10 mo
Salem 2010[81]	291	TheraSphere	BCLC A/B/C	NR	26.9 mo	17.2 mo	7.3-EHD/5.4+EHD mo
Hilgard 2010[82]	108	TheraSphere	BCLC B/C	16.4 mo		16.4 mo	Not reached
Iñarrairaegui 2010[83]	25	SIR-Spheres	BCLC C+PVT	10 mo			10 mo
Iñarrairaegui 2010[84]	72	SIR-Spheres	BCLC A/B/C	13 mo			
Kulik 2008[85]	71	TheraSphere	NR	15.4 mo			
	25	BCLC	C branch PVT	10 mo		10 mo	
	12	BCLC	C main PVT	4.4 mo		4.4 mo	
Salem 2005[86]	43	TheraSphere	Okuda I/II				
			Child–Pugh A	20.5 mo			
			Child–Pugh B	13.8 mo			

Abbreviations: BCLC, Barcelona Clinic Liver Cancer staging system; mo, months; B/C, ??; cTACE, conventional transarterial chemoembolization; nr, not recorded; Std Tx, standard therapy; BSC, best supportive care; PVT, portal vein thrombosis; –EHD/ + EHD: without or with extrahepatic disease.

which, if large enough, will allow SIRT particles to bypass the tumor vasculature and enter the pulmonary circulation. If microparticles are deposited in the lungs, there is both a theoretical and a clinical risk of radiation-induced pneumonitis (RIP). The clinical features of RIP include deteriorating pulmonary function tests in the absence of heart failure, active chest infection, chronic obstructive airway disease, pulmonary embolism, and pulmonary fibrosis. Acute RIP presents as a dry cough and progressive exertional dyspnea occurring approximately 1 to 6 months following SIRT. Treatment usually consists of corticosteroids to decrease the amount of inflammation within the lung parenchyma. Radiologically, RIP is characterized by extensive pulmonary patchy consolidation. Histologically there is edema, congestion, and fibrin exudates in the alveoli with thickening and fibrosis of the alveolar septa, and, although irreversible, it is rarely fatal.[18] Groundglass attenuation may be present in the areas of increased particle deposition, usually in the lung bases.

In order to assess the potential degree of shunting of ^{90}Y microspheres into the lungs during SIRT, 4 to 5 mCi ^{99m}Tc-MAA is initially administered into the liver in a fashion that mimics the anticipated ^{90}Y infusion rate and catheter position. In retrospective analyses, estimated lung doses (assuming uniform distribution of particles) as low as 19.2 Gy have resulted in RIP.[18] However, because the distribution of ^{90}Y microspheres within the lungs is not homogeneous, with activity mainly concentrated at the base and central parts of the lung with the periphery being relatively spared, doses higher than 30 Gy have been well tolerated. Current recommendations from the Radioembolization Brachytherapy Oncology Consortium (REBOC) have advised that the maximum dose of radiation to the lungs, which patients can receive during a single session of SIRT, is 30 Gy.[19] Furthermore, a recent study examining 58 patients who underwent SIRT and received > 30 Gy cumulative lung dose, based on a partition model assuming a uniform lung distribution, demonstrated no clinical or radiographic signs of RIP.[20] Of these 58 patients, 10 patients presented with pleural effusions, atelectasis, and ground-glass attenuation as incidental findings without clinical manifestations of RIP. In situations where there is likely to be an excessive dose of radiation delivered to the lungs (i.e., > 30 Gy assuming a uniform distribution), dose reduction strategies should be considered to prevent RIP. Arbitrary dose reduction, based solely on the percent of lung shunt fraction from the ^{99m}Tc-MAA scan without consideration toward the actual deposited activity in the lung, should be discouraged because there is a greater chance of delivering increased radiation to the lungs in patients with a high body surface area and high tumor index ratio. Hence determination of the required activity during a single session ^{90}Y administration must incorporate safeguards against excessive deposition of radiation into the lungs. However, because all validated activity calculators do not take into account the amount of radioactivity lost to lung shunt, it is the responsibility of the prescribing physician to determine whether there is still an adequate dose of radioactivity being delivered to the target tumors after any activity reduction.

6.7.2 Liver Function

The majority of patients with HCC possess an element of underlying cirrhosis that impairs their baseline liver and regenerative function. Furthermore, the majority of the patients being considered for SIRT will have undergone additional treatments, including TACE, radiofrequency ablation, or surgical resection, further reducing their underlying liver reserve. The preexisting degree of hepatic compromise must be taken into account when considering patients for SIRT because radioembolization-induced liver disease (REILD) presents more commonly in patients with poor liver reserve and will accelerate their risk of developing fulminant liver failure (▶ Fig. 6.3). Liver-dependent factors strongly associated with a 3-month mortality include an infiltrative pattern of HCC (tumor volume > 50% of liver volume), bulky disease, liver transaminases (aspartate aminotransferase [AST] and alanine transaminase [ALT]) more than five times the normal value, albumin < 3 g/dL, and irreversible elevations of total serum bilirubin > 2 mg/dL.[21] Of these, the best pretreatment indicator for the development of liver toxicity following SIRT is the total serum bilirubin.[22] In a multicenter analysis looking at the survival of 325 patients undergoing SIRT, the median overall survival was 24.4 months for BCLC stage A patients, 16.9 months for BCLC stage B patients, and 10 months for BCLC stage C patients.[23] Other poor prognostic factors for survival included an Eastern Cooperative Oncology Group (ECOG) performance status > 1, greater tumor burden (nodules > 5), an INR higher than 1.2, and extrahepatic disease.

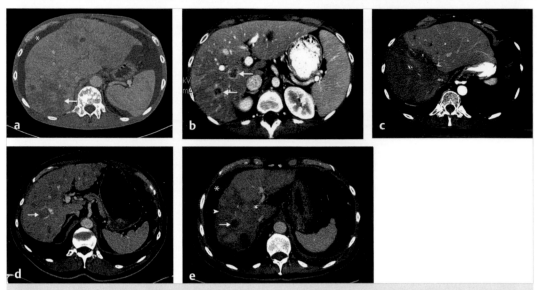

Fig. 6.3 Manifestations of liver parenchymal damage. **(a)** Radioembolization-induced liver disease (REILD) in a patient with prior chemotherapy and whole liver radioembolization with glass microspheres. Axial computed tomographic (CT) image in portovenous phase demonstrates enlargement of the liver with geographic areas of hypoattenuation in keeping with peribiliary edema *(arrow)*. Stigmata of portal hypertension including splenomegaly and ascites *(asterisk)* are also demonstrated. **(b)**. Uniform ring enhancement *(arrows)* representing a hyperemic rim can be seen throughout the liver representing a local inflammatory response. **(c)** Post yttrium-90 differential edema in a lobar distribution with glass microspheres. This is a common appearance following selective internal radiation therapy and is seen in the early inflammatory phase. **(d)** Osttherapy CT demonstrating hypovascular tumor metastases *(arrow)*. **(e)** CT 1 month posttreatment demonstrating differential enhancement in the liver *(arrowhead)* and marked hypovascularity of the tumors due to necrosis *(arrow)*. Note the new ascites *(asterisk)* and the irregular, shrunken appearance of the liver due to REILD.

6.7.3 Vascular Anatomy and Radiation Distribution

The aim of SIRT is to treat as much liver tumor as possible while minimizing nontargeted delivery of ^{90}Y microparticles to healthy tissue, both within and outside of the liver. Consequences of inadvertent delivery of radioactive microparticles to nontarget vessels can result in REILD (liver parenchymal exposure), skin irritation via the falciform artery, gastric mucosal inflammation and necrosis via the right gastric artery (▶ Fig. 6.4), gallbladder ischemia and necrosis via the cystic artery, and small bowel necrosis and perforation via the supra-duodenal or retroduodenal artery.[24] Embolization of extrahepatic vessels is therefore undertaken to protect intestinal organs from nontarget radiation-induced damage while embolization of selective intrahepatic vessels allows internal redistribution within the liver to minimize the delivery of SIRT to normal liver parenchyma. Mesenteric anatomy can be clearly identified on cross-sectional imaging with computed tomography (CT), provided that the slice thickness is 1 mm and the images are reviewed in at least two orthogonal planes to assist with procedural execution. Digital subtraction angiography (DSA) still remains the gold standard for identifying and mapping these vessels; hence all patients undergo an angiographic "mapping" procedure approximately 2 to 4 weeks prior to SIRT, during which time selective extra- or intrahepatic vessels can be catheterized and embolized if required. The aim of embolization is to optimize the arterial hemodynamics to allow the isolation of the precise vascular points for injection of the radioactive microparticles. It is important to recognize the possibility of redistribution and collateralization occurring between the day of the mapping procedure and the day of radioembolization because this may require further embolization at the time of SIRT administration.[25]

A discussion on the specific strategies and principles of vascular optimization is beyond the scope of this chapter; however, the authors encourage

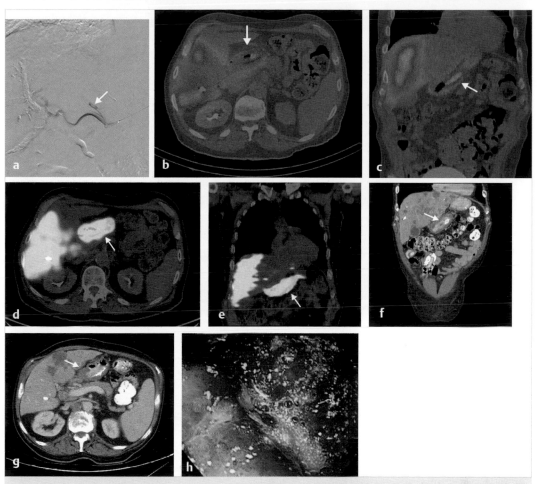

Fig. 6.4 Nontargeted embolization to the right gastric distribution. A 67-year-old man, Childs–Pugh B, diagnosed with nonalcoholic steatohepatitis (NASH) and multicentric hepatocellular carcinoma (HCC), failed attempt at portal vein embolization for surgical resection. Whole liver single-session administration was attempted. **(a)** Postimplantation angiogram demonstrated displacement of the catheter from the selective left lobe implantation and clear visualization of the right gastric artery *(arrow)*. **(b, c)** Postimplantation single-photon emission computed tomography/computed tomography (SPECT-CT) Bremsstrahlung and **(d, e)** three-dimensional time of flight position emission tomography demonstrate accumulation of activity in the antrum of the stomach *(arrows)*. **(f, g)** Contrast-enhanced CT performed 4 weeks after the procedure demonstrates progressive edema and thickening of the antral wall *(arrows)*. **(h)** Endoscopy performed at the same time demonstrates large mucosal ulcer craters within the antrum of the stomach *(arrow)*.

the reader to review Liu et al for a comprehensive overview of techniques and management.[24] Listed following here are some key vessels that should be identified during the mapping procedure and their potential management options.[24]

Cystic Artery

The cystic artery arises from the right hepatic artery in as many as 95% of patients[26] and usually has two branches—a superficial (peritoneal) and a

deep (nonperitoneal) branch. Identification of this artery is required prior to SIRT to assess whether there is a risk that the ^{90}Y microparticles could travel to the gallbladder and cause radiation-induced necrosis. SIRT should therefore be performed distal to the origin of the cystic artery where possible. If the catheter tip is to be placed proximal to the cystic artery, consideration should be made to embolize the artery on the day of treatment with Gelfoam.[27] The overall incidence of radiation-induced cholecystitis is very rare and is restricted to case report series, regardless of whether the cystic artery has been prophylactically embolized.

Right Gastric Artery

The origin of the right gastric artery (▶ Fig. 6.4) has a high degree of variation, but in more than half of cases it will arise from either the common or the proper hepatic artery, with the next most common location being the left hepatic artery.[28] The right gastric artery provides only a minor contribution to the gastric bed; however, if ^{90}Y microparticles travel down this artery they can cause gastric necrosis, ulceration, and perforation. Hence prophylactic embolization of this artery is often performed, but this can be difficult due to tortuosity or orientation of its origin. In some instances, retrograde cannulation of this artery needs to be performed via cannulation of the left gastric artery through the anastomotic arcades (backdoor technique). Although technically successful embolization of the right gastric artery with coils correlates with a decreased incidence of gastric mucosal ulceration, recanalization may occur in as many as 4% of cases.[29]

Pancreaticoduodenal Arcade

The pancreaticoduodenal arcade consists of several vessels and provides a rich collateral vascular network to the head and uncinate process of the pancreas and the duodenal bulb/antrum. This arcade also includes, for the purposes of discussion, the dorsal pancreatic, the supraduodenal, the pancreatica magna, the arc of Buhler, and the arc of Barkow. The understanding of this arcade is therefore necessary in every patient to prevent inadvertent pancreatitis, duodenal ulceration, or perforation following treatment. The dorsal pancreatic artery is the first major pancreatic branch and classically arises from the splenic artery. The supraduodenal artery has a highly variable origin but can be seen in up to 93% of patients[30] and supplies the upper two-thirds of the duodenum (▶ Fig. 6.5). The retroduodenal artery forms part of the posterior arcade and usually tracks along the common duct. Due to the rich degree of collateralization and also the potential for recanalization, detail and attention must be drawn at the time of coil embolization to identify small branch vessels that may result in reestablished flow to nonhepatic circulation.

Falciform Artery

The classic orientation of the falciform artery (see ▶ Fig. 6.5) is in an oblique plane from the left intersegmental fissure to the anterior abdominal wall. It usually arises from the left hepatic artery and can be seen in 2 to 25% of cases. The falciform artery is often seen on the delayed images of prolonged DSA runs as a result of sluggish flow and competitive flow from the internal mammary and superior epigastric arteries.[31] When identified, it is usually embolized in order to prevent a highly localized, midabdominal wall burning sensation, which can last for days or weeks following inadvertent radioembolization. Alternative treatments include placing an ice pack on the patient's abdomen to cause vasoconstriction of the vessel.[32]

6.8 Preprocedural Workup

6.8.1 Clinical Laboratory Results and Preprocedural Medications

The standard assessment of eligibility of patients undergoing SIRT is primarily related to hepatic reserve and function. Base parameters of liver function should be evaluated to minimize the possibility of REILD (to be discussed). In general, liver function, performance status, and tumor morphology must be taken into consideration.

Pre- and periprocedural medications can be divided into two categories: those relating to symptomatic relief and those relating to risk mitigation of REILD, and they are outlined later in the chapter and in Section VII (▶ Table 6.4).

6.8.2 Pre-[90]Y Treatment Imaging

All prospective candidates for SIRT are investigated clinically and then imaged with a combination of cross-sectional imaging and angiography prior to therapy with ^{90}Y microspheres. Patient workup includes a four-phase CT (unenhanced, arterial, portal venous, and delayed phases) and/or gadolinium-enhanced magnetic resonance imaging (MRI) of the liver. The use of CT is advocated due to its superior spatial resolution when compared to MRI. As previously mentioned, if the slice thickness is 1 mm and images can be reconstructed in at least two orthogonal planes, detailed assessment of the intra- and extrahepatic arteries can be made thereby facilitating visceral catheter/

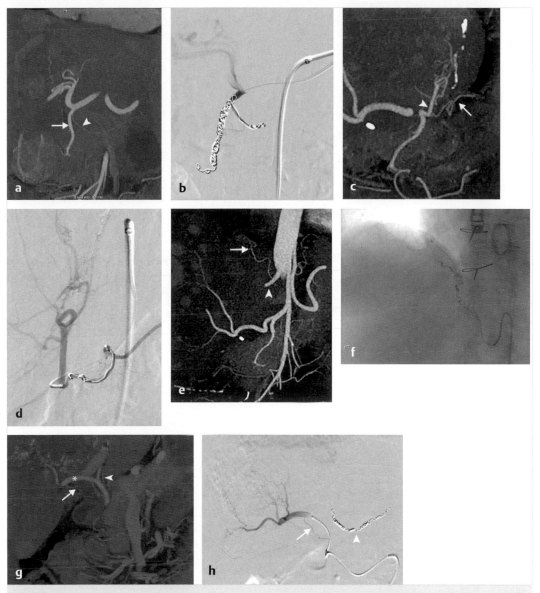

Fig. 6.5 Vascular anatomical variation and the value of high-quality preprocedure computed tomographic angiography (CTA). **(a)** Coronal maximum intensity projection (MIP) reformatted CTA demonstrating the gastroduodenal artery *(arrow)* and right gastric artery *(arrowhead)*. **(b)** Mapping angiogram demonstrating coiling of the gastroduodenal artery (GDA) and right gastric artery RGA in the same patient. **(c)** Coronal MIP CTA demonstrating the RGA *(arrow)* arising off the left hepatic artery *(arrowhead)*. **(d)** Mapping angiogram demonstrating coiling of the RGA in the same patient. **(e)** CTA demonstrating a parasitized right inferior phrenic artery *(arrow)* arising off the proper hepatic artery *(arrowhead)*. **(f)** Mapping angiogram demonstrating coiling of the parasitized inferior phrenic artery. **(g)** CTA demonstrating a supraduodenal artery (long arrow) arising from the right hepatic artery *(asterisk)* and the RGA *(arrowhead)* arising off the left hepatic artery. **(h)** Mapping angiogram demonstrating supraduodenal artery *(arrow)* opacified during a right hepatic artery injection, with coils in the RGA *(arrowhead)*.

Table 6.4 Pre- and periprocedural medications

Symptomatic management	Comment
Proton pump inhibitor (e.g., omeprazole)	For 1 week prior and 30 days following, management of mild forms of radiation gastritis arising from scatter
Systemic oral steroids (e.g., methylprednisolone)	1–2 weeks postadministration rapid taper to address nausea, fatigue, and anorexia
Oral opioid analgesics (e.g., hydrocodone)	Used as needed for management of abdominal pain
Oral antibiotic (e.g., ciprofloxacin)	Empirical prophylaxis for possible biliary tract infection

microcatheter selection during both the mapping and the treatment procedures. The later phases of imaging (portal venous/delayed) allow for a more thorough assessment of the liver parenchyma, patency of the portal vein and the extent of any extrahepatic disease.[33]

By determining the volume of tumor relative to normal liver parenchyma, the percentage of liver involved by tumor can be calculated, which plays a key role in determining the prescribed dose of radiation required for treatment when using all methods of dose and activity determination. Multiphase MRI with Primovist (Gadoxetate acid, Bayer Schering Pharma) and diffusion-weighted imaging (DWI) constitute a useful diagnostic tool when imaging features on CT are indeterminate but are not contributory to evaluation of arterial anatomy.

Once patients are deemed eligible for ^{90}Y treatment, they will undergo a formal angiographic mapping procedure. As previously mentioned, all the vessels that supply both the liver and the tumor are meticulously characterized by catheter angiography. Where required, selected vessels are embolized either to prevent organs from radiation-induced damage or to encourage redistribution of flow to allow for a lower number of potential administration points of ^{90}Y microspheres. At each of these potential ^{90}Y administration points, approximately 5 mCi of ^{99m}Tc-MAA is administered. The thorax and abdomen are then imaged with single-photon emission computed tomography CT (SPECT-CT) to assess for extrahepatic shunting to the lungs or gastrointestinal tract. The detected counts are then used to calculate the lung shunt fraction: (lung counts/lung counts + liver counts) × 100. Recent studies have also shown that SPECT with integrated low-dose CT has increased sensitivity and specificity when compared to SPECT alone in detecting extrahepatic

arterial shunting.[34,35] Furthermore, SPECT-CT has improved spatial resolution and anatomical coregistration. Determination of any theoretical lung shunt is obtained by multiplying the percentage detected shunt by the prescribed activity and then checking that it does not exceed a total distributed dose of 30 Gy to the lungs.

6.9 Determination of Activation/Estimation of Dosimetry

To determine a prescribed activity calculation in patients undergoing SIRT with ^{90}Y, it is important to appreciate the difference between dose and activity.

Dose refers to the amount of energy of radiation that is taken up by the tissue within the body and is measured in gray (Gy). The measure of the health effect on the human body from radiation is measured in sieverts (Sv) and is based on both the absorbed dose and the sensitivity of the tissue being irradiated, thereby representing the stochastic health risk of developing cancer or inducing genetic damage. In general, 1 GBq (27 mCi) delivers a total absorbed dose of 49.7 Gy/kg.

Activity refers to the amount of ionizing radiation and is measured in either curie (Ci) or becquerel (Bq). Because commercially available glass microspheres (TheraSphere) carry more specific activity when compared with resin microspheres (SIR-Spheres), they are delivered to patients in significantly lower numbers. By comparison, the lower specific activity of resin microspheres allows for them to be administered in larger numbers, thereby potentially resulting in a more uniform distribution.[36] There are two widely used methods to estimate the amount of activity delivered by ^{90}Y microspheres to patients using resin microspheres: a BSA model and a (two-compart-ment) partition model. One method of activity determination is used for glass microspheres and is commonly referred to as the medical internal radiation dose (MIRD) single partition model. Because the terms *partition model* (denoting a two-compartment partition in the use of resin microspheres) and *MIRD partition* (denoting a sin-gle-compartment model used with glass micro-spheres) have both been shortened to *partition model* much confusion has been introduced. It is important to note that the partition model and MIRD partition represent distinct and different methods with significant differences in calculated activity.

Body-Surface Area (BSA): SIRT treatment with resin microspheres (SIR-Spheres) uses the BSA model, which has been validated in phase 3 clinical trials investigating metastatic colorectal carcino-ma. BSA is calculated using the following equation:

Equation 6.2

$$BSA(m^2) = 0.20247 \times height(m)0.0725 \\ \times weight(kg)0.42$$

and has been shown to directly correlate with the volume of nontumoral liver as calculated by CT.[37] The BSA method is calculated based on a combina-tion of BSA and the degree of tumor infiltration using the following equation:

Equation 6.3

$$Activity(GBq) = (BSA - 0.2) + \left(\frac{Tumor\ volume}{Total}\right)$$

Limitations using this calculation are encountered if patients are obese or when there is a very large tumor burden.

Partition Model (Two-Compartment): With this method, SIRT activity calculations are based on the two-compartment model, which allowed more accurate optimization of the amount of radiation delivered to tumors with the optimal dose to tumor as >120Gy. A higher degree of complexity is required to arrive at the derivation of the equations relating to the activity (and dose) to the lung, normal liver, and tumor. As a result, this method, although theoretically more sound, has not been widely adopted. Readers are encouraged to review the rationale and methods as described by Ho et al.[38,39]

Clinical studies have demonstrated that back-ground liver parenchyma in cirrhotic patients can tolerate up to 70 Gy of radiation without evidence of radiation-induced hepatitis.[40] Based on this

information the two-compartment partition mod-el has been able to optimize the amount of activity delivered such that tumors received the minimum amount of radiation needed to cause cellular destruction while sparing the background liver from excessive radiation exposure to minimize the risk of inducing REILD.

MIRD Partition Model (Single-Compartment): SIRT treatment with glass microspheres (Thera-Sphere) uses a simplified single-compartment MIRD model based on the size of the entire liver irrespective of the amount of tumor burden with the following formula:

Equation 6.4

$$Activity(GBq) = \frac{(Dose(Gy) \times Mass(Kg))}{49.7}$$

The abbreviated reference to the MIRD Partition Model as the Partition Model has resulted in some confusion regarding compartmental radiation in the tumor versus the normal parenchyma.

All models also rely on the assumption that the tumor vascularity is homogeneous with a regular hierarchy of vessels when in fact angiogenesis results in a heterogeneous vascular supply to the tumor.[41] As a result of this disorganized vascular network, microparticles will tend to cluster in hypervascular areas and in the periphery of tumors, thereby creating an inhomogeneous cloud of radiation covering the tumor, with some areas potentially not receiving enough radiation to kill tumor cells. This effect may be compounded with high specific activity particles, as fewer particles are administered and hence there is the potential for less tumor coverage, especially in tumors that demonstrate greater clustering and thus the need for greater amounts of radiation to create the tumorcidal radioactive cloud. In such cases, lower-specific-activity particles (glass with extended shelf life, EX, or resin) would appear to have a the-oretical advantage of providing greater tumor cov-erage simply by virtue of more microparticles.

Despite this, the single-compartment MIRD model (assuming uniform distribution of activity to both parenchyma and tumor), has been widely adapted in clinical practice and recent publica-tions, under the assumption of noncompartmen-talization of radiation and acceptable safety profile. This methodology likely results in higher doses of radiation being delivered to both the tumor and background liver.[42] At first glance, it may seem beneficial to deliver as much radiation as possible to the tumor; however, if all tumor cells are destroyed above a certain threshold then delivering more radiation above this value will not add any additional value to treatment. In fact, delivering more radiation may indeed be deleterious because the background normal liver will be exposed to higher doses of radiation, thereby increasing the risk for developing REILD, especially in patients with limited functional reserve, and thus adherence to ALARA principles based on underlying physical principles may need to be considered in activity planning with all methods of calculation.

6.10 Equipment and Technique

6.10.1 Commercially Available Microspheres

The two treatment options for the delivery of SIRT to the liver using ^{90}Y include glass microspheres (TheraSphere) and resin microspheres (SIR-Spheres). TheraSphere is made from glass matrix bombarded in a neutron flux reactor and hence has a higher specific gravity resulting in rapid settling. The particles range in size from 23 to 35 µm and carry more radiation per microparticle (i.e., specific activity), resulting in a lower number of microspheres delivered during SIRT (~ 1.2–10 million particles). The high activity per particle may overcome any potential issues of inadequate tumoral coverage due to the known phenomenon of microclustering, whereby the microparticles preferentially cluster in the periphery of tumors.[9] Newer techniques, such as the extended (EX) shelf-life method may address the issue by allowing an increased number of glass microspheres (decayed to the second week of their allowable shelf-life) to be administered for the same planned absorbed dose, thereby allowing better tumoral distribution of the microspheres without causing additional adverse radiation-related events.[43] SIR-Spheres, on the other hand, are made from inert microspheres that are coated with resin and subsequent radioactive labeling performed through a generator. The particles have a lower specific gravity, range in size between 20 and 60 µm, and carry a lower amount of radiation per microparticle; these attributes result in a higher number of resin microparticles administered per treatment (approximately 8–30 million microspheres), translating into a more even distribution of radiation within the targeted area with less overall ^{90}Y activity.[10]

6.10.2 Bilobar versus Unilobar Selective Internal Radiation Therapy

In patients with bilobar disease, whole liver treatment with SIRT is performed, which usually involves an approach whereby SIRT is administered to each liver lobe in sequential sessions separated by approximately 1 month. The sequential lobar approach is the standard of care for glass microsphere administration and the majority of resin microsphere administration for patients with HCC. Treatment can be applied to the whole liver in a single session for multicentric disease, but only with resin microspheres, as demonstrated in 37% of the European Network on Radioembolization with Yttrium-90 Resin Microspheres (ENRY) patient population. [23] A larger number of microparticles can be distributed more homogeneously throughout the liver which, in theory and in practice, reduces the potential for inducing parenchymal damage from excessive radiation exposure as demonstrated by parenchymal fissuring, lobar edema, or compensatory hypertrophy of nontreated liver. In patients with unilobar disease, radiation can be delivered from a proximal location when the disease is multicentric. Alternatively, if there is a large, solitary tumor in a unicentric location the entire dose can be selectively administered into the vessel supplying the affected segment of liver under the assumption that inevitable destruction of all tumor and parenchyma in the distributed area will not result in liver decompensation. The latter approach allows for a large dose of radiation to be concentrated within a single segment, thereby selectively destroying that segment while leaving the remaining liver unaffected, otherwise referred to as a radiation segmentectomy (▶ Fig. 6.6).[44]

6.11 Vascular Optimization

To reduce or even eliminate complications associated with nontargeted deposition of ^{90}Y microspheres, different strategies can be employed to encourage antegrade flow through target vessels while also preventing both retrograde flow and delivery of microparticles into nontarget vessels. The most common technique to protect side-branch vessels that supply important extrahepatic organs (e.g., the stomach, small bowel, and pancreas) is to embolize these nontarget vessels prior to the delivery of ^{90}Y microspheres. Embolization

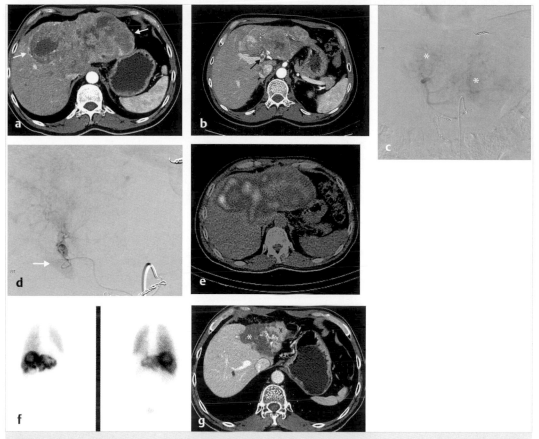

Fig. 6.6 Selective internal radiation therapy (SIRT) sequence of radiation lobectomy. A 51-year-old patient, Childs–Pugh A with hepatitis C, presenting with **(a)** infiltrative expansible hepatocellular carcinoma (HCC) *(arrows)* involving the entire left lobe with **(b)** frank left portal venous tumor thrombus *(arrow)*. **(c)** Mesenteric angiogram demonstrating left hepatic arterial selection with extensive tumor enhancement *(asterisks)*, and **(d)** segment IV angiogram demonstrating portal venous tumor thrombus enhancement *(arrow)*. **(e)** Technetium-99 m macroaggregated serum albumin (^{99m}Tc-MAA) single-photon emission computed tomography/computed tomography (SPECT-CT) demonstrating increased perfusion/uptake within the tumor. **(f)** Anterior and posterior ^{99m}Tc-MAA scintigraphy demonstrates a lung shunt fraction of 24% due to intratumor shunting. A total of 2.1 GBq of glass microspheres using EX protocol was deposited within the left lobe, resulting in 195 Gy estimated dose. **(g)** Three-month post-SIRT CT demonstrating marked devascularization of tumor, and liver parenchymal retraction *(white asterisk)* with a small focus of residual disease *(black asterisk)*.

is performed by superselecting these arteries, usually with a microcatheter platform, and then occluding these vessels, either permanently (i.e., with coils) on the day of the mapping procedure, or temporarily (i.e., with Gelfoam) on the day of the SIRT. Nontarget organ ischemia following embolization does not usually occur due to extensive collateral pathways maintaining organ perfusion. In some circumstances, either the nontarget vessel that arises from the main target vessel cannot be cannulated or the vascular resistance within the target vessel is elevated, thereby predisposing

delivery of ^{90}Y microspheres to reflux. In these circumstances, proximal protection strategies may be warranted. The Surefire catheter (Surefire Medical, Inc.) represents a newer class of device. It consists of a catheter with a funnel-shaped tip, which, when deployed, expands to prevent reflux of particles behind the catheter tip while allowing antegrade flow to continue. Studies have shown its efficacy in cases where there has been no prior prophylactic coil embolization of extrahepatic arterial communications during ^{90}Y administration, with follow-up positron emission tomographic

Table 6.5 Catheter selection

Catheter	Target vessel	Injection rate	Length of injection
4F or 5F base catheter	Celiac axis/SMA	6 mL/s	4 s
4F or 5F base catheter	Common hepatic artery	5 mL/s	4 s
0.018–0.028 in microcatheter	LHA/RHA/Seg IV/GDA/RGA/cystic	1–3 mL/s (the injection rate should be approximately the same rate as the diameter of the vessel)	6–15 s imaged out to the parenchymal phase of opacification

Abbreviations: GDA, gastroduodenal artery; LHA, left hepatic artery; RGA, right gastric artery; RHA, right hepatic artery; ??; SMA, superior mesenteric artery.

(PET) CT demonstrating no nontargeted deposition of radioactive microparticles.[45] Alternatively, a microcatheter occlusion balloon can be transiently inflated in a nontargeted vessel to protect it from unintended embolization while embolotherapy is concurrently performed from a more proximal position.[46]

6.12 Catheter Selection

Catheter selection (▶ Table 6.5) should be based on vessel anatomy; commonly used shapes include Cobra (C2) (Terumo Manufacturing Corporation), Simmons 1/2 (AngioDynamics), SOS Omni 1/2/3 (AngioDynamics), Mickelson, and Rosch left gastric (RLG) catheters.

▶ Table 6.2 serves only as a guide, and the injection rates should be based on both the target vessel diameter and the catheter used.

The injection rate and pressure limit on each microcatheter varies depending on the internal diameter of the catheter. Microcatheter selection is extremely important when planning a case, especially during the mapping, because the inner diameter chosen should serve the dual purpose of coil embolization and adequate injection rates. Too large an inner lumen may cause microcoils to jam in the catheter; conversely too small an inner lumen will limit the injection rate and may lead to poor opacification of target vessels or nonopacification of vessels.

Long, slow injections imaged out to the parenchymal phase of enhancement are recommended in order to visualize lesions in all the phases of enhancement.

If cone beam CT is to be used, the injection rates should be adjusted so that the injection lasts for the duration of the acquisition. It is recommended to obtain a conventional DSA scan prior to cone beam CT acquisition to ensure there is no reflux into nontarget vessels and the segment of liver being assessed can be accurately mapped. Reflux of contrast into nontarget vessels will cause parenchymal enhancement and may alter planning for dose delivery.

The recommended concentration of contrast medium for cone beam CT varies between manufacturers, which should be borne in mind because too dense contrast will cause significant Hounsfield/spray artefact and degrade the image during cone beam CT acquisition.

6.13 Postprocedure Evaluation

The biodistribution of ^{90}Y microspheres within the liver is dependent on the locoregional flow environment distal to the point of injection. This, in turn, is influenced by a myriad of interrelated biophysical variables, such as the catheter tip location, injection rate, proximity to branching vessels, extent of shunting, cardiovascular status, and microparticle load. Despite advances in the techniques used to optimize the delivery of ^{90}Y microspheres to target tumors, the distribution of microparticles remains a significant challenge when assessing the quality of tumor targeting after injection, as well as when performing systematic dosimetry studies.[47] Within the first 24 hours following SIRT, a Bremsstrahlung SPECT scan can be performed to document ^{90}Y deposition within tumor tissue. By indirectly imaging the continuous scatter radiation of ^{90}Y with no definable photopeak, Bremsstrahlung scintigraphy suffers from low spatial resolution, which in turn results in a coarse representation of microsphere deposition.[48,49] To help improve localization of ^{90}Y microspheres, Bremsstrahlung SPECT-CT can be performed. However, distinguishing closely adjacent foci of ^{90}Y Bremsstrahlung activity can be limited due to the diffuse and smooth pattern of activity that lacks sharp margins.[48,50] Despite the latest postprocessing optimization techniques of tissue attenuation, scatter, and collimator-detector response compensation, Bremsstrahlung scintigraphy of ^{90}Y remains quantitatively inaccurate and a poor surrogate for dose-response analysis.[51,52]

Time-of-flight (TOF) PET-CT is a new imaging technique that allows direct imaging of ^{90}Y microspheres and offers both qualitative and quantitative advantages over Bremsstrahlung imaging, including assessment for nontarget activity and tumor vascular thrombosis.[48] Because ^{90}Y microspheres emit β-radiation, coincidence imaging of ^{90}Y is possible due to e−/e + internal pair production as it decays to the ^{90}Z isotope.[53] Recently, several reports have shown encouraging results with ^{90}Y-TOF PET-CT for post-SIRT imaging[54,55,56]; however, viscera closely adjacent to the liver still remain challenging for nontarget activity detection, and this is compounded by a tendency for misregistration. Multiple studies evaluating tumor dose quantification in phantom models with TOF PET-CT have shown promising results producing high-resolution absorbed dose distribution maps, thereby paving the way for future patient-specific PET dosimetry assessments following SIRT.[47,57,58,59,60]

At 30 to 60 days following SIRT, four-phase CT or multiphase MRI is performed, which is repeated at 3-month intervals thereafter to allow accurate evaluation of the response to ^{90}Y treatment. Interval scans are not performed earlier to avoid misinterpretation of transient and partially reversible incidental radiographic findings.[19,61] The most common transient finding on CT is a decrease in the Hounsfield attenuation values within the liver at the site of ^{90}Y microparticle deposition, which is thought to represent congestion, edema, and microinfarction in the treated areas of liver[19] (see ▶ Fig. 6.3). Based on guidelines from the World Health Organization (WHO) and the Response Evaluation Criteria in Solid Tumors (RECIST) group,[62,63] the hallmark feature of a successful treatment response is a reduction in tumor size. However, necrosis, cystic degeneration, hemorrhage, and edema can all increase tumor size. In a recent study, combined size and necrosis criteria were shown to be more accurate in assessing the response to ^{90}Y treatment than the use of size criteria alone.[64] Hence tumor response should also be evaluated with other surrogates, such as the presence of necrosis, the degree of tumor vascularity, metabolic activity of tumors on fludeoxyglucose (FDG)-PET, tumor volume, tumor serum markers, and diffusion weighting on MRI.[65] Maximum response (in the case of complete devascularization and nonrecurrence) may take up to 6 to 9 months to be achieved.

6.14 Side Effects, Complications, and Their Management

The most common side effects and complications following SIRT are summarized in ▶ Table 6.6.

REILD was coined by Sangro and colleagues[11] to refer to a constellation of symptoms resulting from progressive liver decompensation temporally related to SIRT. Historically, REILD has been a poorly understood phenomenon due to its relative rarity; however, the relationship between radiation exposure and hepatic reserve has always been suspected.

Radiation exposure to the tumor, relative to liver parenchyma, is dependent on the distribution of microspheres, which ultimately relies on the complex interaction between tumor hypervascularity and microvascular capacitance. Factors that compromise hepatic reserve and thus increase the probability of developing REILD following SIRT include background cirrhosis, previous surgical resection, NASH, and chemotherapy-associated steatohepatitis (CASH). Supporting this, recent studies stratifying patients based on the Okuda score have shown that patients with lower stages of hepatic compromise tolerate higher doses of radiation without significant liver toxicities [66] Using a single-compartment model, it has been estimated that doses > 150 Gy during a single administration are associated with an increased risk of liver toxicity when glass microspheres are used in HCC populations.[22] However, the benefit of using higher doses of radiation does not appear to provide any clear advantage, with equivalent survival outcomes demonstrated in HCC patients when activity (and dose) reduction algorithms were employed. Indeed, retrospective analysis actually demonstrates a significant reduction in the incidence of REILD in patients who receive dose reduction.[67] Furthermore in non-HCC populations, the phenomenon of "radiation recall" has also been suggested to contribute to REILD; this may result from reactivation of previously

Table 6.6 Common toxicities, incidence and management

Class	Complication/toxicity	Incidence (%)	Management
Constitutional	Fatigue	28–52	Self-limiting Steroid
	Abdominal pain/discomfort	16–19	Self-limiting Steroid Analgesics
	Nausea	6–13	Steroid Antiemetics
Hepatic/tumor vasculature	Gastritis	5	Analgesics Antiemetics Bismuth Motility agent H2 blocker or proton pump inhibitor Partial gastrectomy
	Cholecystitis	3 (1% requiring surgery), case reports	Observation Cholecystectomy
	Radiation pneumonitis	0–6	High-dose steroids
Hepatic parenchyma	Biochemical liver toxicity: grade III or higher (ALP, AST, ALT, bilirubin) (transient)	6–27	Self-limiting
	radioembolization induced liver disease (REILD) or failure	0–20	Diuretics High-dose steroids Defibrotide Low-dose heparin Ursodeoxycholic acid Pentoxifylline
	Portal hypertension; fibrosis	Case reports	Observational TIPS
	Biloma/abscess	1	Observational Drainage
	Ascites	11 (advanced liver disease)	Drainage
	Encephalopathy	3 cases (more common after second treatment)	Lactulose Supportive
	Hemobilia	Single reported case	
Systemic toxicities	Pancytopenia	Case report (likely due to free yttrium-90 unbound to microsphere)	Supportive

Abbreviations: ALP, alkaline phosphatase; ALT, alanene transaminase; AST, aspartate aminotransferase; TIPS, transjugular intrahepatic portosystemic shunt.
Source: Adapted from Liu et al.[68]

administered systemic chemotherapeutic agents (e.g. radiosensitizers) in the presence of radiation therapy, thereby potentiating their effect, which increases the risk of patients developing REILD (► Fig. 6.3).

Clinically, the presentation of REILD is varied, but it is classically described as a rapid deterioration of biochemical markers (i.e., high bilirubin and low albumin) on a background of developing ascites with evidence of perfusion abnormalities within the liver (appearances similar to veno-occlusive disease) and eventual shrinkage of the liver in the final stages. Histopathologically, REILD has been characterized by microscopic veno-occlusive disease and fibrosis on a background of parenchymal congestion and architectural distortion. Upon recognition of REILD, the current standard of treatment includes the use of diuretics for mild cases and sustained high-dose steroids. In more severe and acute situations, sustained low-dose heparin, ursodeoxycholic acid, and pentoxifylline may also warrant consideration (▶ Table 6.6).[68]

Pearls for SIRT

- Understand the vascular anatomy prior to mapping and/or catheterization.
- Full biochemical and radiographic assessment of the liver parenchyma is essential: ALARA and REILD = optimal activity, not maximal activity.
- Proximal protection and redistribution can assist in consolidation of point of delivery: try to consolidate to two-vessel administration where possible.
- Consider the nontargeted delivery of radiation to the nontumorous parenchyma and adjust according to the patient's residual hepatic reserve.
- Recognize the need for adequate distribution of radiation to target tissue and modulate specific activity of the radioembolic accordingly.
- Current evidence suggests an advantageous role for SIRT in the following settings:
  - Advanced disease Childs–Pugh status B (see ▶ Fig. 6.4).
  - Portal vein thrombosis (▶ Fig. 6.6).
  - Downstage to resection (▶ Fig. 6.7).
  - The current literature may bias toward all patient populations to be treated with SIRT; however, current evidence is lacking.
  - Additional benefit of decreased toxicity and (in select cases) outpatient-based single-session whole-liver therapy, paired with decreased frequency of retreatment, may develop into a cost-effective option for Child–Pugh A populations.
- Interval follow-up with imaging should be coupled with an understanding of some of the common findings associated with normal parenchymal and tumor response.
- REILD may present up to 6 months post-SIRT, requiring recognition and rapid initiation of therapy.

Table 6.7 Ranking system for levels of evidence

Level	Criteria
1a	Systematic reviews (with homogeneity) of randomized, controlled trials
1b	Individual randomized, controlled trials (with narrow confidence interval)
1c	All or none randomized, controlled trials
2a	Systematic reviews (with homogeneity) of cohort studies
2b	Individual cohort study or low-quality randomized, controlled trials (< 80% follow-up)
2c	Outcomes research; ecological studies
3a	Systematic review (with homogeneity) of case-control studies
3b	Individual case-control study
4	Case-series (and poor-quality cohort and case-control studies)
5	Expert opinion without explicit critical appraisal, or based on physiology, bench research, or "first principles"

Note: Analysis only includes peer-reviewed data and therefore excludes studies presented at scientific meetings.

6.15 Clinical Data and Outcomes

Summary of Data Supporting SIRT/Radioembolization in Hepatocellular Carcinoma (▶ Table 6.7):

- SIRT/radioembolization should be considered as a valuable treatment option for suitable patients with unresectable/nonablatable HCC, either as an alternative to TACE/transarterial embolization (TAE) or in patients who are not suitable for or who have failed TACE/TAE.
- There are encouraging clinical data from large single-center, multicenter, and comparative studies that SIRT/radioembolization is safe, well tolerated, and effective in unresectable HCC (level 2a/b).
- There are encouraging clinical data that SIRT/radioembolization increases the number of patients with unresectable/nonablatable HCC that can be downsized to enable radical therapy (resection, ablation, or liver transplantation) (level 2b).
- The following subgroups of HCC patients have been shown to be particularly suitable for treatment with SIRT/radioembolization (level 2a/b):

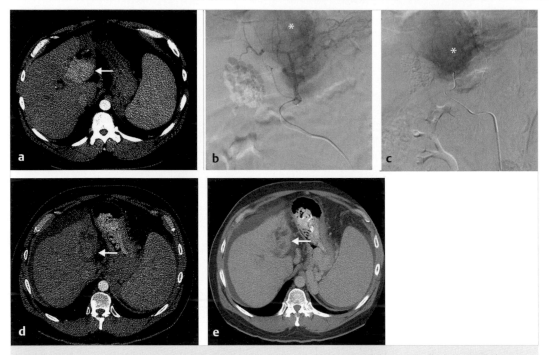

Fig. 6.7 Downstaging of tumor prior to transplantation. A 62-year-old woman, Childs–Pugh B with long-standing hepatitis B, cirrhosis, and hepatocellular carcinoma in the left lobe of the liver. **(a)** Axial computed tomographic (CT) scan in arterial phase demonstrates hypervascular tumor in segments 2/4a of the liver *(arrow)*. **(b, c)** Selective catheterization of the left lobe hepatic artery demonstrates the hypervascular tumor (asterisk). TheraSphere (3 GBq) were selectively injected into segment 2/4a of the liver, representing approximately 324 Gy administered to the segment (radiation segmentectomy). **(d)** Posttherapy CT images in arterial and **(e)** portovenous phases demonstrate marked reduction in tumor enhancement and volume *(arrows)* in keeping with a satisfactory response.

○ Unresectable/nonablatable patients that are typical candidates for TACE: BCLC stage A or stage B with unilobar disease and/or a limited number of nodules (1–5).

○ Patients that are poor candidates for TACE: BCLC stage B with bilobar disease or a large number of nodules (> 5, typically an uncountable number).

○ Patients that have previously failed TACE/TAE.

○ Patients that are contraindicated for TACE: BCLC stage C, portal vein thrombosis.

○ Patients receiving SIRT/radioembolization experience fewer complications and spend fewer days in hospital compared with those receiving TACE (level 3b).

References

[1] American Cancer Society. Cancer facts and figures 2013. Atlanta, GA: American Cancer Society; 2013

[2] Sanyal AJ, Yoon SK, Lencioni R. The etiology of hepatocellular carcinoma and consequences for treatment. Oncologist 2010; 15 Suppl 4: 14–22

[3] De Minicis S, Marzioni M, Saccomanno S et al. Cellular and molecular mechanisms of hepatic fibrogenesis leading to liver cancer. Transl Gastrointest Cancer 2012; 1: 88–94

[4] Pons F, Varela M, Llovet JM. Staging systems in hepatocellular carcinoma. HPB (Oxford) 2005; 7(1): 35–41

[5] Hsieh YH, Hsu JL, Su IJ, Huang W. Genomic instability caused by hepatitis B virus: into the hepatoma inferno. Front Biosci (Landmark Ed) 2011; 16: 2586–2597

[6] Fung J, Lai CL, Yuen MF. Hepatitis B and C virus-related carcinogenesis. Clin Microbiol Infect 2009; 15(11): 964–970

[7] Kennedy A, Coldwell D, Sangro B, Wasan H, Salem R. Radioembolization for the treatment of liver tumors general principles. Am J Clin Oncol 2012; 35(1): 91–99

[8] Jackson A, Ten Haken RK, Robertson JM, Kessler ML, Kutcher GJ, Lawrence TS. Analysis of clinical complication data for radiation hepatitis using a parallel architecture model. Int J Radiat Oncol Biol Phys 1995; 31(4): 883–891

[9] Kennedy AS, Nutting C, Coldwell D, Gaiser J, Drachenberg C. Pathologic response and microdosimetry of (90)Y microspheres in man: review of four explanted whole livers. Int J Radiat Oncol Biol Phys 2004; 60(5): 1552–1563

[10] Kritzinger J, Klass D, Ho S et al. Hepatic embolotherapy in interventional oncology: technology, techniques, and applications. Clin Radiol 2013; 68(1): 1–15

[11] Bilbao JI, de Martino A, de Luis E et al. Biocompatibility, inflammatory response, and recannalization characteristics of nonradioactive resin microspheres: histological findings. Cardiovasc Intervent Radiol 2009; 32(4): 727–736

[12] Koukourakis MI. Tumour angiogenesis and response to radiotherapy. Anticancer Res 2001; 21 6B: 4285–4300

[13] Das U. A radical approach to cancer. Med Sci Monit 2002; 8 (4): RA79–RA92

[14] Fleming ID. AJCC/TNM cancer staging, present and future. J Surg Oncol 2001; 77(4): 233–236

[15] Llovet JM. Updated treatment approach to hepatocellular carcinoma. J Gastroenterol 2005; 40(3): 225–235

[16] Llovet JM, Fuster J, Bruix J, Barcelona-Clinic Liver Cancer G.. The Barcelona approach: diagnosis, staging, and treatment of hepatocellular carcinoma. Liver Transpl 2004; 10(2) Suppl 1: S115–S120

[17] Salem R, Lewandowski RJ, Kulik L et al. Radioembolization results in longer time-to-progression and reduced toxicity compared with chemoembolization in patients with hepatocellular carcinoma. Gastroenterology 2011; 140(2): 497–507.e2

[18] Leung TW, Lau WY, Ho SK et al. Radiation pneumonitis after selective internal radiation treatment with intraarterial 90yttrium-microspheres for inoperable hepatic tumors. Int J Radiat Oncol Biol Phys 1995; 33(4): 919–924

[19] Kennedy A, Nag S, Salem R et al. Recommendations for radioembolization of hepatic malignancies using yttrium-90 microsphere brachytherapy: a consensus panel report from the radioembolization brachytherapy oncology consortium. Int J Radiat Oncol Biol Phys 2007; 68(1): 13–23

[20] Salem R, Parikh P, Atassi B et al. Incidence of radiation pneumonitis after hepatic intra-arterial radiotherapy with yttrium-90 microspheres assuming uniform lung distribution. Am J Clin Oncol 2008; 31(5): 431–438

[21] Goin JE, Salem R, Carr BI et al. Treatment of unresectable hepatocellular carcinoma with intrahepatic yttrium 90 microspheres: a risk-stratification analysis. J Vasc Interv Radiol 2005; 16(2 Pt 1): 195–203

[22] Goin JE, Salem R, Carr BI et al. Treatment of unresectable hepatocellular carcinoma with intrahepatic yttrium 90 microspheres: factors associated with liver toxicities. J Vasc Interv Radiol 2005; 16(2 Pt 1): 205–213

[23] Sangro B, Carpanese L, Cianni R et al. European Network on Radioembolization with Yttrium-90 Resin Microspheres (ENRY). Survival after yttrium-90 resin microsphere radioembolization of hepatocellular carcinoma across Barcelona clinic liver cancer stages: a European evaluation. Hepatology 2011; 54(3): 868–878

[24] Liu DM, Salem R, Bui JT et al. Angiographic considerations in patients undergoing liver-directed therapy. J Vasc Interv Radiol 2005; 16(7): 911–935

[25] Abdelmaksoud MH, Hwang GL, Louie JD et al. Development of new hepaticoenteric collateral pathways after hepatic arterial skeletonization in preparation for yttrium-90 radioembolization. J Vasc Interv Radiol 2010; 21(9): 1385–1395

[26] Ottery FD, Scupham RK, Weese JL. Chemical cholecystitis after intrahepatic chemotherapy. The case for prophylactic cholecystectomy during pump placement. Dis Colon Rectum 1986; 29(3): 187–190

[27] McWilliams JP, Kee ST, Loh CT, Lee EW, Liu DM. Prophylactic embolization of the cystic artery before radioembolization: feasibility, safety, and outcomes. Cardiovasc Intervent Radiol 2011; 34(4): 786–792

[28] Yamagami T, Nakamura T, Iida S, Kato T, Nishimura T. Embolization of the right gastric artery before hepatic arterial infusion chemotherapy to prevent gastric mucosal lesions: approach through the hepatic artery versus the left gastric artery. Am J Roentgenol 2002; 179(6): 1605–1610

[29] Inaba Y, Arai Y, Matsueda K, Takeuchi Y, Aramaki T. Right gastric artery embolization to prevent acute gastric mucosal lesions in patients undergoing repeat hepatic arterial infusion chemotherapy. J Vasc Interv Radiol 2001; 12(8): 957–963

[30] Bianchi HF, Albanèse EF. The supraduodenal artery. Surg Radiol Anat 1989; 11(1): 37–40

[31] Gibo M, Hasuo K, Inoue A, Miura N, Murata S. Hepatic falciform artery: angiographic observations and significance. Abdom Imaging 2001; 26(5): 515–519

[32] Wang DS, Louie JD, Kothary N, Shah RP, Sze DY. Prophylactic topically applied ice to prevent cutaneous complications of nontarget chemoembolization and radioembolization. J Vasc Interv Radiol 2013; 24(4): 596–600

[33] Murthy R, Nunez R, Szklaruk J et al. Yttrium-90 microsphere therapy for hepatic malignancy: devices, indications, technical considerations, and potential complications. Radiographics 2005; 25 Suppl 1: S41–S55

[34] Ahmadzadehfar H, Sabet A, Biermann K et al. The significance of 99mTc-MAA SPECT/CT liver perfusion imaging in treatment planning for 90Y-microsphere selective internal radiation treatment. J Nucl Med 2010; 51(8): 1206–1212

[35] Hamami ME, Poeppel TD, Müller S et al. SPECT/CT with 99mTc-MAA in radioembolization with 90Y microspheres in patients with hepatocellular cancer. J Nucl Med 2009; 50 (5): 688–692

[36] Gulec SA, Sztejnberg ML, Siegel JA, Jevremovic T, Stabin M. Hepatic structural dosimetry in (90)Y microsphere treatment: a Monte Carlo modeling approach based on lobular microanatomy. J Nucl Med 2010; 51(2): 301–310

[37] Urata K, Kawasaki S, Matsunami H et al. Calculation of child and adult standard liver volume for liver transplantation. Hepatology 1995; 21(5): 1317–1321

[38] Ho S, Lau WY, Leung TW et al. Partition model for estimating radiation doses from yttrium-90 microspheres in treating hepatic tumours. Eur J Nucl Med 1996; 23(8): 947–952

[39] Kao YH, Hock Tan AE, Burgmans MC et al. Image-guided personalized predictive dosimetry by artery-specific SPECT/CT partition modeling for safe and effective 90Y radioembolization. J Nucl Med 2012; 53(4): 559–566

[40] Andrews JC, Walker SC, Ackermann RJ, Cotton LA, Ensminger WD, Shapiro B. Hepatic radioembolization with yttrium-90 containing glass microspheres: preliminary results and clinical follow-up. J Nucl Med 1994; 35(10): 1637–1644

[41] Jain RK. Normalizing tumor vasculature with anti-angiogenic therapy: a new paradigm for combination therapy. Nat Med 2001; 7(9): 987–989

[42] Salem R, Lewandowski RJ, Sato KT et al. Technical aspects of radioembolization with 90Y microspheres. Tech Vasc Interv Radiol 2007; 10(1): 12–29

[43] Lewandowski RJ, Minocha J, Memon K et al. Sustained safety and efficacy of extended-shelf-life (90)Y glass microspheres: long-term follow-up in a 134-patient cohort. Eur J Nucl Med Mol Imaging 2014; 41(3): 486–493

[44] Riaz A, Gates VL, Atassi B et al. Radiation segmentectomy: a novel approach to increase safety and efficacy of radioembolization. Int J Radiat Oncol Biol Phys 2011; 79(1): 163–171

[45] van den Hoven AF, Prince JF, Samim M et al. Posttreatment PET-CT-confirmed intrahepatic radioembolization performed without coil embolization, by using the antireflux Surefire Infusion System [published correction appears in Cardiovasc Intervent Radiol 2013;36(6):1721. Zonneberg, Bernard A corrected to Zonnenberg, Bernard A. Cardiovasc Intervent Radiol 2014; 37(2): 523–528

[46] Itagaki MW. Temporary distal balloon occlusion for hepatic embolization: a novel technique to treat what cannot be selected. Cardiovasc Intervent Radiol 2014; 37(4): 1073–1077

[47] Carlier T, Eugène T, Bodet-Milin C et al. Assessment of acquisition protocols for routine imaging of Y-90 using PET/CT. EJNMMI Res 2013; 3(1): 11

[48] Kao YH, Steinberg JD, Tay YS et al. Post-radioembolization yttrium-90 PET/CT - part 1: diagnostic reporting. EJNMMI Res 2013; 3(1): 56

[49] Minarik D, Sjögreen Gleisner K, Ljungberg M. Evaluation of quantitative (90)Y SPECT based on experimental phantom studies. Phys Med Biol 2008; 53(20): 5689–5703

[50] Salem R, Lewandowski RJ, Gates VL et al. Technology Assessment Committee. Interventional Oncology Task Force of the Society of Interventional Radiology. Research reporting standards for radioembolization of hepatic malignancies. J Vasc Interv Radiol 2011; 22(3): 265–278

[51] Fabbri C, Sarti G, Cremonesi M et al. Quantitative analysis of 90Y Bremsstrahlung SPECT-CT images for application to 3D patient-specific dosimetry. Cancer Biother Radiopharm 2009; 24(1): 145–154

[52] Ito S, Kurosawa H, Kasahara H et al. (90)Y bremsstrahlung emission computed tomography using gamma cameras. Ann Nucl Med 2009; 23(3): 257–267

[53] Selwyn RG, Nickles RJ, Thomadsen BR, DeWerd LA, Micka JA. A new internal pair production branching ratio of 90Y: the development of a non-destructive assay for 90Y and 90Sr. Appl Radiat Isot 2007; 65(3): 318–327

[54] Lhommel R, Goffette P, Van den Eynde M et al. Yttrium-90 TOF PET scan demonstrates high-resolution biodistribution after liver SIRT. Eur J Nucl Med Mol Imaging 2009; 36(10): 1696

[55] Kao YH, Tan EH, Ng CE, Goh SW. Yttrium-90 time-of-flight PET/CT is superior to Bremsstrahlung SPECT/CT for postradioembolization imaging of microsphere biodistribution. Clin Nucl Med 2011; 36(12): e186–e187

[56] Wissmeyer M, Heinzer S, Majno P et al. 90Y Time-of-flight PET/MR on a hybrid scanner following liver radioembolisation (SIRT). Eur J Nucl Med Mol Imaging 2011; 38(9): 1744–1745

[57] Willowson K, Forwood N, Jakoby BW, Smith AM, Bailey DL. Quantitative (90)Y image reconstruction in PET. Med Phys 2012; 39(11): 7153–7159

[58] Goedicke A, Berker Y, Verburg FA, Behrendt FF, Winz O, Mottaghy FM. Study-parameter impact in quantitative 90-Yttrium PET imaging for radioembolization treatment monitoring and dosimetry. IEEE Trans Med Imaging 2013; 32(3): 485–492

[59] Elschot M, Vermolen BJ, Lam MG, de Keizer B, van den Bosch MA, de Jong HW. Quantitative comparison of PET and Bremsstrahlung SPECT for imaging the in vivo yttrium-90 microsphere distribution after liver radioembolization. PLoS ONE 2013; 8(2): e55742

[60] D'Arienzo M, Chiaramida P, Chiacchiararelli L et al. 90Y PET-based dosimetry after selective internal radiotherapy treatments. Nucl Med Commun 2012; 33(6): 633–640

[61] Marn CS, Andrews JC, Francis IR, Hollett MD, Walker SC, Ensminger WD. Hepatic parenchymal changes after intraarterial Y-90 therapy: CT findings. Radiology 1993; 187(1): 125–128

[62] Miller AB, Hoogstraten B, Staquet M, Winkler A. Reporting results of cancer treatment. Cancer 1981; 47(1): 207–214

[63] Therasse P, Arbuck SG, Eisenhauer EA et al. New guidelines to evaluate the response to treatment in solid tumors. European organization for research and treatment of cancer, national cancer institute of the united states, national cancer institute of canada. J Natl Cancer Inst 2000; 92(3): 205–216

[64] Keppke AL, Salem R, Reddy D et al. Imaging of hepatocellular carcinoma after treatment with yttrium-90 microspheres. Am J Roentgenol 2007; 188(3): 768–775

[65] Atassi B, Bangash AK, Bahrani A et al. Multimodality imaging following 90Y radioembolization: a comprehensive review and pictorial essay. Radiographics 2008; 28(1): 81–99

[66] Young JY, Rhee TK, Atassi B et al. Radiation dose limits and liver toxicities resulting from multiple yttrium-90 radioembolization treatments for hepatocellular carcinoma. J Vasc Interv Radiol 2007; 18(11): 1375–1382

[67] Gil-Alzugaray B, Chopitea A, Iñarrairaegui M et al. Prognostic factors and prevention of radioembolization-induced liver disease. Hepatology 2013; 57(3): 1078–1087

[68] Liu DM, Cade D, Klass D, Loh C, McWilliams JP, Valenti D. Interventional oncology: avoiding common pitfalls to reduce toxicity in hepatic radioembolization. J Nucl Med Radiat Ther 2011;2

[69] Gramenzi A, Golfieri R, Mosconi C et al. BLOG (Bologna Liver Oncology Group). Yttrium-90 radioembolization vs sorafenib for intermediate-locally advanced hepatocellular carcinoma: a cohort study with propensity score analysis. Liver Int 2014

[70] Moreno-Luna LE, Yang JD, Sanchez W et al. Efficacy and safety of transarterial radioembolization versus chemoembolization in patients with hepatocellular carcinoma. Cardiovasc Intervent Radiol 2013; 36(3): 714–723

[71] Iñarrairaegui M, Pardo F, Bilbao JI et al. Response to radioembolization with yttrium-90 resin microspheres may allow surgical treatment with curative intent and prolonged survival in previously unresectable hepatocellular carcinoma. Eur J Surg Oncol 2012; 38(7): 594–601

[72] Lance C, McLennan G, Obuchowski N et al. Comparative analysis of the safety and efficacy of transcatheter arterial chemoembolization and yttrium-90 radioembolization in patients with unresectable hepatocellular carcinoma. J Vasc Interv Radiol 2011; 22(12): 1697–1705

[73] Kooby DA, Egnatashvili V, Srinivasan S et al. Comparison of yttrium-90 radioembolization and transcatheter arterial chemoembolization for the treatment of unresectable hepatocellular carcinoma. J Vasc Interv Radiol 2010; 21(2): 224–230

[74] Carr BI, Kondragunta V, Buch SC, Branch RA. Therapeutic equivalence in survival for hepatic arterial chemoembolization and yttrium 90 microsphere treatments in unresectable hepatocellular carcinoma: a two-cohort study. Cancer 2010; 116(5): 1305–1314

[75] D'Avola D, Iñarrairaegui M, Bilbao JI et al. A retrospective comparative analysis of the effect of Y90-radioembolization on the survival of patients with unresectable hepatocellular carcinoma. Hepatogastroenterology 2009; 56(96): 1683–1688

[76] Lewandowski RJ, Kulik LM, Riaz A et al. A comparative analysis of transarterial downstaging for hepatocellular carcinoma: chemoembolization versus radioembolization. Am J Transplant 2009; 9(8): 1920–1928

[77] Woodall CE, Scoggins CR, Ellis SF et al. Is selective internal radioembolization safe and effective for patients with inoperable hepatocellular carcinoma and venous thrombosis? J Am Coll Surg 2009; 208(3): 375–382

[78] Chow PK, Poon DY, Khin MW et al. Asia-Pacific Hepatocellular Carcinoma Trials Group. Multicenter phase II study of sequential radioembolization-sorafenib therapy for inoperable hepatocellular carcinoma. PLoS ONE 2014; 9(3): e90909

[79] Khor AY, Toh Y, Allen JC, et al. Survival and pattern of tumor progression with yttrium-90 microsphere radioemboliza-

tion in predominantly hepatitis B Asian patients with hepatocellular carcinoma. Hepatol Int 2014

[80] Mazzaferro V, Sposito C, Bhoori S et al. Yttrium-90 radioembolization for intermediate-advanced hepatocellular carcinoma: a phase 2 study. Hepatology 2013; 57(5): 1826–1837

[81] Salem R, Lewandowski RJ, Mulcahy MF et al. Radioembolization for hepatocellular carcinoma using Yttrium-90 microspheres: a comprehensive report of long-term outcomes. Gastroenterology 2010; 138(1): 52–64

[82] Hilgard P, Hamami M, Fouly AE et al. Radioembolization with yttrium-90 glass microspheres in hepatocellular carcinoma: European experience on safety and long-term survival. Hepatology 2010; 52(5): 1741–1749

[83] Iñarrairaegui M, Thurston KG, Bilbao JI et al. Radioembolization with use of yttrium-90 resin microspheres in patients with hepatocellular carcinoma and portal vein thrombosis. J Vasc Interv Radiol 2010; 21(8): 1205–1212

[84] Iñarrairaegui M, Martinez-Cuesta A, Rodríguez M et al. Analysis of prognostic factors after yttrium-90 radioembolization of advanced hepatocellular carcinoma. Int J Radiat Oncol Biol Phys 2010; 77(5): 1441–1448

[85] Kulik LM, Carr BI, Mulcahy MF et al. Safety and efficacy of 90Y radiotherapy for hepatocellular carcinoma with and without portal vein thrombosis. Hepatology 2008; 47(1): 71–81

[86] Salem R, Lewandowski RJ, Atassi B et al. Treatment of unresectable hepatocellular carcinoma with use of 90Y microspheres (TheraSphere): safety, tumor response, and survival. J Vasc Interv Radiol 2005; 16(12): 1627–1639

Chapter 7

Colorectal Hepatic Metastatic Disease: Ablation

7 Colorectal Hepatic Metastatic Disease: Ablation

Muneeb Ahmed

7.1 Introduction

Percutaneous image-guided tumor ablation can be used to effectively treat hepatic metastases from primary colorectal cancer. Specific advantages of percutaneous tumor ablation include the ability to treat patients with limited disease who are not candidates for surgical resection based on medical comorbidities, generally reduced morbidity and mortality compared to surgical therapies, relative cost-effectiveness, and equivalent or near-equivalent long-term outcomes in well-selected patient populations. This chapter reviews how to perform percutaneous ablation, specifically focusing on case selection, patient evaluation, technical considerations in performing ablation, potential complications, and clinical outcomes.

7.2 Clinical Indications

Percutaneous image-guided thermal ablation is commonly indicated for the treatment of liver-dominant or limited metastatic disease from primary colorectal cancer. Use of thermal ablation for colorectal liver metastases has the best long-term outcomes in patients who have undergone resection of their primary colorectal tumor and have liver-only metastases, and when liver metastases are small and few in number (< 3 cm diameter, and < 3 in number).[1] However, thermal ablation can be offered in greater disease burden (tumors > 3 cm or > 3 in number) in select cases. Patients must be evaluated in the context of their disease burden as a whole, and a comprehensive treatment plan developed that considers timing of resection of the primary cancer, use of adjuvant (and neoadjuvant) chemotherapy, staged hepatic resection combined with ablation, and treatment of other potential sites of metastases (e.g., lung metastases) either with additional ablation or surgery. Thus indications for thermal ablation can be broadly divided into (1) limited liver-only metastases with thermal ablation as the primary and singular treatment (i.e., curative intent) in situations where tumors are unresectable, patients are medically inoperable or lack sufficient hepatic reserve, or patients prefer this option; and (2) more extensive metastatic disease with thermal ablation as one of several treatments to control disease in combination with systemic therapy, additional locoregional treatment (transarterial therapies or stereotactic radiation), or extensive or staged surgical resection. Ultimately, the overall intent of treatment should be curative (i.e., treatment of all visible sites of metastases) because the benefit of palliative treatment of some metastases (either through ablation of some metastases or through partial/incomplete ablation of large metastases) has not been proven.

7.3 Contraindications

Contraindications to ablation are largely relative, according to patient and tumor characteristics. Patient characteristics that might preclude ablation include very poor performance status (e.g., Eastern Cooperative Oncology Group (ECOG) performance status ≥ 2) or unrelated advanced/severe medical comorbidities (such that overall life expectancy is limited and thermal ablation would not confer significant survival benefit), uncorrectable coagulopathy, absolute contraindications to intravenous (IV) contrast (limiting evaluation of treatment margins during or after treatment), or an inability to tolerate moderate sedation or general anesthesia. Technical contraindications include an inability to ablate the entire lesion, either due to location or to the risk of nontarget thermal ablation that cannot be addressed by adjunctive techniques (to be described). For example, proximity to central biliary ducts (within 1 cm) can place patients at higher risk for developing main right or left hepatic duct strictures.[2] Patients with more extensive disease (larger tumors, > 5 tumors in number) should be evaluated for other therapies (e.g., transarterial yttrium-90 radioembolization). Finally, there is currently no evidence that use of ablation for large tumor debulking has any benefit in overall survival.

7.4 Patient Selection and Preprocedure Evaluation

Multiple potential treatment options are available for patients with hepatic colorectal metastases, often necessitating the need for determining optimal order and combination of treatment (e.g., preoperative or preablation chemotherapy, combination ablation and surgical resection). As such, a prospective multidisciplinary review of patients with metastatic colorectal cancer is strongly recommended and should involve medical oncologists, colorectal and hepatobiliary surgeons, and interventional radiologists. This will help in planning the best patient-specific treatment course, and it also allows the interventional radiologist to present ablation as a treatment option early in the disease course (where it is most beneficial).

7.4.1 Initial Clinical Evaluation

All patients should undergo careful evaluation prior to any procedure, including a thorough history and physical examination.[3] This should include a formal initial outpatient clinic visit that allows the physician to carefully evaluate the patient for procedure suitability, plan the procedure itself, discuss ablation in detail with the patient (including a thorough discussion of likelihood of outcome and potential complications), obtain informed consent, and map out the course for postprocedure care and follow-up imaging.

During an initial clinical evaluation, a detailed history and physical examination should be performed.[3] First, a detailed oncological history should be obtained, including initial presentation, symptoms related to the tumor and/or treatment, current staging and extent of the tumor involvement, and treatment to date (e.g., systemic chemotherapy regimens and number of cycles administered, primary tumor resection, or hepatic resection). Next, an assessment of overall performance status should be performed. ECOG and Karnofsky scoring systems are commonly used oncological tools to grade the impact of the patient's disease and overall functional status.[4,5] Overall, a falling performance status score is indicative of a poor prognosis and should be considered when an ablative procedure is planned in the context of the overall goals of care. Third, a clinical review should focus on issues that will affect if and how ablation can be performed. This includes a review of medical comorbidities that will influence the level of procedure complexity (such as prior hepatic or biliary surgery), choice of moderate sedation or general anesthesia use, patient positioning (e.g., prior back or joint surgeries), and use of contrast (medical diseases that predispose to chronic renal insufficiency, such as diabetes and hypertension). Medications and allergies should also be reviewed, specifically screening for use of anticoagulation (e.g., antiplatelet agents, Coumadin [Bristol-Myers Squibb Company], and heparin),

medications that need to be stopped periprocedurally (e.g., metformin), and prior reactions to contrast.

Preprocedure laboratory testing should be obtained in all patients, including a complete blood count (CBC), serum chemistry profile, renal function tests, coagulation tests, and liver function tests. Some degree of hepatic dysfunction can be common in patients treated with systemic chemotherapy. Chemotherapy-associated steatohepatitis (CASH) can occur in up to 20% of patients who undergo treatment with regimens that include oxaliplatin and irinotecan.[6] Aberrant coagulation needs to be identified and corrected appropriately prior to the procedure to minimize bleeding complications. Carcinoembryonic antigen (CEA) levels are elevated in patients with colorectal cancer–related hepatic metastases, and baseline levels should be established prior to ablation because this can identify patients who have responded to initial chemotherapy, stratify those in whom early use of ablation may yield better outcomes,[7] and make it possible to follow trends after treatment and to detect development of new metastases.[8]

Finally, all available imaging should be reviewed to determine the overall number of tumors and exclude evidence of extrahepatic disease. Prior to the procedure, all patients should have undergone recent (within the last 2 weeks) contrast-enhanced cross-sectional computed tomographic (CT) or magnetic resonance imaging (MRI) scans. Knowing the original extent of intrahepatic disease (including tumor size and number), some of which may be smaller or not visible on most recent imaging studies, is important in planning the extent of ablation required. Additionally, imaging should be reviewed to plan probe placement and identify factors (central location, subcapsular tumor, nearby organs such as the gallbladder or colon) that might make tumor targeting more difficult.

7.4.2 Neoadjuvant/Adjuvant Chemotherapy

Neoadjuvant chemotherapy can be given in patients who are not suitable candidates for ablation on initial assessment, with interval follow-up to assess for potential downstaging of their tumor burden for resection/ablation. One study has reported a 5-year survival of 34% with use of neoadjuvant chemotherapy followed by radiofrequency ablation (RFA).[9] However, ablation of residual tumor may be difficult given tumor shrinkage and reduced visibility in the setting of global CASH-related changes, and larger ablative margins are often required to treat nonvisible microscopic residual tumor at the margins. Ablating tumors that have completely disappeared with chemotherapy can be very challenging, and close surveillance may be required with plans to treat tumors that reemerge at those sites.[10] Based on studies suggesting some benefit for adjuvant chemotherapy surrounding hepatic resection, adjuvant chemotherapy postablation has also been reported and likely confers some benefit. Studies have reported median survival times of up to 48 months after RFA followed by adjuvant chemotherapy for unresectable colorectal liver metastases. Others have similarly reported improvement in overall survival with RFA followed by adjuvant chemotherapy of 9 months (28 vs. 19 months after laparoscopic ablation),[11] and 10-year survival of 18% using RFA with adjuvant 5-fluorouracil (5-FU)/ irinotecan.[1] Given low morbidity associated with percutaneous ablation, adjuvant chemotherapy can be started shortly after (within 2 weeks), or if patients are on chemotherapy, it can be continued through the periablation period. In summary, ablation with chemotherapy is generally preferred over either alone (if tolerated).

7.4.3 Choice of Sedation

Hepatic ablation procedures can be performed under conscious sedation or general anesthesia. In general, uncomplicated procedures can be performed under conscious sedation. However, thermal ablation (particularly heat-based modalities using radiofrequency and microwave) within the liver can be quite uncomfortable and may not be adequately managed with moderate sedation in some cases. Use of general anesthesia should be considered in (1) patients with significant medical comorbidities, corresponding to an American Society of Anesthesiologists (ASA) physical status score of IV[3]; (2) patients who have a high tolerance for pain or are routinely taking narcotic pain medications; (3) procedures that are likely to cause procedural pain that will not be well controlled with moderate sedation, as for subcapsular tumors or tumors adjacent to the diaphragm; (4) patients with a difficult airway, placing them at risk for airway compromise with moderate sedation, as denoted by a Mallampati airway classification of IV[12]; (5) patients with specific comorbidities that require careful airway and ventilator management during sedation (e.g., morbid obesity, large pleural effusions, or sleep apnea); and (6) ablations with a predicted long procedure time or complicated technical elements (e.g., requiring multiple electrodes, repositioning, and/or overlapping ablations).[13] The procedure plan should be discussed beforehand with the anesthesiologist so that the choice of anesthesia is matched to the needs of the procedure. This should include discussing the use of monitored anesthesia care (MAC) or general anesthesia with endotracheal intubation, the use of paralytics (necessary for breath holds), patient positioning, and the use of regional paravertebral blocks.[3,14,15]

7.4.4 Preprocedure Antibiotics

Although the benefit of preprocedural antibiotics remains unclear, administering single-dose antibiotics immediately before the procedure is likely indicated.[16] A specific subset of patients are at higher risk, including those who have had prior hepatic abscesses or diabetes mellitus or who have undergone surgical biliary reconstructive or biliary-enteric bypass procedures (e.g., hepaticojejunostomies).[3] Different pre- and postablation antibiotic regimens for preventing hepatic abscess in patients with biliary-enteric anastomoses have been reported with mixed success. At our institution, we use one of two regimens that have had reported success in small series for transarterial chemoembolization (a population with similarly increased risk of posttreatment abscess) either using (1) a combination of bowel preparation and IV antibiotics (IV piperacillin/tazobactam or cefotetan with IV metronidazole)[17] or (2) oral moxifloxacin (an agent with broad-spectrum gram-negative coverage and biliary excretion) given 3 days before to 21 days after treatment.[18]

7.5 Hepatic Ablation Technique

Performing successful hepatic ablations requires being familiar with what the overall goals of ablation therapy are (including definitions of a successful treatment), available ablation modalities and energy sources, common methods of intraprocedural imaging guidance, planning probe placement, and immediate postprocedure imaging evaluation.

7.5.1 Key Objectives of Hepatic Ablation

First, the main goal of hepatic ablation is inducing focal cytotoxic injury (by placing needle-like applicators at the center of the tumor to generate high temperatures [>60°C]) throughout the entire target tumor.[19] An appropriate "ablative" margin is necessary to adequately treat a rim of apparently "normal" tissue around the tumor, which often contains microscopic invasion of malignant cells at the tumor periphery. For hepatic colorectal metastases, this rim should be 10 mm thick extending circumferentially beyond the edge of visible tumor.[20] This means that for 3 to 5 cm tumors, a single ablation treatment may not be sufficient to entirely encompass the target volume.[21] In these cases, multiple overlapping ablations or simultaneous use of multiple applicators may be required to successfully treat the entire tumor and achieve an ablative margin.[22] Additionally, if metastases have decreased in size from chemotherapy before ablation is being performed, the ablation zone should be sufficiently large to include the area originally involved by the tumor. The second objective is to ensure accuracy and minimize damage to nontarget normal tissue, an advantage over surgical resection. This is particularly important in patients who have undergone extensive hepatic resections for liver metastases and then develop new tumors in the remaining liver remnant. Third, tumor ablation should be performed to treat the entire target while simultaneously minimizing the potential for nontarget thermal injury to nearby structures both inside and outside the liver. Careful planning is required to ensure that each of these three objectives is met.

7.5.2 Selection of Ablation Modality

A detailed discussion of different types of ablation modalities is beyond the scope of this chapter. However, it is important to be familiar with two types of ablation platforms that are most commonly used for hepatic ablation of colorectal metastases—radiofrequency (RF) or microwave (MW) energies. Both types of ablation elevate tissue temperatures sufficient to create zones of irreversible cellular damage. RF energy is easy to generate, but it suffers in areas of high blood flow or high tissue impedance and requires use of electrode switching or multiple-applicator use to achieve large ablation zones in a time-efficient manner. MW heating is fast and efficient and thus appears better equipped to overcome heat sinks and treat large tumor volumes. In current clinical practice, RF-based platforms are most commonly used and have the largest set of relevant long-term clinical data (i.e., studies were performed with systems still used in clinical practice). However, there are now a number of commercially available MW-based systems, with data increasingly demonstrating at least equivalency to RFA, and potentially superiority for larger tumors. This is particularly relevant in treating colorectal liver metastases, where the need to achieve a 10 mm ablative margin necessitates larger ablation zones (e.g., 5 cm ablations for 3 cm tumors). Finally, operator technique likely has as much influence on performance as device technology; for example, multiple applicators can be used to increase heating rather than switching to a different energy source.

7.5.3 Intraprocedural Image Guidance and Monitoring

Hepatic ablation procedures are commonly performed under ultrasound (US), CT (with or without fluoroscopy), or combination US and CT guidance (preferred in our practice) (▶ Fig. 7.1). Selection of the appropriate imaging modality depends on optimal tumor visibility. Real-time US guidance is very useful in electrode placement and positioning during the procedure but may provide limited visibility of tumors in certain locations, such as the hepatic dome. Additionally, US provides limited information on monitoring success of the procedure as the area of treatment becomes obscured by echogenic foci of gas generated by the ablation. CT with or without fluoroscopy can be helpful in targeting deep tumors or in cases where a difficult access trajectory is required. However, target tumors are often difficult to visualize on noncontrast CT images. IV contrast can also be administered at the time of the procedure to confirm target location.

7.5.4 Probe Placement

Probe positioning requires careful planning to ensure that the end ablation zone sufficiently encompasses the target tumor. This includes planning initial placement and/or repositioning of the probe or placement of multiple probes simultaneously, with appropriate consideration of the size of ablation zone that will be achieved around each probe. It is important to remember that a number of overlapping ablations will be required to adequately cover the three-dimensional volume of larger tumors.[21] The use of multiple probes requires attention to parallel probe orientation

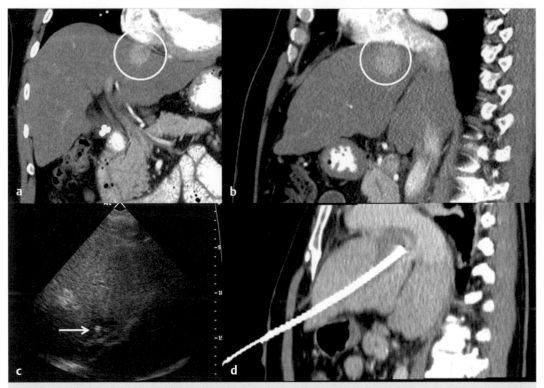

Fig. 7.1 Combined ultrasound/computed tomography (US/CT) targeting a difficult-to-reach liver tumor. Multimodality imaging for guidance and targeting during hepatic ablation can be particularly helpful in treating difficult-to-reach tumors. **(a, b)** A liver tumor is seen with the superiormost aspect of the left hepatic lobe abutting the pericardium *(white circles)*. **(c)** Combined real-time US guidance *(white arrow)* and **(d)** confirmatory needle position with multiplanar CT imaging was critical to successful ablation.

and appropriate spacing, and it is specific to device type. In cases where a biopsy is necessary, a guiding needle can be used through which both biopsy and ablation can be performed, especially beneficial in deep and difficult to access tumors, while minimizing the number of punctures/passes that are needed. For RF devices, care should be taken to ensure that the guiding needle is either electrically insulated or short enough that the active RF electrode tip does not touch the guiding needle (which would result in electrical short-circuiting).

7.5.5 Immediate Postablation Assessment

Once the ablation has been completed, including any overlapping ablations for a single tumor or ablation of multiple tumors, contrast-enhanced imaging is required to determine adequacy of treatment. Either contrast-enhanced CT (using multiphasic arterial and portal venous phase

imaging) or contrast-enhanced US can be used to accurately evaluate for entire coverage of the target tumor.[20] Given the need to achieve a 10 mm ablative margin in all directions surrounding a three-dimensional tumor, careful evaluation of the ablation zone on multiplanar (axial, sagittal, and coronal) imaging is important in determining that ablation has been complete[23] (▶ Fig. 7.2). Postablation imaging should be reviewed for any evidence of residual tumor on contrast enhancement and appropriate coverage in relationship to nearby structures (e.g., key vascular bifurcations). If there is concern for residual tumor, repeat ablation should be performed in the same setting and repeat evaluation with contrast-enhanced imaging performed to document complete ablation. Multiple rounds of contrast-enhanced imaging can be performed easily with redosing of US contrast. With iodinated CT contrast, given concerns for nephrotoxicity with larger (> 200 mL) doses of contrast, lower volumes of contrast (~ 70 mL) can be

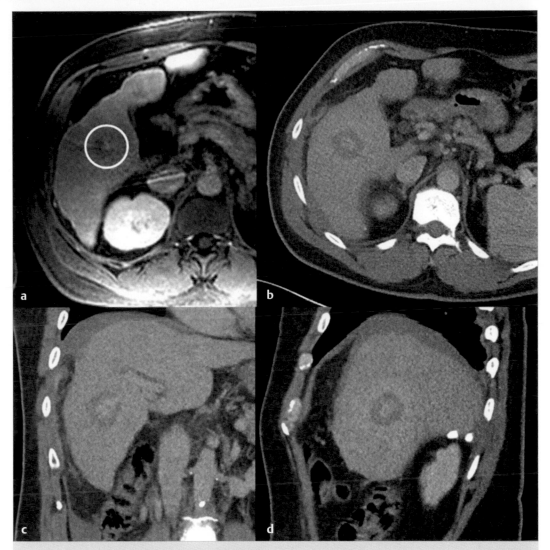

Fig. 7.2 Multiplanar imaging assessment immediately after ablation is required to ensure an appropriate ablative margin is achieved circumferentially around the target tumor. **(a)** A 2 cm primary liver tumor was identified on portal venous phase magnetic resonance imaging *(white circle)*. Percutaneous computed tomography/ultrasound–guided radio-frequency ablation (RFA) was performed. On subsequent immediate post-RFA images, adequate coverage of the tumor (including an ablative margin) was confirmed in **(b)** axial, **(c)** sagittal, and **(d)** coronal planes.

used for each round of imaging. Finally, every imaging series should be closely surveyed for evidence of complications (e.g., hemorrhage or pneumothorax).

7.6 Strategies for Treating Difficult Tumors

Tumors in certain locations present technical challenges by virtue of difficult access to the tumor,

adjacent nontarget structures, higher rates of complications, or difficult underlying anatomy (e.g., near large blood vessels). Several strategies can be used to facilitate completion of percutaneous ablation for these difficult-to-treat tumors.

7.6.1 Adjunctive Techniques

Structures near the ablation zone, such as the colon, stomach, gallbladder, diaphragm, and abdominal wall, can be injured by adjacent heating. Often, creating a sufficient separation between the anticipated edge of the ablation zone and the nearby critical structure is required to complete the ablation safely. Ideally, a 5 to 10 mm distance is required, though this may vary when fat or air insulation is present around the ablation zone (e.g., for exophytic tumors surrounded by mesenteric or retroperitoneal fat). There are several techniques that can be used to successfully create a margin of safety around the ablation zone, referred to as either displacement or dissection. This can be done through placement of a separate 18- to 19-gauge needle into the gap between the two structures followed by injection of air (either room air or CO_2) or fluid until an appropriate distance is achieved. When RFA is being used, only nonionic fluids should be injected (sterile water or 5% dextrose in water) to prevent asymmetric transmission of electrical current. Contrast (usually 2–5%) can be added to improve fluid visibility and demonstrate adequate tissue separation.[24] Artificial ascites can be created using a Yueh needle placed into the perihepatic space under US guidance. Careful monitoring during the procedure is required, with reinjection as necessary to maintain the distance throughout the procedure. Finally, balloon catheters can also be placed over a wire to assist with mechanical displacement when fluid or air dissection is insufficient.[25] Use of 18- to 19-gauge needles for initial air/fluid injection allows placement of 0.035 inch wires and over-the-wire balloon catheter placement if needed.

7.6.2 Difficult-to-Treat Locations

Central hepatic tumors located near the hepatic hilum are often difficult to treat (or untreatable) with thermal ablation. Stricture-inducing thermal injury to central biliary structures can occur more frequently with central tumors, and once strictures occur, are often difficult to treat with percutaneous intervention. Furthermore, blood vessels > 3 mm in diameter adjacent to the tumor act as a heat sink and limit completeness of tumor heating.[26] Strategies to minimize complications include careful selection of patients to avoid hilar tumors. For expandable electrodes, tines can occasionally be positioned within a large blood vessel, preferentially drawing RF current and limiting heating around the remaining electrodes. This can be seen if, at the start of or during the procedure, impedance levels are abnormally low, and it can be addressed by withdrawing the tines, rotating

the needle 45 degrees, and redeploying the expandable electrode. Given the location geometry of these tumors (often positioned between two blood vessels), a needle-type electrode may be easier to both visualize and confirm position.

Subcapsular tumors have been associated with a higher risk of tumor seeding and hemorrhage for some tumor types (e.g., hepatocellular carcinoma). These tumors should be approached through the liver when at all possible. If puncture through an involved capsule is necessary, electrode positioning should be performed with a single puncture, and the capsule should also be ablated. If the tumor is exophytic, the proximal/central portion of the tumor can be targeted first to ablate the tumor blood supply before treating the peripheral exophytic component. Finally, probe choice can be tailored to the tumor. If the tumor is round, an expandable electrode shape may provide a better ablation zone, whereas if the tumor is located close to the hepatic capsule in two locations (e.g., in the inferior tip of the right hepatic lobe), a needle probe may be easier to position.

Organs (e.g., gallbladder and colon) abutting or within 5 mm of the ablation zone are at a higher risk of nontarget thermal injury. Dissection and displacement techniques as already described can be used to create sufficient separation. When the colon abuts the ablation zone, operators should pay particular attention to achieving an appropriate space using multiplanar imaging (noncontrast CT with coronal or sagittal reconstructions) because nontarget colonic thermal injuries leading to perforation are associated with significant morbidity and mortality.[2] For tumors adjacent to the gallbladder, several studies have reported safe and successful RFA of pericholecystic tumors.[27] Technique (parallel insertion of the electrode with respect to the gallbladder), tumor size (< 3 cm in diameter), and location (slightly away from the gallbladder compared to immediately abutting it) are associated with higher complete treatment rates. The risk of nontarget thermal injury of the gallbladder wall can be reduced using pneumo- or hydrodissection alone or with gallbladder aspiration or gallbladder contraction (IV cholecystokinin) to reduce gallbladder distention[28,29] (▶ Fig. 7.3).

Tumors located within the superiormost aspects of the liver, often abutting the diaphragm, can also pose a significant treatment challenge. The adjacent aerated right lung base obscures visualization on US, and respiratory motion can interfere with probe positioning under CT guidance. Introduction

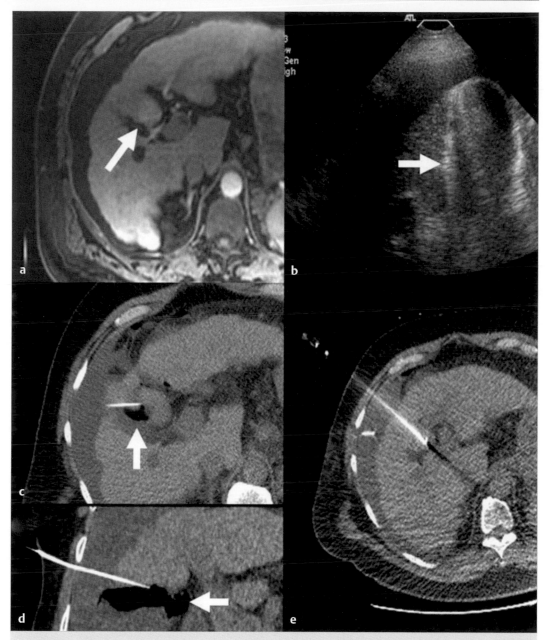

Fig. 7.3 Pneumodissection can be used to create a plane of separation for safe ablation of a pericholecystic tumor. **(a)** A 55-year-old man with a primary liver tumor abutting the gallbladder *(white arrow)*. **(b)** A 21-gauge spinal needle was placed in the plane between the gallbladder and liver using ultrasound guidance *(white arrow points to needle tip)*. **(c, d)** Air was injected under intermittent computed tomographic fluoroscopy to create a plane of separation between the edge of the tumor and the gallbladder *(white arrows)*, followed by **(e)** percutaneous radiofrequency ablation.

of artificial ascites can often separate the liver from the adjacent diaphragm, improve visualization, and reduce the risk of nontarget diaphragmatic thermal injury, though this strategy can be limited by peritoneal adhesions or if tumors are located in the bare area. Use of the epicardial fat pad or a transpulmonary approach without or with creation of an artificial pneumothorax (to shift the right lower lobe up from the diaphragm) can also be performed.

117

7.7 Postprocedure Care and Follow-Up

7.7.1 Immediate Postprocedure Care

Percutaneous hepatic ablation can easily and routinely be performed as an outpatient procedure. After the procedure, patients should be monitored in a dedicated procedural recovery area for several hours (including close observation, dedicated nursing care, and the ability to monitor physiological parameters). Most patients have some postprocedural pain, often manageable with oral pain medication or limited additional doses of IV pain medications. Using adjuvant anti-inflammatory agents (e.g., IV ketorolac) can be particularly effective in managing immediate postprocedure pain. Patients should be monitored for early signs of complications. Set discharge criteria should be used that incorporate standard guidelines for anesthesia recovery along with appropriate transition to oral pain and antiemetic medications, oral intake, and urination. A subset of patients may require hospital admission to an inpatient unit. Common reasons for postprocedure admission (in our practice, this occurs in 15% of cases) include postprocedure pain management, anesthesia-related side effects (e.g., urinary retention), observation for complications (e.g., bleeding or pneumothorax), and nonmedical social indications. Following discharge, early follow-up within the first week should be performed to ensure that patients are recovering well from any procedure-related symptoms. A follow-up outpatient clinic visit should also be scheduled 4 weeks after the procedure to review imaging (or earlier if complications occur).

7.7.2 Definitions of Ablation Success

Familiarity with key standardized definitions of ablation success and failure is essential to prospectively determining treatment plans and follow-up, and adequately interpreting and applying published clinical data.[30] *Technical success* is achieved when a tumor is treated according to the prospective plan/protocol and covered completely (i.e., ablation zone completely overlaps or encompasses target tumor plus an ablative margin) as determined at the time of the procedure. A predefined *course of treatment* may include several ablation

procedures spaced out over time. Primary technical success should be determined on the first follow-up imaging study after completion of the predetermined course of treatment. Distinction between *technical success* and *technique efficacy* must be made for each treated tumor. Efficacy can be demonstrated only with appropriate clinical follow-up. *Technique efficacy* should therefore refer to a prospectively defined time point (i.e., 1 month after treatment) at which point *complete ablation* of macroscopic tumor as evidenced by imaging follow-up (or another specified end point) was achieved. *Primary efficacy* is achieved for those target tumors successfully eradicated following the initial procedure or a defined course of treatment, whereas *secondary* or *assisted efficacy* refers to those tumors that have undergone successful repeat ablation following identification of local tumor progression. The term *retreatment* should be reserved for describing ablation of locally progressive tumor, in cases where complete ablation was initially thought to have been achieved based on imaging demonstrating adequate ablation of the tumor. When initial follow-up imaging demonstrates residual tumor at the ablative margin, this is referred to as *residual unablated tumor. Local tumor progression* describes the appearance of tumor foci at the edge of the ablation zone, after at least one contrast-enhanced follow-up study has documented adequate ablation and an absence of viable tissue in the target tumor and surrounding ablation margin by imaging criteria. This term applies regardless of when tumor foci were discovered, either early or late in the course of imaging follow-up.

7.7.3 Long-Term Clinical Follow-Up

Follow-up imaging is required at regular intervals to determine completeness of ablation and screen for local tumor progression or new intra- or extra-hepatic tumors. A commonly used follow-up regimen includes imaging at 1 month and then every 3 months after the procedure indefinitely, given the potential for local tumor progression or new tumor development. Either a CT or MRI scan with multiphasic contrast enhancement (including noncontrast, hepatic arterial, portal venous, and delayed phases) can be sufficient. Finally, detecting residual tumor with conventional contrast-enhanced imaging can be challenging and dependent on changes that occur over several follow-up imaging studies, which can delay reintervention. Here, fludeoxyglucose positron emission tomography–computed tomography (FDG-PET-CT) can be helpful in early confirmation of suspected recurrence on conventional contrast-enhanced imaging. Posthepatic ablation imaging findings have been described in detail elsewhere and are beyond the scope of this chapter.[31]

7.8 Side Effects and Complications

As with any image-guided procedure, thermal ablation entails a small but significant range of potential procedure-related complications. Livraghi et al, in the largest study to date reporting hepatic RFA-related complications, reported six deaths (0.3%) and 50 (2.2%) additional major complications in 3,554 tumors treated with RFA.[32] The majority of complications, such as pleural effusions, can be managed with medical supportive care and without the need for surgical intervention. Key complications are reviewed here.

RFA-related hemorrhage occurs in < 2% of cases (a 0.5% incidence of intraperitoneal hemorrhage in a large multicenter study). Risk factors include an elevated international normalized ratio (INR) and a superficial or subcapsular location. Finally, larger-caliber electrodes and multiple attempts at electrode insertion also increase the risk of bleeding. Fluid collections within the ablation zone can represent sterile bilomas (5%) or intrahepatic abscess (0.3–1.7%)[33] (▶ Fig. 7.4). A key risk factor for postablation infection is biliary stenting or biliary-enteric anastomoses. Post-RFA hepatic abscesses can be asymptomatic or present with low-grade fever with or without abdominal pain (often 3–6 weeks after RFA). Treatment includes IV antibiotics with or without percutaneous image-guided drainage. In one large series, several patients with hepatic abscesses received subsequent chemotherapy, leading to septicemia and shock, suggesting that careful evaluation is required in patients with suspected hepatic abscesses before administering potentially immunosuppressive therapy.

Complications from nontarget thermal injury to organs adjacent to the liver, such as gallbladder, colon, or diaphragm, can also occur. Thermal injury to adjacent bowel, and particularly the colon, can lead to perforation and is a reported cause of ablation-related deaths. Risk factors for bowel wall injury include < 1 cm interposing distance between the target tumor edge and bowel wall, and in patients with a history of prior abdominal surgery, possibly from the presence of peritoneal adhesions. Additionally, the colon appears more susceptible to injury than either the stomach (protected by its greater wall thickness, fewer peritoneal adhesions, and greater vascularity) or the small bowel (protected by its greater mobility). The gallbladder is also at risk for nontarget thermal injury from RFA of adjacent tumors. Mild, iatrogenic cholecystitis from treating tumors near or abutting the gallbladder is often self-limited and can be managed conservatively (pain control, IV fluids, antibiotics as needed). Regardless, several studies confirm that RFA near or adjacent to the gallbladder is technically feasible and safe, with minimal additional self-limited morbidity. Nontarget heating of the diaphragm can cause significant moderate to severe right shoulder pain lasting 2 to 14 days (in 70%). Artificial ascites can be used to reduce the potential for this injury.

Larger multicenter studies have reported the incidence of tumor seeding along the probe tract at 0.3 to 0.5%.[2,32] Specific factors that increased the risk of seeding included subcapsular location (~ 11-fold higher risk), multiple treatment sessions (~ two fold higher risk), and multiple electrodes (~ 1.4-fold higher risk). Tract seeding is often detected as an enhancing soft tissue nodule 7 to 10 months after the procedure. Strategies to minimize this risk include identification of those patients who are at higher risk prior to the procedure, with careful, optimal electrode positioning at first pass in these patients (preferably through nontumor liver parenchyma rather than the capsular surface). Additionally, maintaining a heated RF electrode during withdrawal (a technique referred to as needle tract ablation) can also be applied to coagulate the tract and may reduce, but not completely eliminate, this risk.[32]

Postablation syndrome is a constellation of flu-like symptoms, including fever (can be up to 103° F), malaise, and chills, similar to that described after intravascular embolization procedures, and can occur in up to 30% of patients.[34] This starts several days postprocedure, resolves in 7 to 10 days, is self-limited, and requires supportive measures only. If a fever persists, other etiologies (e.g., abscess, urinary tract infection, pneumonia, pleural effusion, or atelectasis) should be excluded.

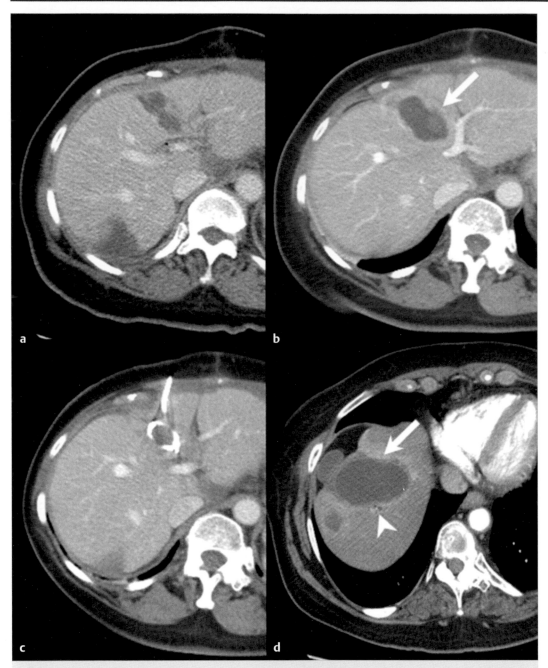

Fig. 7.4 Postablation fluid collections. **(a)** A 64 year-old-woman with a prior hepaticojejunostomy and a liver metastasis underwent hepatic resection (segment VII) and image-guided ablation (segment IV). **(b)** She had persistent fevers and chills 10 days later, and follow-up imaging demonstrated an enlarging fluid collection in the ablation bed *(white arrow)* compared to the initial postablation study, successfully treated with **(c)** percutaneous drainage. **(d)** In contrast, a 73 year-old-woman is asymptomatic 6 months after computed tomographically guided radiofrequency ablation of a colorectal metastasis. Follow-up imaging demonstrates a persistent large biloma adjacent to the ablation site *(white arrow)*, likely from a small ductal injury. Note adjacent dilated segmental duct *(white arrowhead)*.

7.9 Clinical Data and Outcomes

Approximately 30% of patients with colorectal cancer develop synchronous or metachronous hepatic metastases. Although newer chemotherapy regimens (e.g., oxaliplatin, irinotecan, and the anti-vascular endothelial growth factor antibody bevacizumab) have improved traditionally poor survival median times to 20 to 22 months, 5-year survival with chemotherapy alone remains dismally low (< 10%). As such, for patients with "liver-only" disease, "curative" treatment with surgical resection or "surgical-equivalent" thermal ablation remains the standard treatment for colorectal metastases. The optimal 5-year survival after surgical resection in well-selected patients is as high as 40 to 50%, with poor prognosis associated with hepatic metastases numbering more than three, extrahepatic disease, tumor diameter > 5 cm, and a positive resection margin. When tumor is left behind after surgery, overall survival is similar to that for the unresected group. Generally, extrahepatic disease is considered a contraindication to surgical intervention, with the exception being patients with liver and lung-only metastases, in whom some studies have demonstrated 5-year survival rates upward of 30% when treated with localized resection in both organs. A very common approach to patients with initially unresectable disease is to pursue downstaging with chemotherapy followed by aggressive, staged surgical resection (with or without portal vein embolization). However, 5-year survival for such resection combined with adjunctive measures is only 25%.[35] Some of these patients will be eligible for ablation with comparable (or better) 5-year survival, and much more likely to tolerate one or two staged ablation treatments than the long, often complicated and expensive route of surgery with adjunctive measures (where patients drop out at every stage). Finally, 40 to 70% of patients will develop new sites of disease after resection.

The largest experience using thermal ablation therapies for hepatic metastases has been in patients with colorectal "liver-only" disease who do not meet criteria for surgical resection but would still benefit from liver-directed therapy, or who have developed new sites of tumor after having undergone resection, or who underwent RFA as an adjunct to staged hepatectomy. Patients with unresectable but limited disease who undergo RFA have better outcomes compared to those who undergo chemotherapy alone.[36] Initial studies using RFA for hepatic colorectal metastases had relatively poor 5-year survival rates (~ 15%) compared to those achieved with surgical resection. Subsequent studies have reported improved 5-year survival outcomes more closely approximating surgical resection, in part due to improvements in patient selection, more accurate and improved follow-up, advances in chemotherapy regimens, and immediate retreatment of persistent or untreated tumor.[1] A review of the existing literature on RFA for hepatic colorectal metastases remains mixed because many studies comparing percutaneous therapy to surgical resection contain inherent selection biases (RFA is often performed in nonsurgical patients). Nevertheless, Gillams and Lees report their long-term outcomes in a subset of well-selected patients (tumors < 5 cm, tumor number < 5, no extrahepatic disease) where 5-year survival was between 24 and 33%, approaching that of surgical resection.[37] Although higher rates (~ 15–20%) of local tumor progression can occur after RFA compared to surgical resection, this is compensated for with the ability to easily retreat residual tumor, resulting in equivalent 5-year survival rates (48–51%). Finally, Solbiati et al recently reported their 10-year survival data in 99 patients who underwent RFA for small colorectal liver metastases (< 3 cm, < 5 in number), with excellent results (48% at 5 years, 25% at 7 years, and 18% at 10 years) easily comparable to ► Fig. 7.5.[1]

In a classic study in the ablation literature, Livraghi et al applied a "test-of-time" approach using RFA as first-line treatment in patients who were otherwise eligible for surgery.[38] Patients with solitary hepatic metastases < 4 cm in diameter underwent initial RFA, rather than surgical resection. The authors found a significant portion of their patients developed new intra- and extrahepatic disease, and, as such, 50% were spared noncurative surgery, 26% were spared surgery due to curative RFA, and no patients lost eligibility for hepatic resection. More recently, in 309 patients with RFA for hepatic colorectal metastases, patients with < 5 metastases and tumors < 5 cm with no extrahepatic disease had 3- and 5-year survival rates of 63% and 34%, respectively.[37] In a smaller series of 40 patients by the same group, treating smaller tumors (mean 2.3 cm) had even better outcomes (1-, 3-, and 5-year survival rates of 97%, 84%, and 40%, respectively).

Ultimately, in any discussion of comparative efficacy between resection and ablation, it is important to recognize that, in almost all studies, the two techniques are applied selectively, with

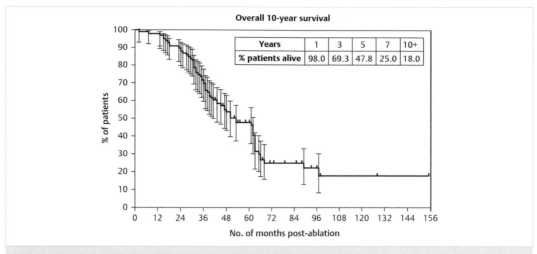

Fig. 7.5 Kaplan–Meier overall survival curve for hepatic radiofrequency ablation for solitary small colorectal metastases. Solbiati et al reported long-term 10-year results in 99 patients with small (<3 cm), limited (<5 tumors) colorectal hepatic metastases. (Reproduced from Solbiati et al with permission from Radiology.[1])

ablation being used in patients who are expected to fare less well. More often than not, ablation arms have more disease (including extrahepatic disease), the patients are older with more comorbidities, or attempts have been made to ablate larger tumors (which were unlikely to succeed). When ablation has been applied as first-line therapy to patients with resectable disease, the 5-year survival results have been very similar to those for surgical series.[1] At least five retrospective studies have demonstrated similar outcomes for ablation in well-selected populations (tumors <3 cm, <3–5 in number). Building a clinical ablation practice mandates regular participation in multidisciplinary oncology conferences ("tumor board") with specialists from multiple disciplines. Successful participation in this setting requires that the interventionalist be familiar with efficacy data and limitations for all other treatments beyond ablation, and understand the reasons why there may be a lack of comparative studies.[39]

7.10 Conclusion

In conclusion, this chapter is a comprehensive and practical guide to performing thermal ablation in colorectal hepatic metastases. This has included a review of the current clinical circumstances in which RFA is performed and information on patient selection. Patient preparation prior to the procedure, the technique of performing thermal ablation, and postprocedure patient management

and complications are also covered, including strategies to successfully treat more difficult cases. Finally, a summary of current clinical literature has been presented.

> **Pearls**
>
> - Tumor ablation for colorectal liver metastases is most efficacious with limited intrahepatic tumor (tumors <3 cm in diameter, <3 in number).
> - Ablation of colorectal liver metastasis requires a 10 mm ablative margin in all dimensions.
> - Patients with biliary-enteric bypass procedures (surgical or stents) are at high risk for intrahepatic abscesses and should get antibiotic prophylaxis before and after treatment.
> - Adjunctive techniques (using air/fluid dissection or mechanical separation) can reduce the risk of nontarget thermal injury.
> - Follow-up imaging should be obtained (contrast-enhanced CT or MRI) 1 month postablation, then every 3 months.
> - RFA should be followed with adjuvant chemotherapy if possible.

References

[1] Solbiati L, Ahmed M, Cova L, Ierace T, Brioschi M, Goldberg SN. Small liver colorectal metastases treated with percuta-

neous radiofrequency ablation: local response rate and long-term survival with up to 10-year follow-up. Radiology 2012; 265(3): 958–968

[2] Rhim H, Yoon KH, Lee JM et al. Major complications after radio-frequency thermal ablation of hepatic tumors: spectrum of imaging findings. Radiographics 2003; 23(1): 123–134, discussion 134–136

[3] Brennan IM, Faintuch S, Ahmed M. Preparation for percutaneous ablation procedures. Tech Vasc Interv Radiol 2013; 16 (4): 209–218

[4] Karnofsky DA, Burchenal H. The clinical Evaluation of chemotherapeutic agents in cancer. In: MacLeod CM, ed. Evaluation of Chemotherapeutic Agents. New York, NY: Columbia University Press; 1949:196

[5] Oken MM, Creech RH, Tormey DC et al. Toxicity and response criteria of the Eastern Cooperative Oncology Group. Am J Clin Oncol 1982; 5(6): 649–655

[6] Pilgrim CH, Thomson BN, Banting S, Phillips WA, Michael M. The developing clinical problem of chemotherapy-induced hepatic injury. ANZ J Surg 2012; 82(1–2): 23–29

[7] Stang A, Oldhafer KJ, Weilert H, Keles H, Donati M. Selection criteria for radiofrequency ablation for colorectal liver metastases in the era of effective systemic therapy: a clinical score based proposal. BMC Cancer 2014; 14: 500

[8] White RR, Avital I, Sofocleous CT et al. Rates and patterns of recurrence for percutaneous radiofrequency ablation and open wedge resection for solitary colorectal liver metastasis. J Gastrointest Surg 2007; 11(3): 256–263

[9] Knudsen AR, Kannerup AS, Mortensen FV, Nielsen DT. Radiofrequency ablation of colorectal liver metastases downstaged by chemotherapy. Acta Radiol 2009; 50(7): 716–721

[10] van Vledder MG, de Jong MC, Pawlik TM, Schulick RD, Diaz LA, Choti MA. Disappearing colorectal liver metastases after chemotherapy: should we be concerned? J Gastrointest Surg 2010; 14(11): 1691–1700

[11] Siperstein AE, Berber E, Ballem N, Parikh RT. Survival after radiofrequency ablation of colorectal liver metastases: 10-year experience. Ann Surg 2007; 246(4): 559–565, discussion 565–567

[12] Mallampati SR, Gatt SP, Gugino LD et al. A clinical sign to predict difficult tracheal intubation: a prospective study. Can Anaesth Soc J 1985; 32(4): 429–434

[13] Mulier S, Ni Y, Jamart J, Ruers T, Marchal G, Michel L. Local recurrence after hepatic radiofrequency coagulation: multivariate meta-analysis and review of contributing factors. Ann Surg 2005; 242(2): 158–171

[14] Gazzera C, Fonio P, Faletti R et al. Role of paravertebral block anaesthesia during percutaneous transhepatic thermoablation. Radiol Med (Torino) 2014; 119(8): 549–557

[15] Sabo B, Dodd GD, III, Halff GA, Naples JJ. Anesthetic considerations in patients undergoing percutaneous radiofrequency interstitial tissue ablation. AANA J 1999; 67(5): 467–468

[16] Venkatesan AM, Kundu S, Sacks D et al. Society of Interventional Radiology Standards of Practice Committee. Practice guidelines for adult antibiotic prophylaxis during vascular and interventional radiology procedures. Written by the Standards of Practice Committee for the Society of Interventional Radiology and Endorsed by the Cardiovascular Interventional Radiological Society of Europe and Canadian Interventional Radiology Association [corrected]. J Vasc Interv Radiol 2010; 21(11): 1611–1630, quiz 1631

[17] Geschwind JF, Kaushik S, Ramsey DE, Choti MA, Fishman EK, Kobeiter H. Influence of a new prophylactic antibiotic therapy on the incidence of liver abscesses after chemoembolization treatment of liver tumors. J Vasc Interv Radiol 2002; 13(11): 1163–1166

[18] Khan W, Sullivan KL, McCann JW et al. Moxifloxacin prophylaxis for chemoembolization or embolization in patients with previous biliary interventions: a pilot study. Am J Roentgenol 2011; 197(2): W343–5

[19] Ahmed M, Brace CL, Lee FT, Jr, Goldberg SN. Principles of and advances in percutaneous ablation. Radiology 2011; 258(2): 351–369

[20] Wang X, Sofocleous CT, Erinjeri JP et al. Margin size is an independent predictor of local tumor progression after ablation of colon cancer liver metastases. Cardiovasc Intervent Radiol 2013; 36(1): 166–175

[21] Chen MH, Yang W, Yan K et al. Large liver tumors: protocol for radiofrequency ablation and its clinical application in 110 patients—mathematic model, overlapping mode, and electrode placement process. Radiology 2004; 232(1): 260–271

[22] Dodd GD, III, Frank MS, Aribandi M, Chopra S, Chintapalli KN. Radiofrequency thermal ablation: computer analysis of the size of the thermal injury created by overlapping ablations. Am J Roentgenol 2001; 177(4): 777–782

[23] Passera K, Selvaggi S, Scaramuzza D, Garbagnati F, Vergnaghi D, Mainardi L. Radiofrequency ablation of liver tumors: quantitative assessment of tumor coverage through CT image processing. BMC Med Imaging 2013; 13: 3

[24] Campbell C, Lubner MG, Hinshaw JL, Muñoz del Rio A, Brace CL. Contrast media-doped hydrodissection during thermal ablation: optimizing contrast media concentration for improved visibility on CT images. Am J Roentgenol 2012; 199 (3): 677–682

[25] Ginat DT, Saad WE. Bowel displacement and protection techniques during percutaneous renal tumor thermal ablation. Tech Vasc Interv Radiol 2010; 13(2): 66–74

[26] Lu DS, Raman SS, Limanond P et al. Influence of large peritumoral vessels on outcome of radiofrequency ablation of liver tumors. J Vasc Interv Radiol 2003; 14(10): 1267–1274

[27] Orlacchio A, Chegai F, Del Giudice C et al. Radiofrequency thermoablation of HCC larger than 3 cm and less than 5 cm proximal to the gallbladder without gallbladder isolation: a single center experience. Biomed Res Int 2014; 2014: 896527

[28] Levit E, Bruners P, Günther RW, Mahnken AH. Bile aspiration and hydrodissection to prevent complications in hepatic RFA close to the gallbladder. Acta Radiol 2012; 53(9): 1045–1048

[29] Tewari SO, Petre EN, Osborne J, Sofocleous CT. Cholecystokinin-assisted hydrodissection of the gallbladder fossa during FDG PET/CT-guided liver ablation. Cardiovasc Intervent Radiol 2013; 36(6): 1704–1706

[30] Ahmed M, Solbiati L, Brace CL et al. International Working Group on Image-guided Tumor Ablation. Interventional Oncology Sans Frontières Expert Panel. Technology Assessment Committee of the Society of Interventional Radiology. Standard of Practice Committee of the Cardiovascular and Interventional Radiological Society of Europe. Image-guided tumor ablation: standardization of terminology and reporting criteria—a 10-year update. Radiology 2014; 273(1): 241–260

[31] Lencioni R, Cioni D, Bartolozzi C. Percutaneous radiofrequency thermal ablation of liver malignancies: techniques, indications, imaging findings, and clinical results. Abdom Imaging 2001; 26(4): 345–360

[32] Livraghi T, Solbiati L, Meloni MF, Gazelle GS, Halpern EF, Goldberg SN. Treatment of focal liver tumors with percutaneous radio-frequency ablation: complications encountered in a multicenter study. Radiology 2003; 226(2): 441–451

[33] Chang IS, Rhim H, Kim SH et al. Biloma formation after radiofrequency ablation of hepatocellular carcinoma: incidence, imaging features, and clinical significance. Am J Roentgenol 2010; 195(5): 1131–1136

[34] Dodd GD, III, Napier D, Schoolfield JD, Hubbard L. Percutaneous radiofrequency ablation of hepatic tumors: postablation syndrome. Am J Roentgenol 2005; 185(1): 51–57

[35] Pamecha V, Glantzounis G, Davies N, Fusai G, Sharma D, Davidson B. Long-term survival and disease recurrence following portal vein embolisation prior to major hepatectomy for colorectal metastases. Ann Surg Oncol 2009; 16(5): 1202–1207

[36] Abdalla EK, Vauthey JN, Ellis LM et al. Recurrence and outcomes following hepatic resection, radiofrequency ablation, and combined resection/ablation for colorectal liver metastases. Ann Surg 2004; 239(6): 818–825, discussion 825–827

[37] Gillams AR, Lees WR. Five-year survival in 309 patients with colorectal liver metastases treated with radiofrequency ablation. Eur Radiol 2009; 19(5): 1206–1213

[38] Livraghi T, Solbiati L, Meloni F, Ierace T, Goldberg SN, Gazelle GS. Percutaneous radiofrequency ablation of liver metastases in potential candidates for resection: the "test-of-time approach". Cancer 2003; 97(12): 3027–3035

[39] Doyle MB, Chapman WC. Radiofrequency ablation for resectable colorectal hepatic metastases: is it time for a randomized controlled trial? Ann Surg 2010; 251(5): 804–806

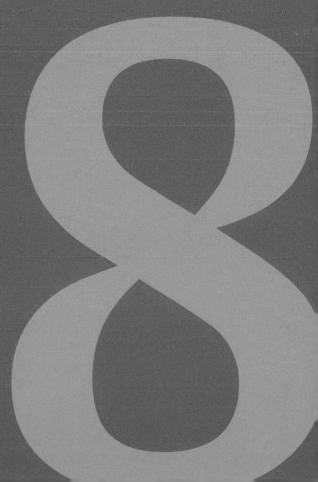

Chapter 8

Colorectal Cancer Hepatic Metastatic Disease: Intra-arterial Therapies

8 Colorectal Cancer Hepatic Metastatic Disease: Intra-arterial Therapies

Govindarajan Narayanan, and Prasoon P. Mohan

8.1 Introduction

Colon cancer is the second leading cause of death from cancer in the United States.[1] The prognosis of colorectal carcinoma primarily depends on the presence of distant metastases.[2,3] There were an estimated 142,820 new cases of colon cancer and 50,830 deaths attributed to the disease in the United States in 2013.[4] Liver-only metastasis affects approximately 50% of patients.[1] Liver is the most common site, and about 40% of patients die with the liver as their only site of metastasis.[5] Hepatic metastases are initially resectable in about 25% of cases, and resection of liver metastases has been shown to improve long-term survival.[1,6]

For patients with nonresectable liver metastasis, systemic chemotherapy remains the standard first-line therapy. However, despite significant improvements in modern systemic regimens containing both conventional and molecular targeted agents, most patients eventually develop progressive disease within months.[7,8] Over the last 2 decades, several intra-arterial locoregional therapies for the treatment of liver-only or liver-dominant hepatic colorectal cancer (hmCRC) have been developed. These therapies take advantage of the fact that the tumor vascularity is derived nearly 100% from the hepatic artery, whereas normal liver parenchyma derives only 30% of its blood supply from the hepatic artery and 70% from the portal vein. This chapter covers the intra-arterial treatment options for hmCRC, including transarterial chemoembolization (TACE) using either emulsions of ethiodized oil and chemotherapy solution (conventional TACE), TACE using drug-eluting beads loaded with irinotecan (DEBIRI-TACE), and radioembolization with microspheres labeled with the β emitter yttrium-90 (^{90}Y).

8.2 Chemoembolization

Chemoembolization combines transarterial local delivery of high-dose chemotherapy and local ischemia by means of embolization. The embolic particles slow the passage of chemotherapy agents through the hepatic circulation, and the drug concentrations in the tumor can reach levels up to 25 times greater than levels reached with standard intravenous (IV) infusion. The drugs also remain within tumor cells for as long as 1 month after infusion, greatly augmenting the therapeutic effect.[9,10,11,12] Embolization also causes ischemia, resulting in tumor hypoxia, which has been shown to augment the effects of cytotoxic drugs by increasing their uptake and retention by tumor cells.[13]

8.2.1 Indications

Patients with unresectable or nonablatable liver-only or liver-dominant metastases, or those who cannot undergo surgery due to comorbidities, are potential candidates for both transarterial embolization techniques. Candidates should have a life expectancy of more than 3 months with an Eastern Cooperative Oncology Group (ECOG) status ≤ 2. Patients should also have sufficient functional liver reserve. Although there is no consensus on the optimal functional reserve of liver, a bilirubin level of > 2 mg/dL, an albumin level of < 3 g/dL, and an international normalized ratio of 1.6 or higher are considered indicators of insufficient liver functional reserve.[14]

8.2.2 Contraindications

Patients with contraindications to angiography, such as anaphylactoid reaction to iodinated contrast or uncorrectable coagulopathy, are excluded from treatment. Patients who cannot receive chemotherapy due to severe thrombocytopenia (< 50,000), leucopenia (absolute neutrophil count < 1,000), severe renal insufficiency (creatinine > 2 mg/dL), or severe cardiac dysfunction (American Heart Association [AHA] class III–IV failure) are also excluded from therapy. Hepatic encephalopathy or other signs of liver failure are also considered contraindications.

Portal vein occlusion is a relative contraindication. However, these patients can be treated safely as long as there are sufficient collaterals with hepatopetal flow.[15] Biliary obstruction is another relative contraindication. Even with a normal bilirubin level, the presence of biliary ductal dilatation puts patients at risk for bile duct necrosis and biloma formation. The presence of a bilioenteric anastomosis, a biliary stent, or prior sphincterotomy causes colonization of the bile ducts with enteric bacteria. These patients are at high risk of developing liver abscess following treatment. Aggressive prophylactic antibiotic regimens can reduce the incidence of this complication.[16]

8.2.3 Preprocedure Workup

Patients for TACE (whether conventional TACE or DEBIRI-TACE) should be evaluated in the interventional oncology clinic. A detailed oncological history should be obtained, including the tissue diagnosis, prognostic markers such as *KRAS* and *BRAF*, presence of synchronous versus metchronous metastasis, time interval from diagnosis of primary cancer to the appearance of metastasis and details of prior treatment (chemotherapy, surgery or radiation therapy). It is important to emphasize the palliative role of intra-arterial therapies during the clinic visit, and both the physician and the patient should agree on clear, realistic goals.

The imaging workup should include triple phase computed tomography (CT) or magnetic resonance imaging (MRI), which needs to be evaluated for tumor burden, distribution, status of the portal vein and biliary tree, and presence and extent of extrahepatic disease. Patients with > 70% liver volume involvement with tumor are unlikely to benefit from TACE and should be discouraged from pursuing chemoembolization.

Laboratory evaluation should include complete blood count (CBC), coagulation studies, renal function tests, liver function tests, and carcinoembryonic antigen (CEA) level.

8.2.4 Conventional Transarterial Chemoembolization

At present, there is no standardized protocol for conventional TACE for the treatment of hmCRC. The chemotherapy agents used vary between centers. Studies comparing different chemotherapy regimens have not revealed a superior combination.[17] Combination therapy with cisplatin, doxorubicin, and mitomycin C is the most commonly used regimen in the United States, whereas monotherapy with doxorubicin is most frequently used worldwide.[18] All of these drugs have shown significantly higher target drug concentration when administered intra-arterially compared to intravenously.[19]

Many agents are used to achieve embolization in conventional TACE. Pharmacokinetic data suggest that the chemotherapeutic drugs in the aqueous phase of the solution will wash out unless efflux is simultaneously blocked by the particles.[18] The materials used include polyvinyl alcohol, gelatin sponge, starch microspheres, and collagen particles. Most protocols include Ethiodol, or ethiodized oil, an iodinated ethyl ester of poppy seed oil (Guerbet). Some regimens involve delivery of the chemotherapeutic agents and oil emulsion followed by particulate embolization.

8.2.5 Technique

Patients are admitted to the interventional radiology service on the morning of the procedure following overnight fasting. Vigorous IV hydration is important. Premedication with prophylactic IV antibiotics and antiemetics is preferred, and both are continued until discharge. However, the use of antibiotic prophylaxis is not strictly evidence based. The procedure is performed under conscious sedation.

The procedure starts with detailed diagnostic visceral arteriography.[20] Power-injected digital subtraction angiograms of the superior mesenteric and celiac angiograms are obtained to identify variant anatomy, such as replaced or accessory hepatic arteries, nontarget branches to the viscera, hepatic branch anatomy, and patency of the portal vein. If nontarget branches are identified, these vessels must be either embolized using coils or avoided by placing the catheter tip well beyond their origin. Cone-beam CT is a valuable adjunct to identify target and nontarget tissue perfusion, and its routine use has been demonstrated to improve clinical outcomes in chemoembolization.[21] Complete mesenteric arteriography needs to be performed prior to only the first session. Subsequent chemoembolizations usually require detailed angiography of only the specific vessel(s) supplying the segments to be treated.

Once the arterial anatomy and tumor supply are clearly identified, a microcatheter is advanced superselectively into the right or left hepatic arterial branches. Whole-liver chemoembolization is not recommended due to unacceptable toxicity.[22] Segmental or subsegmental delivery of the chemoembolic agent is preferred when liver function is marginal. Once the catheter is positioned for treatment, a final arteriogram is performed to delineate the vascular territory prior to the chemotherapy injection.

The chemoembolic mixture or emulsion is injected in 1 to 5 mL increments until near stasis.

Excessive embolization must be avoided, particularly for patients in whom repeated chemoembolizations are anticipated. After satisfactory treatment, the vessels should appear as a "tree in winter," with no tumor blush, but with preservation of flow in the segmental and lobar branches. For bilobar disease, patients will require two to four treatments, depending on the arterial supply.

8.2.6 Side Effects and Complications

Postembolization syndrome occurs in approximately 67% of patients undergoing TACE, with patients complaining of varying degrees and combinations of abdominal pain, nausea, fever, fatigue, and elevated liver enzymes.[14] Because the hepatic arteries are the main supply for the biliary tree, bile duct injury occurs in 5.3 to 11.3% of cases.[23,24] Patients whose right hepatic artery is chemoembolized proximal to the cystic artery may experience a prolonged postembolization syndrome and may develop sterile ischemic chemical cholecystitis that resolves with conservative treatment.[25] The incidence of major complications after chemoembolization is 2 to 7%.[26] Major complications of hepatic embolization include hepatic insufficiency or infarction, abscess, biliary necrosis, and nontarget embolization of the gut. Other complications occur < 1% of the time, including periprocedural cardiac events, renal insufficiency, anemia requiring transfusion, and complications related to angiography. Thirty-day mortality rates have been reported to be 1 to 4%.

8.2.7 Outcomes of Conventional Transarterial Chemoembolization

Studies assessing conventional TACE for the treatment of hmCRC show significant heterogeneity in the patient population. Currently, conventional TACE is used as salvage therapy in patients with tumors refractory to other treatments, and patients selected for TACE often have more complex and extensive disease.

Three of the largest studies on survival data following conventional TACE for hmCRC permit subgroup analyses. Vogl et al[17] reported a 10-year series of 564 patients chemoembolized with either mitomycin alone (43%), mitomycin and gemcitabine (27%), mitomycin and irinotecan (15%), or mitomycin, irinotecan, and cisplatin (15%), depending on their prior systemic therapy, with

Lipiodol and starch microspheres. All patients had progressed or become intolerant of systemic chemotherapy. Patients with liver involvement of > 70%, or ECOG performance status > 1 were excluded. The mean number of embolizations per patient was 6, with a range of 3 to 29. Partial response by Response Evaluation Criteria in Solid Tumors (RECIST) was seen in 17%, with disease control in 65%. Median survival from time of chemoembolization was 14.3 months, with no difference among the drug regimens. Eighty-four patients (15%) were downstaged to potentially curative resection or ablation, which was predictive of better survival. The presence of extrahepatic disease did not affect survival (median 13.8 mo vs. 12 mo, $p = 0.68$).

Vogl reported separately on a subset of 224 patients with up to five metastases with none > 5 cm, who were chemoembolized, followed 1 month later by thermal ablation with magnetic resonance (MR)-guided laser thermometry.[27] Only 2 of 464 ablated metastases developed local recurrence. The median time to progression of disease was 8 months, almost entirely due to the appearance of new metastases. Additional chemoembolizations and ablations were performed as indicated for recurrences. The median survival from initiation of chemoembolization was 23 months, with actuarial survival of 88% at 1 year, 49% at 2 years, and 19% at 5 years.

Albert et al reported a retrospective series of 121 patients chemoembolized with CAM (Cisplatin, Adriamycin and Mitomycin), Lipiodol, and polyvinyl alcohol (PVA).[28] The disease control rate was 43%, with a median survival of 2 months from diagnosis of metastases and 9 months from the time of chemoembolization. ECOG performance status > 0 and prior treatment with more than two lines of systemic therapy were negative prognostic factors, but the presence of extrahepatic disease was not.

8.3 DEBIRI-TACE

Drug–eluting beads allow for controlled release of a fixed dose of chemotherapy agents that are loaded onto microspheres. They achieve simultaneous embolization and delivery of chemotherapeutic agent to the target tumor. Irinotecan is the most common drug that is loaded onto the microspheres. Irinotecan is a camptothecin derivative that inhibits the production of the enzyme topoisomerase I, which is essential to DNA replication in cancer cells. Irinotecan is used as a second-line treatment for advanced colorectal cancer as part of FOLFIRI (5-fluorouracil [5-FU], leucovorin, and irinotecan) (FOLFIRI) or as a single agent in patients who have failed an established 5-FU-containing treatment regimen.

DC Beads (Biocompatibles), known as LC Beads in the United States, is the most extensively studied drug-eluting embolic. It is a soft, deformable material composed of PVA hydrogel with sulfonate groups. Positively charged drugs like irinotecan interact with the anionic charge in the sulfonate group by an ion-exchange mechanism. The elution of the drug from the beads happens in the presence of counterions, such as sodium, potassium, or calcium (Na, K, or Ca) in the plasma. The beads are approved in Europe for embolization and loading with doxorubicin. In the United States, the addition of the chemotherapeutic agent is considered an off-label application. The size varies from 70 to 900 μm, and the spheres are stored in a phosphate packaging solution.

8.3.1 Chemotherapy Loading

Loading is done in the pharmacy under aseptic conditions. Beads come in 10 mL sterile vials containing 2 mL of sedimented beads in phosphate-buffered saline. The saline is removed from the vial and irinotecan is loaded from 5 mL vials of Campto (Pfizer Inc.) containing 100 mg of irinotecan hydrochloride in liquid form. Loading time is variable, depending on the size of the beads. Average loading time is 2 hours. Smaller beads need shorter loading times due to the greater surface area.[29] During the process, the beads must be shaken for effective loading. If the beads have been correctly loaded with irinotecan, the color changes to turquoise. At the end of the loading time, excess solution must be removed from the vial and discarded.

The loaded beads can be stored up to 14 days under refrigerated conditions (2–8°C). The loaded beads are mixed with contrast during the procedure and are used immediately because some drug elution is initiated in the process. Because the drug release is driven by ion exchange, nonionic contrast should be used.[30] Saline is not recommended for preparing suspensions of loaded beads. Prior to usage, any supernatant containing irinotecan should be removed from the vial of before mixing with 5 mL of nonionic contrast medium and 5 mL of sterile water. The syringe is then gently inverted to obtain an even suspension of beads. For a standard procedure, 100 to 300 μm DC beads are recommended. Each vial contains 2 mL of beads and is loaded with 100 mg irinotecan (loading dose, 50 mg irinotecan/mL of beads).

8.4 Peri- and Intraprocedural Management

Compared to conventional TACE, DEBIRI-TACE is associated with a higher incidence of pain and other adverse effects, such as nausea and vomiting. Patients are typically admitted the night before the procedure, and IV hydration is started with normal saline at the rate of 100 mL/h. Esomeprazole 40 mg is administered intravenously on the day of admission, 30 minutes prior to the procedure, and a second dose is given the day after the procedure. Palonosetron 0.25 mg is started intravenously 30 minutes prior to the procedure. IV morphine 10 mg is administered prior to injection of the beads and is followed by a second dose 6 hours after the procedure. Other medications include IV dexamethasone 20 mg 30 minutes prior to chemotherapy, ondansetron 8 mg IV 30 minutes prior to chemotherapy, and 8 mg IV 6 hours postchemoembolization. Antibiotic coverage is with cefazolin 1 gram intravenously IVPB 6 hours prior to chemotherapy, and Flagyl (Pfizer) 500 mg IVPB every 8 hours, continued while the patient is admitted. The medications are listed in ▶ Table 8.1.

8.4.1 Technique

Initial catheterization and angiographic techniques for DEBIRI-TACE are the same as already described for conventional TACE. Embolization is started after the microcatheter is positioned in the target vessel. An injection rate of approximately 1 mL/min of the beads–contrast suspension is recommended. Injection of intra-arterial lidocaine (4–10 mL split before and near the end of DEBIRI administration) has been shown to reduce the postprocedure pain and length of hospital stay.[31] It is important to realize that the goal of transcatheter treatment with DEBIRI is to deliver the planned dose of anticancer agent, not to occlude the vessel. In a multi-institutional registry, achievement of complete stasis was an independent predictor of adverse events and significantly greater hospital length of stay.[31]

It is important to maintain forward flow into the vessel throughout the procedure. If "near stasis" is observed during the injection (i.e., the contrast column does not clear within 2–5 heartbeats) before the full planned dose has been administered, the injection should be stopped at that time,

Table 8.1 Peri- and postprocedural medications: DEBIRI-TACE

Day 0 (day before TACE)	Day 1 (day of TACE)	Day 2 (day after TACE)
Esomeprazole 40 mg, IV	Esomeprazole 40 mg, IV (30 minutes prior to TACE)	Esomeprazole 40 mg, IV
Intravenous hydration with normal saline @100 mL/h	Intravenous hydration with normal saline @100 mL/h	Intravenous hydration with normal saline @100 mL/h (until adequate oral intake)
	Ondansetron 8 mg, IV (30 minutes prior to TACE and 6 hours after the procedure)	Ondansetron 8 mg, IV, every 6 hours, as needed
	Metronidazole 500 mg, IV every 8 hours	Metronidazole 500 mg, IV every 8 hours (until discharge)
	Dilaudid PCA postprocedure	Dilaudid PCA postprocedure (as needed)
	Morphine 10 mg, IV (prior to injection of beads and 6 hours after the procedure)	
	Dexamethasone 20 mg, IV (30 minutes prior to TACE)	
	Palonosetron 0.25 mg, IV (30 minutes prior to TACE)	
	Cefazolin 1 g, IV (preprocedure prophylactic antibiotic)	

Abbreviations: DEBIRI, drug-eluting beads with irinotecan; IV, intravenous; PCA, patient-controlled analgesia; TACE, transarterial chemoembolization.

regardless of the amount of beads that have been actually delivered, to avoid reflux of embolic material. Additional embolic material of any kind should not be injected following the delivery of DEBIRI, even if the full dose has been delivered with maintained forward flow.

Transarterial delivery of the beads is performed in a lobar fashion. In patients with unilobar disease, two lobar treatments are planned, each with 100 mg irinotecan loaded in one vial of 100 to 300 μ (micron) DC Beads. Repeat treatment is separated by 3 to 4 weeks after ensuring that the liver enzymes have returned to baseline. In patients with bilobar disease four lobar treatments should be planned, each with 100 mg irinotecan loaded in one DC Bead vial separated by a minimum interval of 2 weeks.

8.4.2 Outcomes of DEBIRI-TACE

Many prospective trials have shown that DEBIRI-TACE is safe and effective in hmCRC. Fiorentini reported a prospective, multi-institutional, double-arm study of 74 patients randomized to receive DEBIRI ($n = 36$) or systemic chemotherapy (FOLFIRI) ($n = 38$).[32] Overall response rate Complete response [CR] + Partial response [PR] in the liver in the DEBIRI group was 68.6% ($n = 24$) compared with 20% ($n = 7$) in the systemic treatment group. Median survival was 22 months for DEBIRI and 15 months for FOLFIRI. At 50 months, overall survival was significantly longer for patients treated with DEBIRI than for those treated with FOLFIRI. Progression-free survival was 7 months in the DEBIRI group compared to 4 months in the FOLFIRI group.

Martin et al reported a prospective, multi-institutional, single-arm study of 55 patients treated with DEBIRI. Ninety-nine DEBIRI treatments were performed, with a median of 2 (range 1–5) per patient.[33] Response rates were 66% at 6 months and 75% at 12 months. Overall median progression-free survival (PFS) was 11 months with a median hepatic-specific PFS of 15 months and a median overall survival of 19 months.

Richardson et al reported a comprehensive review of five observational studies and one randomized, controlled trial (RCT) describing the use of DEBIRI in the treatment of hmCRC (total of 235 patients).[34] The median survival time in this systemic review was 15 to 25 months. There was an improvement in disease-free survival associated with DEBIRI. The response rate (CR + PR) varied from 36 to 78%. Patients with response at 6 months showed a durable response up to 12 months.

Narayanan et al reported a retrospective study of 28 patients treated with 47 DEBIRI-TACE procedures. Three patients (15%) had a complete response, six (30%) had a partial response, four (20%) had stable disease, and disease progression was recorded in seven (35%); CT scans were unavailable for eight patients.[35] The median time from diagnosis of liver metastases to initial DEBIRI treatment was 19.6 months. The median overall survival from first treatment was 13.3 months.

8.4.3 Postprocedure Management and Follow-up after Transarterial Chemoembolization

Postprocedure management and follow-up are the same for both conventional TACE and DEBIRI-TACE. Patients are admitted overnight following the procedure. IV hydration, IV patient-controlled analgesia, antiemetics, and IV antibiotics are maintained during the stay. The patient may be discharged once oral intake of fluids is adequate and parenteral narcotic analgesia is no longer required. Average hospital length of stay is 1 to 2 days. Patients are discharged with prescriptions for oral antibiotics for 5 days, antiemetics, and oral narcotic analgesics as necessary. The patient returns to the interventional radiology clinic for follow-up with cross-sectional imaging and laboratory evaluation 1 month following the procedure. If multiple sessions are needed, it is not necessary to reimage the liver until all tumor has been treated. Patients who respond to treatment are followed every 3 months, and retreatment is considered for responders who develop intrahepatic recurrence.

8.5 Radioembolization of Hepatic Colorectal Cancer Metastasis

8.5.1 Introduction

Normal liver parenchyma has poor tolerance to radiation, which limits the use of external beam radiation in treating metastasis. It has also been shown that external beam radiation in patients with diffuse liver metastasis does not improve

survival.[36] The aim of radioembolization is to provide high-dose radiation to the target tumor while limiting the dose to the normal liver. This is achieved by intra-arterial delivery of microspheres carrying a high-energy radiation source (yttrium-90 [^{90}Y], 0.97 MeV). These microspheres are trapped in the capillary bed and deliver a high dose of radiation (100–1,000 + Gy) to the immediate surrounding tissues (mean tissue penetration 2.5 mm; maximum 11 mm) for a limited time (half-life of ^{90}Y is 64.2 h). There has been a growing body of evidence in the last decade supporting the use of radioembolization in hmCRC.

There are two types of radioactive microspheres available in the United States. One is made from biocompatible resin (SIR-Spheres, Sirtex Medical Inc.) and the other is made of glass (TheraSphere, Nordion Inc.). The resin microspheres have full premarket approval by the Food and Drug Administration (FDA) for the treatment of unresectable hmCRC.[37] The glass microspheres have a humanitarian device exemption from the FDA for treatment of unresectable hepatocellular carcinoma.[38]

8.5.2 Indications

Prior to being considered for radioembolization, patients should have CT- or MRI-proven liver metastases that are not amenable to curative surgery or ablation.[39] Ideal candidates have liver only or liver dominant metastasis.[40] Patients with ECOG performance status of ≤ 2 with a life expectancy of 12 weeks or more are considered for treatment. Generally, candidates are not excluded on the basis of age alone.[39]

8.5.3 Contraindications

The presence of significant vascular shunting is a contraindication to radioembolization. Patients with arteriovenous communications that allow more than 20% of the microspheres to pass through the liver capillary bed to the lungs, leading to a total lung dose of more than 30 Gy in single administration or 50 Gy in multiple administrations are excluded from treatment. Lung shunting is assessed by technetium-99 m macroaggregated albumin (^{99m}Tc-MAA) study, which is described elsewhere in the chapter. Similarly, the inability to safely isolate the liver arterial tree from gastric and small bowel branches is another contraindication.[39] Adequate liver reserve is an important prerequisite for radioembolization. The presence of ascites, or abnormal synthetic function of the liver suggested by albumin level of ≤ 3 g/dL or total bilirubin of > 2 mg/dL are indicators of inadequate liver reserve. Other relative contraindications are included in the following list.[39]

8.5.4 Relative Contraindications to Radioembolization

- Portal venous compromise
- Prior radiation therapy to the liver
- Excessive tumor burden with limited hepatic reserve
- Abnormal organ or bone marrow function as determined by the following:
  ○ Leukocytes < 2,500/μL
  ○ Absolute neutrophil count < 1,500/μL
  ○ Platelets < 60,000/μL
  ○ Aspartate aminotransferase (AST)/ Alanine aminotransferase (ALT) > 5 times the institutional upper limit of normal
  ○ Elevated total bilirubin level > 2 mg/dL
  ○ Serum albumin < 3 g/dL
  ○ Creatinine > 2.5 mg/dL

8.5.5 Preprocedure Workup

Patients are initially seen in the interventional radiology clinic for a detailed assessment, including history and physical examination, laboratory evaluation, and cross-sectional imaging. Laboratory workup includes liver function tests (LFTs), CBC, coagulation parameters, and metabolic panel. All patients undergo a triple-phase contrast CT or contrast-enhanced MRI. Tumor and nontumor volume, portal vein patency, and the extent of extrahepatic disease are assessed on imaging. The primary aim of the next stage of the workup is the detailed assessment of the hepatic vasculature. The hepatic arterial tree is then skeletonized to prevent nontarget embolization to the gastrointestinal tract. Finally, the amount of shunting to the lungs is quantified using ^{99m}Tc-MAA scintigraphy.

The second stage of the workup starts with meticulous angiography, which maps the hepatic vasculature supplying the tumor, and also any vessels that could potentially carry microspheres away from the liver to the stomach, duodenum, or gallbladder. At first, an aortogram is performed to identify parasitized extrahepatic branches supplying the tumor. Commonly parasitized vessels include the right inferior phrenic and right T8 to T11 intercostal arteries.[41,42] Once identified, these vessels are embolized with coils or large particles. The aim of this embolization is not to induce

tumor ischemia but to restore arterial supply from intrahepatic braches to the tumor so that ^{90}Y particles could be delivered to the tumor during treatment.[42] Angiography is then performed with the catheter positioned in the common hepatic artery to carefully identify branches that may supply extrahepatic parenchyma. Many authors recommend routine embolization of gastroduodenal and right gastric branches unless the planned selective embolization is far distal to the origin of these vessels.[43] Cystic artery embolization has been shown to be safe and effective prior to radioembolization.[44] Other branches that are often embolized to prevent nontarget embolization include supraduodenal, pancreaticoduodenal, and falciform arteries.[43] Contrast-enhanced cone-beam CT, with the catheter tip at the anticipated treatment location, is valuable in confirming the completeness of the hepatic artery skeletonization. The CT also gives a better idea of the distribution of the ^{90}Y microspheres.[43]

Following the completion of prophylactic embolization, 200 to 400 MBq of ^{99m}Tc-MAA is administered intra-arterially through a catheter positioned at the planned microsphere delivery site. Because the size of ^{99m}Tc-MAA particles closely mimics ^{90}Y, it is assumed that the distribution of the two will be identical, and this concept is used to assess the splanchnic and pulmonary shunting. The lung-shunting fraction (LSF) is defined as the percent shunt fraction of microspheres from liver to lung (i.e., lung counts/[lung counts + liver counts]). LSF is calculated from planar scintigraphy. If LSF is deemed to be high, appropriate reduction is made in the overall dose administered. Up to 20% of hepatocellular carcinomas and < 5% of those with liver metastases may have a lung-shunt fraction > 20%.[40] Patients also undergo single-photon emission CT (SPECT) imaging to evaluate for possible extrahepatic deposition and prediction of intrahepatic microsphere distribution. It is important to correlate the findings of angiography to the findings of the ^{99m}Tc-MAA scan because the proximity of the gastrointestinal tract to the liver may complicate the findings of nuclear medicine scans.[45]

8.5.6 Dose Calculation

Dose calculation for SIR-Spheres is based on whole-liver infusion. The calculated activity in GBq of the whole liver is multiplied by the ratio of the target volume to the whole-liver volume. The most widely used method is based on body-surface area (BSA) and is calculated as follows[46]:

Equation 8.1

$$A = (BSA - 0.2) + (\% \text{ tumor})$$

Where A is the activity in GBq, BSA is the body-surface area in meters squared (m²), and % of tumor burden is the percentage of the liver that is involved by tumor.[46] As per manufacturer instructions, to minimize the risk of radiation pneumonitis, dose reduction should be considered when the LSF is between 10 and 20%, and radioembolization should not be performed when the LSF is > 20%.[37]

Dose calculation for TheraSphere is based on the weight of liver to be treated. The volume of the liver to be infused in cubic centimeters is calculated using three-dimensional reconstruction through commercially available software. This value is used to calculate the mass of infused liver tissue in grams by multiplying it by a factor of 1.03 mg/mL. The activity administered to the target volume of the liver (A) in GBq, assuming uniform distribution of microspheres, is calculated using the following formula[46]:

$A = D \times m/50$, where D is the administered dose in Gy and m is the mass in kilograms.

Dose delivered to the treated mass also depends on the percent residual activity (R) in the vial after treatment and the LSF, which is calculated beforehand using the ^{99m}Tc-MAA scan. These factors are accounted for in the following formula[46]:

Equation 8.2

$$D = A \times 50 \times (1 - LSF) \times \frac{(1 - R)}{m}$$

8.5.7 Technique

For further details on dosimetry and technique of ^{90}Y administration, please refer to the radioembolization technique section in Chapter 6.

8.5.8 Postprocedure Management and Follow-up Evaluation

Following treatment, most centers discharge the patients on the same day. Patients are discharged on proton pump inhibitors (for prevention of gastric ulceration), antiemetics, and oral analgesics. Many centers use a short tapering course of corticosteroids to minimize postradioembolization syndrome.[43] Postradioembolization syndrome is usually mild and occurs in about 50% of patients.[47] It consists of fatigue, abdominal discomfort, nausea, and anorexia lasting for up to 2 weeks.

Patients are followed up in clinic 2 to 4 weeks following therapy. Laboratory follow-up includes CBC, LFT, coagulation parameters, and CEA levels. Laboratory tests are repeated at 2, 4, 8, and 12 weeks postprocedure.[43]

Patients are seen in the clinic following treatment, and imaging studies are essential in the assessment of response. Positron emission tomography (PET) scan is recommended 6 to 12 weeks from treatment.[48] A CT scan is obtained at 6 to 12 weeks from treatment, and then every 3 months for the first year. If there is no sign of recurrence at 1 year, scans should be continued at 6-month intervals for 5 years.[48] Modified RECIST criteria are used for assessment of response.

8.5.9 Side Effects and Complications

Postradioembolization syndrome (PRS) is usually mild and consists of the following symptoms: fatigue, nausea, vomiting, anorexia, fever, abdominal discomfort, and cachexia. The incidence ranges from 20 to 55%, and hospitalization is usually not required.[47] Patients are given a short tapering course of steroids along with oral analgesics and antiemetics for treatment.

Radioembolization-induced liver disease (REILD) occurs in up to 4% of patients.[49] This is often manifested as abnormal liver function tests with ascites and/or jaundice typically occurring 1 to 2 months after treatment in the absence of disease progression. REILD results from the exposure of normal liver parenchyma to high doses of radiation and is seen most often in patients with preexisting liver function abnormalities and prior exposure to multiple systemic chemotherapeutic agents.[50]

The incidence of biliary sequelae after radioembolization is < 10%.[51] These complications likely result from the embolic or radiation effect of the therapy on the biliary structures. Most biliary complications do not manifest clinically. Radiation cholecystitis requiring surgery occurs in < 1% of cases.[47] With the use of standard dosimetry models, the incidence of radiation pneumonitis is < 1%. It manifests as a restrictive ventilatory dysfunction. The management is medical, and steroids may have a role in treatment.[52]

The incidence of gastrointestinal ulceration is < 5% if appropriate techniques are used.[47] Gastrointestinal ulceration is secondary to nontarget embolization of the gastrointestinal tract. Careful

Table 8.2 Studies assessing outcomes of ^{90}Y radioembolization in hepatic metastasis from colorectal cancer

Study and year	No. of patients	Study design	Response				Median survival (m)	Progression-free survival (m)
			Complete	Partial	Stable disease	Progressive disease		
Seidensticker et al, 2012[57]	20	Retrospective	1	41	17	38	8.3	5.5
Nace et al, 2011[58]	29	Retrospective	0	13	64	23	10.2	NR
Chua eta al, 2011[59]	140	Retrospective	1	31	31	37	9	NR
Hendlisz et al, 2010[56]	46	RCT	0	10	80	10	10	4.5
Cosimelli et al, 2010[60]	50	Prospective	2	24	26	48	12.6	3.7
Cianni et al, 2009[61]	41	Retrospective	5	41	34	20	12	9.3
Mulcahy et al, 2009[62]	72	Prospective	0	40	45	15	14.5	NR
van Hazel et al, 2009[63]	25	Prospective	0	48	39	13	12.2	6
Jakobs et al, 2008[64]	41	Retrospective	0	19	70	11	10.5	NR
Stubbs et al, 2006[65]	100	Retrospective	1	73	20	6	11	NR
Kennedy et al, 2006[66]	208	Retrospective	0	36	55	10	10.5	NR
Mancini et al, 2006[67]	35	Retrospective	0	36	55	13	NR	NR
Lim et al, 2005[68]	32	Retrospective	0	31	28	41	NR	NR
Lewandowski et al, 2005[69]	27	Prospective	0	35	52	13	9.3	NR
van Hazel et al, 2004[55]	21	RCT	0	91	9	0	29.4	18.6
Gray et al, 2001[54]	35	RCT	6	40	37	9	15.9	NR

Abbreviations: NR, not reported; RCT, randomized, controlled trial.

pretreatment evaluation of the vascular anatomy and skeletonization of hepatic vessels is of paramount importance in preventing this complication. Unlike a normal ulcer that develops at the mucosal surface, ^{90}Y-induced ulcers originate from the serosal surface, which makes them difficult to treat. Surgery may be required for nonhealing ulcers. Lymphopenia is another possible complication of ^{90}Y treatment. Lymphocytes are extremely radiosensitive, and > 25% reduction in lymphocytes is seen in the majority of the patients. However, there are no reports of opportunistic infections in the literature.[53]

8.5.10 Outcome Data

There have been three randomized, controlled trials on the use of radioembolization in mCRC.[54,55,56] The current available literature on radioembolization for mCRC is quite heterogeneous and consists mostly of observational cohort studies obtained from salvage situations with or without the use of systemic chemotherapy. Gray et al conducted a randomized, controlled trial comparing the use of a surgically implanted arterial infusion pump of floxuridine with or without radioembolization with ^{90}Y. The median time to disease progression was significantly longer in the radioembolization group (9.7 vs. 15.9 mo). Overall survival was also better for the combined treatment group with 1-, 2-, and 3-year survival rates of 72%, 39%, and 17%, respectively, in the radioembolization group, as compared with 68%, 29%, and 6.5%, respectively, for the hepatic artery infusion chemotherapy alone group.[54] The same group of authors conducted another smaller randomized, controlled trial comparing the use of systemic 5-FU chemotherapy with or without additional radioembolization in patients with advanced colorectal liver metastases. In that study with 21 patients, both time to progression (18.6 vs. 3.6 mo) and median survival (29.4 vs. 12.8 mo) were significantly longer for patients receiving the combined treatment.[55]

The latest randomized, controlled trial was conducted by Hendlisz et al, which compared the combination of radioembolization with 5-FU versus protracted IV infusion of 5-FU alone in 46 patients with unresectable, chemotherapy-refractory, liver-limited metastatic colorectal cancer. The primary end point was time to liver progression, which was better for the combination therapy (2.1 vs. 4.5 mo). Median overall survival was also better for the combination treatment, but the difference did not reach statistical significance (10 vs. 7.3 mo; $p = 0.80$).[56] Most other studies on the subjects are prospective or retrospective cohort studies, and these are summarized in ▶ Table 8.2.

Pearls ■

- A multidisciplinary approach ensures the best results in hmCRC. Cases should be discussed in a multidisciplinary tumor board consisting of an interventional radiologist, an oncologist, a diagnostic radiologist, a hepatologist, and colorectal/liver surgeons.
- Patients should be seen in the interventional radiology clinic prior to treatment where a detailed history and physical examination along with a review of laboratory and imaging data are performed.
- Imaging data reviewed should include recent triple-phase CT or MRI and PET scan.
- Ideal patients should have liver-only or liver-dominant metastasis with adequate liver reserve and performance status.
- It is extremely important to stress the palliative nature of arterial liver-directed therapies. Patients and physicians should agree on realistic treatment goals.
- For DEBIRI-TACE, in unilobar disease, two lobar treatments with 100 mg of irinotecan each and in bilobar disease four lobar treatments with two doses of 100 mg of irinotecan for each lobe should be performed. Each treatment should be separated by an interval of 3 to 4 weeks.
- Patients should be followed up in the interventional radiology clinic with appropriate imaging.
- Repeat treatments are planned based on the response and patient tolerance.

References

[1] Engstrom PF, Arnoletti JP, Benson AB, III et al. National Comprehensive Cancer Network. NCCN Clinical Practice Guidelines in Oncology: colon cancer. J Natl Compr Canc Netw 2009; 7(8): 778–831

[2] Steinberg SM, Barkin JS, Kaplan RS, Stablein DM. Prognostic indicators of colon tumors. The Gastrointestinal Tumor Study Group experience. Cancer 1986; 57(9): 1866–1870

[3] Chafai N, Chan CL, Bokey EL, Dent OF, Sinclair G, Chapuis PH. What factors influence survival in patients with unresected synchronous liver metastases after resection of colorectal cancer? Colorectal Dis 2005; 7(2): 176–181

[4] Stat Fact Sheets SEER. Colon and Rectum Cancer. seer.cancer.gov/statfacts/html/colorect/html. Accessed August 3, 2014

[5] Frankel TL, D'Angelica MI. Hepatic resection for colorectal metastases. J Surg Oncol 2014; 109(1): 2–7

[6] Tan MC, Butte JM, Gonen M et al. Prognostic significance of early recurrence: a conditional survival analysis in patients with resected colorectal liver metastasis. HPB (Oxford) 2013; 15(10): 803–813

[7] Macedo LT, da Costa Lima AB, Sasse AD. Addition of bevacizumab to first-line chemotherapy in advanced colorectal cancer: a systematic review and meta-analysis, with emphasis on chemotherapy subgroups. BMC Cancer 2012; 12: 89

[8] Köhne CH, Lenz HJ. Chemotherapy with targeted agents for the treatment of metastatic colorectal cancer. Oncologist 2009; 14(5): 478–488

[9] Nakamura H, Hashimoto T, Oi H, Sawada S. Transcatheter oily chemoembolization of hepatocellular carcinoma. Radiology 1989; 170(3 Pt 1): 783–786

[10] Sasaki Y, Imaoka S, Kasugai H et al. A new approach to chemoembolization therapy for hepatoma using ethiodized oil, cisplatin, and gelatin sponge. Cancer 1987; 60(6): 1194–1203

[11] Konno T. Targeting cancer chemotherapeutic agents by use of lipiodol contrast medium. Cancer 1990; 66(9): 1897–1903

[12] Egawa H, Maki A, Mori K et al. Effects of intra-arterial chemotherapy with a new lipophilic anticancer agent, estradiol-chlorambucil (KM2210), dissolved in lipiodol on experimental liver tumor in rats. J Surg Oncol 1990; 44(2): 109–114

[13] Kruskal JB, Hlatky L, Hahnfeldt P, Teramoto K, Stokes KR, Clouse ME. In vivo and in vitro analysis of the effectiveness of doxorubicin combined with temporary arterial occlusion in liver tumors. J Vasc Interv Radiol 1993; 4(6): 741–747

[14] Mahnken AH, Pereira PL, de Baère T. Interventional oncologic approaches to liver metastases. Radiology 2013; 266 (2): 407–430

[15] Pentecost MJ, Daniels JR, Teitelbaum GP, Stanley P. Hepatic chemoembolization: safety with portal vein thrombosis. J Vasc Interv Radiol 1993; 4(3): 347–351

[16] Kim W, Clark TW, Baum RA, Soulen MC. Risk factors for liver abscess formation after hepatic chemoembolization. J Vasc Interv Radiol 2001; 12(8): 965–968

[17] Vogl TJ, Gruber T, Balzer JO, Eichler K, Hammerstingl R, Zangos S. Repeated transarterial chemoembolization in the treatment of liver metastases of colorectal cancer: prospective study. Radiology 2009; 250(1): 281–289

[18] Solomon B, Soulen MC, Baum RA, Haskal ZJ, Shlansky-Goldberg RD, Cope C. Chemoembolization of hepatocellular carcinoma with cisplatin, doxorubicin, mitomycin-C, ethiodol, and polyvinyl alcohol: prospective evaluation of response and survival in a U.S. population. J Vasc Interv Radiol 1999; 10(6): 793–798

[19] Gaba RC. Chemoembolization practice patterns and technical methods among interventional radiologists: results of an online survey. Am J Roentgenol 2012; 198(3): 692–699

[20] Liu DM, Salem R, Bui JT et al. Angiographic considerations in patients undergoing liver-directed therapy. J Vasc Interv Radiol 2005; 16(7): 911–935

[21] Iwazawa J, Ohue S, Hashimoto N, Muramoto O, Mitani T. Survival after C-arm CT-assisted chemoembolization of unresectable hepatocellular carcinoma. Eur J Radiol 2012; 81 (12): 3985–3992

[22] Borner M, Castiglione M, Triller J et al. Considerable side effects of chemoembolization for colorectal carcinoma metastatic to the liver. Ann Oncol 1992; 3(2): 113–115

[23] Yu JS, Kim KW, Jeong MG, Lee DH, Park MS, Yoon SW. Predisposing factors of bile duct injury after transcatheter arterial chemoembolization (TACE) for hepatic malignancy. Cardiovasc Intervent Radiol 2002; 25(4): 270–274

[24] Kim HK, Chung YH, Song BC et al. Ischemic bile duct injury as a serious complication after transarterial chemoembolization in patients with hepatocellular carcinoma. J Clin Gastroenterol 2001; 32(5): 423–427

[25] Leung DA, Goin JE, Sickles C, Raskay BJ, Soulen MC. Determinants of postembolization syndrome after hepatic chemoembolization. J Vasc Interv Radiol 2001; 12(3): 321–326

[26] Brown DB, Cardella JF, Sacks D et al. SIR Standards of Practice Committee. Quality improvement guidelines for transhepatic arterial chemoembolization, embolization, and chemotherapeutic infusion for hepatic malignancy. J Vasc Interv Radiol 2009; 20(7) Suppl: S219–S226, 226.e1–226.e10

[27] Vogl TJ, Jost A, Nour-Eldin NA, Mack MG, Zangos S, Naguib NN. Repeated transarterial chemoembolisation using different chemotherapeutic drug combinations followed by MR-guided laser-induced thermotherapy in patients with liver metastases of colorectal carcinoma. Br J Cancer 2012; 106 (7): 1274–1279

[28] Albert M, Kiefer MV, Sun W et al. Chemoembolization of colorectal liver metastases with cisplatin, doxorubicin, mitomycin C, ethiodol, and polyvinyl alcohol. Cancer 2011; 117 (2): 343–352

[29] Lewis AL, Gonzalez MV, Leppard SW et al. Doxorubicin eluting beads - 1: effects of drug loading on bead characteristics and drug distribution. J Mater Sci Mater Med 2007; 18(9): 1691–1699

[30] Jones RP, Dunne D, Sutton P et al. Segmental and lobar administration of drug-eluting beads delivering irinotecan leads to tumour destruction: a case-control series. HPB (Oxford) 2013; 15(1): 71–77

[31] Martin RC, Howard J, Tomalty D et al. Toxicity of irinotecan-eluting beads in the treatment of hepatic malignancies: results of a multi-institutional registry. Cardiovasc Intervent Radiol 2010; 33(5): 960–966

[32] Fiorentini G, Aliberti C, Tilli M et al. Intra-arterial infusion of irinotecan-loaded drug-eluting beads (DEBIRI) versus intravenous therapy (FOLFIRI) for hepatic metastases from colorectal cancer: final results of a phase III study. Anticancer Res 2012; 32(4): 1387–1395

[33] Martin RC, Joshi J, Robbins K et al. Hepatic intra-arterial injection of drug-eluting bead, irinotecan (DEBIRI) in unresectable colorectal liver metastases refractory to systemic chemotherapy: results of multi-institutional study. Ann Surg Oncol 2011; 18(1): 192–198

[34] Richardson AJ, Laurence JM, Lam VW. Transarterial chemoembolization with irinotecan beads in the treatment of colorectal liver metastases: systematic review. J Vasc Interv Radiol 2013; 24(8): 1209–1217

[35] Narayanan G, Barbery K, Suthar R, Guerrero G, Arora G. Transarterial chemoembolization using DEBIRI for treatment of hepatic metastases from colorectal cancer. Anticancer Res 2013; 33(5): 2077–2083

[36] Russell AH, Clyde C, Wasserman TH, Turner SS, Rotman M. Accelerated hyperfractionated hepatic irradiation in the management of patients with liver metastases: results of the RTOG dose escalating protocol. Int J Radiat Oncol Biol Phys 1993; 27(1): 117–123

[37] SIRTeX Medical. SIR-Spheres Yttrium-90 microspheres package insert O. http://www.sirtex.com/files/SSL-US-09. pdf. Accessed August 2, 2014

[38] BTG. TheraSphere Yttrium-90 microspheres package insert, US ed. http://www.therasphere.com/physicians-package-insert/package-insert-us.pdf. Accessed August 2, 2014

[39] Coldwell D, Sangro B, Wasan H, Salem R, Kennedy A. General selection criteria of patients for radioembolization of liver

tumors: an international working group report. Am J Clin Oncol 2011; 34(3): 337–341

[40] Kennedy A, Nag S, Salem R et al. Recommendations for radioembolization of hepatic malignancies using yttrium-90 microsphere brachytherapy: a consensus panel report from the radioembolization brachytherapy oncology consortium. Int J Radiat Oncol Biol Phys 2007; 68(1): 13–23

[41] Abdelmaksoud MH, Louie JD, Kothary N et al. Consolidation of hepatic arterial inflow by embolization of variant hepatic arteries in preparation for yttrium-90 radioembolization. J Vasc Interv Radiol 2011; 22(10): 1364–1371.e1

[42] Abdelmaksoud MH, Louie JD, Kothary N et al. Embolization of parasitized extrahepatic arteries to reestablish intrahepatic arterial supply to tumors before yttrium-90 radioembolization. J Vasc Interv Radiol 2011; 22(10): 1355–1362

[43] Wang DS, Louie JD, Sze DY. Intra-arterial therapies for metastatic colorectal cancer. Semin Intervent Radiol 2013; 30(1): 12–20

[44] McWilliams JP, Kee ST, Loh CT, Lee EW, Liu DM. Prophylactic embolization of the cystic artery before radioembolization: feasibility, safety, and outcomes. Cardiovasc Intervent Radiol 2011; 34(4): 786–792

[45] Ahmadzadehfar H, Sabet A, Biermann K et al. The significance of 99mTc-MAA SPECT/CT liver perfusion imaging in treatment planning for 90Y-microsphere selective internal radiation treatment. J Nucl Med 2010; 51(8): 1206–1212

[46] Memon K, Lewandowski RJ, Kulik L, Riaz A, Mulcahy MF, Salem R. Radioembolization for primary and metastatic liver cancer. Semin Radiat Oncol 2011; 21(4): 294–302

[47] Riaz A, Lewandowski RJ, Kulik LM et al. Complications following radioembolization with yttrium-90 microspheres: a comprehensive literature review. J Vasc Interv Radiol 2009; 20(9): 1121–1130, quiz 1131

[48] Kennedy A, Coldwell D, Sangro B, Wasan H, Salem R. Radioembolization for the treatment of liver tumors general principles. Am J Clin Oncol 2012; 35(1): 91–99

[49] Kennedy AS, McNeillie P, Dezarn WA et al. Treatment parameters and outcome in 680 treatments of internal radiation with resin 90Y-microspheres for unresectable hepatic tumors. Int J Radiat Oncol Biol Phys 2009; 74(5): 1494–1500

[50] Sangro B, Gil-Alzugaray B, Rodriguez J et al. Liver disease induced by radioembolization of liver tumors: description and possible risk factors. Cancer 2008; 112(7): 1538–1546

[51] Ng SS, Yu SC, Lai PB, Lau WY. Biliary complications associated with selective internal radiation (SIR) therapy for unresectable liver malignancies. Dig Dis Sci 2008; 53(10): 2813–2817

[52] Salem R, Parikh P, Atassi B et al. Incidence of radiation pneumonitis after hepatic intra-arterial radiotherapy with yttrium-90 microspheres assuming uniform lung distribution. Am J Clin Oncol 2008; 31(5): 431–438

[53] Salem R, Lewandowski RJ, Atassi B et al. Treatment of unresectable hepatocellular carcinoma with use of 90Y microspheres (TheraSphere): safety, tumor response, and survival. J Vasc Interv Radiol 2005; 16(12): 1627–1639

[54] Gray B, Van Hazel G, Hope M et al. Randomised trial of SIR-Spheres plus chemotherapy vs. chemotherapy alone for treating patients with liver metastases from primary large bowel cancer. Ann Oncol 2001; 12(12): 1711–1720

[55] Van Hazel G, Blackwell A, Anderson J et al. Randomised phase 2 trial of SIR-Spheres plus fluorouracil/leucovorin chemotherapy versus fluorouracil/leucovorin chemotherapy alone in advanced colorectal cancer. J Surg Oncol 2004; 88(2): 78–85

[56] Hendlisz A, Van den Eynde M, Peeters M et al. Phase III trial comparing protracted intravenous fluorouracil infusion alone or with yttrium-90 resin microspheres radioembolization for liver-limited metastatic colorectal cancer refractory to standard chemotherapy. J Clin Oncol 2010; 28(23): 3687–3694

[57] Seidensticker R, Denecke T, Kraus P et al. Matched-pair comparison of radioembolization plus best supportive care versus best supportive care alone for chemotherapy refractory liver-dominant colorectal metastases. Cardiovasc Intervent Radiol 2012; 35(5): 1066–1073

[58] Nace GW, Steel JL, Amesur N et al. Yttrium-90 radioembolization for colorectal cancer liver metastases: a single institution experience. Int J Surg Oncol 2011; 2011: 571261

[59] Chua TC, Bester L, Saxena A, Morris DL. Radioembolization and systemic chemotherapy improves response and survival for unresectable colorectal liver metastases. J Cancer Res Clin Oncol 2011; 137(5): 865–873

[60] Cosimelli M, Golfieri R, Cagol PP et al. Italian Society of Locoregional Therapies in Oncology (SITILO). Multi-centre phase II clinical trial of yttrium-90 resin microspheres alone in unresectable, chemotherapy refractory colorectal liver metastases. Br J Cancer 2010; 103(3): 324–331

[61] Cianni R, Urigo C, Notarianni E et al. Selective internal radiation therapy with SIR-spheres for the treatment of unresectable colorectal hepatic metastases. Cardiovasc Intervent Radiol 2009; 32(6): 1179–1186

[62] Mulcahy MF, Lewandowski RJ, Ibrahim SM et al. Radioembolization of colorectal hepatic metastases using yttrium-90 microspheres. Cancer 2009; 115(9): 1849–1858

[63] van Hazel GA, Pavlakis N, Goldstein D et al. Treatment of fluorouracil-refractory patients with liver metastases from colorectal cancer by using yttrium-90 resin microspheres plus concomitant systemic irinotecan chemotherapy. J Clin Oncol 2009; 27(25): 4089–4095

[64] Jakobs TF, Hoffmann RT, Dehm K et al. Hepatic yttrium-90 radioembolization of chemotherapy-refractory colorectal cancer liver metastases. J Vasc Interv Radiol 2008; 19(8): 1187–1195

[65] Stubbs RS, O'Brien I, Correia MM. Selective internal radiation therapy with 90Y microspheres for colorectal liver metastases: single-centre experience with 100 patients. ANZ J Surg 2006; 76(8): 696–703

[66] Kennedy AS, Coldwell D, Nutting C et al. Resin 90Y-microsphere brachytherapy for unresectable colorectal liver metastases: modern USA experience. Int J Radiat Oncol Biol Phys 2006; 65(2): 412–425

[67] Mancini R, Carpanese L, Sciuto R et al. Italian Society of Locoregional Therapies in Oncology. A multicentric phase II clinical trial on intra-arterial hepatic radiotherapy with 90yttrium SIR-spheres in unresectable, colorectal liver metastases refractory to i.v. chemotherapy: preliminary results on toxicity and response rates. In Vivo 2006; 20(6A) 6a: 711–714

[68] Lim L, Gibbs P, Yip D et al. A prospective evaluation of treatment with Selective Internal Radiation Therapy (SIR-spheres) in patients with unresectable liver metastases from colorectal cancer previously treated with 5-FU based chemotherapy. BMC Cancer 2005; 5: 132

[69] Lewandowski RJ, Thurston KG, Goin JE et al. 90Y microsphere (TheraSphere) treatment for unresectable colorectal cancer metastases of the liver: response to treatment at targeted doses of 135–150 Gy as measured by [18F]fluorodeoxyglucose positron emission tomography and computed tomographic imaging. J Vasc Interv Radiol 2005; 16(12): 1641–1651

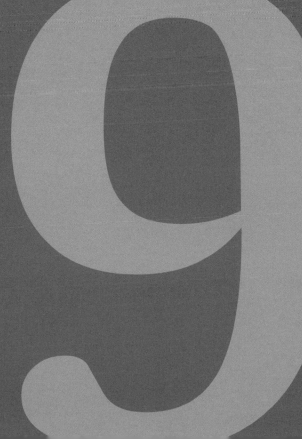

Chapter 9

**Carcinoid and Neuroendocrine
Tumors: Intra-arterial Therapies**

9 Carcinoid and Neuroendocrine Tumors: Intra-arterial Therapies

Elena N. Petre, Karen Brown, and Constantinos Sofocleous

9.1 Introduction

Neuroendocrine tumors (NETs) are rare, typically slow-growing tumors that are frequently found only when the disease becomes metastatic, with the liver being the most common site of involvement.[1,2,3] The incidence in the United States in 2004 was 1.25% of all malignancies and has been rising 3 to 10% per year since then. These tumors may be functional or nonfunctional, and disease-specific survival ranges from 70 to 95% at 5 years.[4] If functional, these tumors may secrete a variety of vasoactive or hormonal substances, such as serotonin, glucagon, gastrin, or insulin. The development of hepatic metastases from functional NETs is accompanied by release of these hormonal substances into the systemic circulation that lead to a constellation of symptoms, such as flushing, hypertension, diarrhea, and electrolyte disorders, known as the carcinoid syndrome. The development of these symptoms often brings the patient to medical attention. Symptoms can result in significant morbidity and can negatively impact the patient's quality of life. Nonfunctional NETs metastatic to the liver may first be diagnosed incidentally on an imaging study obtained for something unrelated or when the metastases cause "bulk-related" symptomatology, such as pain, discomfort, and dyspnea, usually in the latest stages of the disease, due to significant hepatomegaly.

Similar to other liver metastases, such as colorectal adenocarcinoma, surgical resection of NET liver metastases has been associated with improved survival in carefully selected patients. Five-year survival rates of 60 to 80% have been reported.[5,6,7,8,9] Unfortunately, < 10% of patients are initially seen with resectable tumors.[10,11,12,13] For untreated patients, 5-year survival ranges from 17 to 54%.[14] Inoperable tumors can be managed by the administration of pharmacological antagonists of tumor metabolites, nonsurgical liver-directed therapies, or a combination of these treatments.[1,2,3,10,11,12,13,15,16] More than 80% of patients express somatostatin receptors and increased availability of long-acting somatostatin analogue (SSA) has allowed relatively good medical management of NETs, with SSA being a cytostatic agent as well as controlling hormonal symptoms.[17] A 5-year overall survival rate of 75% has been reported in a recent retrospective study that comprised 146 patients with midgut NETs who had received SSA treatment.[18] Unfortunately, over time patients frequently become refractory to this treatment. At this stage, transarterial therapies (hepatic arterial embolization [HAE], transarterial chemoembolization [TACE], and radioembolization [RAE]) are useful for treating both hormone-producing and nonfunctional tumors, thus reducing hormonal symptoms and pain.[19,20,21,22,23,24,25,26,27]

NET metastases derive ~ 90% of their blood supply from the hepatic artery, whereas nutritional supply to normal hepatic parenchyma originates predominantly from the portal venous system. Therefore, transarterial therapies (TATs) allow for selective treatment of the tumor while preserving the blood supply to the organ.[28,29] In 1983, Moertel demonstrated that 80% of patients with carcinoid syndrome responded to hepatic artery ligation alone.[11] During HAE with particles alone, occlusion of the intratumoral blood supply results in ischemia and selective tumor necrosis.[28,29,30] This is achieved with the use of spherical embolic agents (particles) small enough to reach and occlude such vessels. TACE combines the effects of HAE with chemotherapeutic agents, based on the theoretical advantage of delivering concentrated drug to a tumor sensitized by embolization-induced ischemia. Chemotherapeutic dwell time in the tumor is thought to be prolonged, and the systemic effects are minimized.[31] Drug-eluting bead transarterial chemoembolization (DEB-TACE) has been more recently used as a form of chemoembolization in which embolic microspheres are loaded with anthracycline drugs, such as doxorubicin, acting as a direct carrier and resulting in a more favorable drug-release profile,[32,33,34] despite the fact that doxorubicin has never demonstrated activity against NETs. Unfortunately, higher complication rates have been reported with DEB-TACE for metastatic NETs[35,36]; we do not use DEB-TACE for metastatic NETs and do not recommend it. Radioembolization using yttrium-90 (^{90}Y) microspheres allows targeted radiotherapy to be delivered to the tumor. It is not intended as an embolic treatment

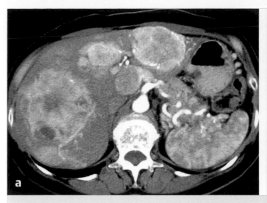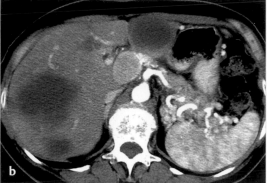

Fig. 9.1 Computed tomographic images obtained **(a)** before and **(b)** 3 months after right and left hepatic artery embolization in a patient who progressed while on somatostatin analogues *and* did not respond to chemotherapy.

but rather a means of delivering internal radiation to the tumor.

Until recently there has not been any effective systemic therapy for NETs metastatic to the liver, and external beam radiation is not useful for diffuse hepatic metastases; thus TAT has formed the mainstay of therapy. This is changing, and appropriate treatment for the patient is now based on knowledge of the site of the primary as well as the grade of the tumor. Tumors with the primary arising in the pancreas are known as pancreatic neuroendocrine tumors (pNETs), whereas those arising outside the pancreas—typically in the aerodigestive tract—are called carcinoids. They are further classified by degree of differentiation and grade. Poorly differentiated high-grade tumors are considered aggressive and treated with platinum-based therapy, so histology is important, and biopsy should be performed before initiating TAT if tissue has not already been obtained.

9.2 Indications

Due to the "hypervascular" nature of hepatic NET metastases and the dual vascular supply of the liver, TATs have been used for symptomatic relief with the hope of improving survival in unresectable patients.[19,20,21,22,23,24,25,26,27,30,37,38,39,40,41,42,43,44,45,46,47,48,49,50] Indications for embolization include rapid progression of liver disease in the face of stable or absent extrahepatic disease, progression of liver disease while on SSA (▶ Fig. 9.1), and symptoms related to hepatic tumor bulk or to hormonal excess that is refractory to SSA.[51] Control of hepatic metastases may allow prolonged survival when compared with patients who are

not treated.[1,52] For the uncommon situation of a relatively small (< 5 cm) solitary lesion or not more than three NET deposits, TAT can be combined with radiofrequency ablation or other ablation techniques to maximize tumor necrosis and improve local disease control.[25]

Rarely, embolization can be used in patients with large hepatic deposits to decrease the tumor load and render a previously inoperable patient a surgical candidate. With tumor reduction the previously inoperable or borderline patient may become a surgical candidate,[1] or, based on response to embolization, a decision may be made to resect the patient's primary tumor (▶ Fig. 9.2). It is probably more common, at least at our institution, for surgery to *precede* embolization for patients with bulky metastases that can be resected, leaving behind a lower volume of metastases to be controlled with HAE (▶ Fig. 9.3).

9.3 Contraindications

There is a limited number of relative contraindications to hepatic embolization for the treatment of hepatic NET metastases. Involvement of > 75% of the liver parenchyma by tumor renders a patient vulnerable to embolization and at high risk for the development of liver failure. Any treatment should proceed with caution, and embolization should be performed in stages.[22,38,51] Instead of treating a hemi-liver, either the anterior *or* the posterior division of the right liver, *or* the lateral segment of the left liver could be treated initially, and after seeing how this treatment is tolerated by the patient, further embolization could be performed.

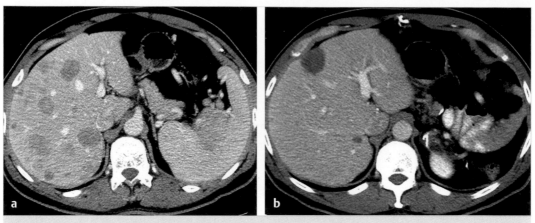

Fig. 9.2 Computed tomographic images obtained **(a)** before and **(b)** 10 months after hepatic arterial embolization. The patient had such a good response to embolization that the surgeon resected the pancreatic tail primary. Note the absence of the pancreatic tail and spleen in **(b)**.

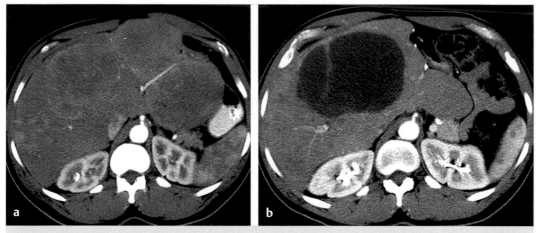

Fig. 9.3 (a) Large masses essentially replacing the left lateral segment on the preoperative image. **(b)** After resection and right hepatic arterial embolization, note the absence of the left lateral segment, necrotic tumor in the right liver, and hypertrophy of the caudate.

Renal insufficiency is a contraindication unless the patient is already undergoing hemodialysis and plans have been made for hemodialysis before and after the procedure. Mild renal insufficiency (creatinine > 1.5 but < 2 mg/dL) can be managed with good hydration; we also infuse sodium bicarbonate (3 mL/kg/h of a solution of sodium bicarbonate, 154 mEq/L administered over a 1-hour period before the procedure and 1 mL/kg/h infused for 6 hours during/after the procedure) in an attempt to prevent deterioration in renal function. The volume of contrast material should be kept to a minimum. Patients with allergies to contrast agents are premedicated with 50 mg of prednisone administered orally 13, 8, and 1 hour before the procedure.

Patients with elevated bilirubin, leukopenia, thrombocytopenia, or coagulopathy should be carefully evaluated because liver dysfunction is uncommon in this group of patients and abnormalities here should make one consider the possibility of underlying cirrhosis. Patients with metastatic NET are as likely to suffer from nonalcoholic fatty liver disease as the rest of the U.S. population, or they may have hepatitis B, hepatitis C, or drink alcohol excessively. If the laboratory abnormalities are due to replacement of the liver by tumor, the disease is probably too advanced to consider TAT. Additional considerations apply to RAE. Absolute contraindications include significant hepatopulmonary shunting and uncorrectable extrahepatic shunting to the gastroduodenal tract, which may result in extrahepatic deposition of microspheres and cause complications related to nontarget radiation. At our institution, patients are treated with RAE only if they fail HAE.

9.4 Patient Selection and Preprocedure Workup

Prior to transarterial therapy, patients undergo hepatic and renal function tests, complete blood count, and coagulation studies. It is critical that, prior to any embolization procedure, optimal imaging of the liver be performed to depict the anatomy and the characteristics of the tumor to be embolized. Multiphase computed tomography (CT) or magnetic resonance imaging (MRI), ideally obtained within 1 month of treatment, is essential for documenting the extent of disease, demonstrating arterial anatomy, evaluating the portal venous system, and looking for nonhepatic blood supply to the tumor (▶ Fig. 9.4). We prefer multiphase CT because we find it easier to assess the nonhepatic blood supply to the tumor, as well as to identify landmarks that might be helpful during embolization, such as metallic clips from previous surgery. This study serves as the basis for a treatment plan. The extent and distribution of the tumor are laid out, arterial blood supply to the tumor is evident, and contribution from the nonhepatic vasculature, such as the phrenic or internal mammary arteries, can be seen. On the day of the procedure, the plan need only be executed.

When RAE is chosen for treatment, preprocedure "mapping" is performed 2 to 4 weeks before treatment to (1) delineate the hepatic vasculature, including any variant anatomy, and to assess the tumor vascular supply; (2) prophylactically embolize any extrahepatic vessels with hepatofugal flow to prevent inadvertent delivery of ^{90}Y in extrahepatic sites; and (3) inject technetium-99 m macroaggregated serum albumin (^{99m}Tc-MAA) to vascular territories to be treated in order to detect extrahepatic activity (e.g., extrahepatic shunting to the gastrointestinal tract) and to estimate the percentage of shunting to the lungs.

Patients are to receive nothing by mouth after midnight. They are admitted to the hospital the morning of the procedure and have an intravenous line started. Patients with impaired renal function receive sodium bicarbonate (see earlier mention). Hydration is begun in all patients with normal saline. Patients with allergies to contrast receive 50 mg of prednisone orally 1 hour before the procedure (they have already received two other doses of prednisone). All patients are given 4 mg of ondansetron (Zofran, GlaxoSmithKline) and 1 g of cefazolin (Ancef, GlaxoSmithKline) intravenously and 250 μg of octreotide subcutaneously. The SSA is administered to *all* NET patients, even those without hormonal symptoms. We have found these tumors capable of making low levels of vasoactive or hormonal substances that may be clinically silent but become clinically significant when cells undergo uniform and rapid cell death and release intracellular contents.[38] For this reason we also have 250 μg of octreotide available in the procedure room to be administered intravenously during the procedure if necessary. It is very important in this group of patients to screen for bilioenteric bypass because patients with pNET may have undergone a Whipple for treatment of a pancreatic primary. These patients are at extremely high risk for developing a liver abscess. In a review of almost 1,000 patients undergoing more than 2,000 embolization procedures, the risk of liver abscess in patients with a contaminated biliary tree was found to be up to 30 times higher than the baseline risk.[53] Patients who do not have an intact sphincter of Oddi receive cefotetan (B. Braun), 2 g intravenously. Patients without an intact sphincter of Oddi are treated prophylactically with an antibiotic expected to cover biliary flora, such as cefotetan (Cefotan 2 g), before embolization, rather than the customary Ancef. The cefotetan is given intravenously for as long as the patient is in the hospital. Oral metronidazole (Flagyl, Pfizer) and ciprofloxacin (Cipro, Bayer) are continued for 1 week postdischarge. Despite this, liver abscess may still occur.

9.5 Technique

Visceral angiography is always performed before embolization, studying the celiac axis and superior mesenteric artery (SMA). Imaging is carried out

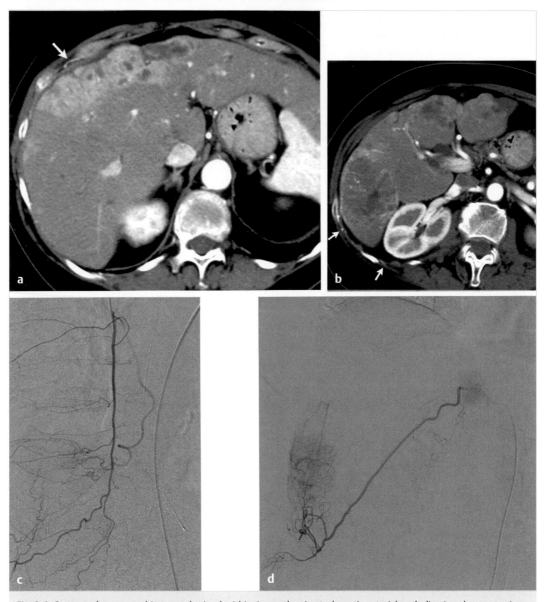

Fig. 9.4 Computed tomographic scan obtained within 1 month prior to hepatic arterial embolization demonstrating conspicuous enlarged branches of **(a)** the internal mammary *(arrow)* and **(b)** intercostal vessels *(arrows)*. **(c)** Corresponding images from the internal mammary angiogram and **(d)** T11 intercostal angiogram showing parasitized blood supply to the tumor.

into the portal venous phase, not as much for assessing portal vein patency, which is rarely an issue in this patient population, as for determining direction of flow. Common or proper hepatic angiography is then performed using 4 or 5F selective catheters, such as Cobras (Terumo Medical Corporation) and reverse-curve catheters (Simmons or Sos catheters, AngioDynamics), through a vascular sheath placed in the common femoral artery. Coaxial microcatheters are used when necessary for subselective embolization. Conventional nonionic contrast material is typically used.

When treating patients with multifocal, bilobar disease, we usually treat the lobe with the most disease at the first sitting. Initially, arteriography is performed with the catheter positioned selectively in the right or left hepatic artery, followed by embolization. Coaxial catheters might be used to avoid nontarget embolization, or in other situations when necessary. For HAE, spherical embolic agents are used, typically tris-acryl gelatin microspheres (Embosphere Microspheres, Merit Medical Systems Inc.), beginning with the smallest microspheres (40–120 µm) unless patients are felt to be at risk for nontarget pulmonary embolization.[54] Those would be patients with large (≥ 10 cm) very vascular tumors, particularly high in the dome of the liver adjacent to the hemidiaphragm, or with systemic blood supply (phrenic). In such cases we begin embolization with 100 to 300 µm tris-acryl gelatin microspheres. When TACE is used, antineoplastic agents such as doxorubicin, cisplatin, gemcitabine, and/or mitomycin are used in combination with Lipiodol (Guerbet) and embolic agents. In DEB-TACE, embolic beads loaded with doxorubicin are infused to a total dose of no more than 150 mg, with 100 mg being more widely used today.

RAE is performed selectively based on preprocedure planning. Most patients have bilobar disease, and the side with the most lesions is treated first, with administration to the contralateral lobe performed 4 to 6 weeks later in a separate session. Patients who have undergone right or left hepatectomy receive treatment to the whole remnant liver in a single session. Targeted therapy is performed in a sublobar, selective manner whenever feasible for patients with disease limited to one segment to further minimize toxicity to uninvolved liver parenchyma. This is relatively uncommon in this patient population, who generally have more widespread disease.

For HAE the desired end point of the procedure is stasis in the target vessel defined as absence of antegrade flow, such that even slow administration of contrast material results in reflux, or retrograde flow. For TACE the end point is a bit more variable, with some authors advocating a "pruned tree" appearance and many stating that complete stasis should be avoided. When embolization is complete, a final angiogram is obtained to document occlusion of the target vessel and identify any supply to the target area from other vessels, which may then be selected and embolized. Finally, arteriography will show stasis in the embolized vessels, with preservation of antegrade blood flow to nontarget vessels, such as the gastroduodenal and the cystic artery.

RAE is not intended to be an "embolic" therapy and is not intentionally performed to stasis. Radiation-induced cell death requires normal oxygen tension[55]; therefore transarterial delivery of the ^{90}Y loaded spheres is concluded when the calculated dose has been administered or when stasis occurs. Stasis that limited the total administered activity has been documented to occur in up to 38% of the cases in one series.[56]

9.6 Postprocedural Management and Follow-up Evaluation

After HAE, patients are observed in the postanesthesia care unit for several hours. Requirement for pain medication is monitored, and patient-controlled analgesia is initiated when warranted. Blood pressure is stabilized, and patients are transferred to the floor when stable. Clear liquids are allowed for the first 24 hours, and the diet is then advanced as tolerated. Intravenous antibiotics are administered for 24 hours when the sphincter of Oddi is intact or for the duration of hospital stay when not. Antipyretics are administered as needed; if the temperature exceeds 38.5°C, blood is drawn for culture. Patients are discharged from the hospital when they are taking adequate nutrition by mouth, when pain is adequately controlled with oral narcotics, and when the temperature is maintained below 38.5°C for 24 hours.

Follow-up multiphase imaging is performed 2 to 6 weeks after treatment is complete. In the case of patients requiring more than one embolization for complete treatment this is 2 to 4 weeks after the final treatment. The follow-up CT scan is reviewed for any evidence of persistent untreated disease. If there is no evidence of enhancement of the treated tumor, these patients are monitored with triple-phase CT every 3 months for the first year and every 6 months thereafter. When there is evidence of significant untreated, recurrent, or new disease elsewhere within the liver, the patient is scheduled for retreatment.

9.7 Side Effects and Complications

Postembolization syndrome (PES) occurs in approximately 80% of patients and consists of pain, fever, nausea, and/or vomiting. The patient may experience any one or all of those symptoms. PES

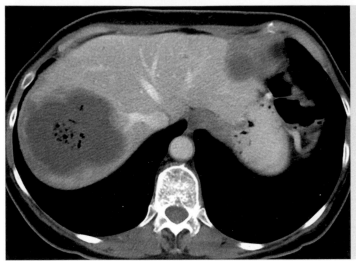

Fig. 9.5 Higher level of computed tomography in the same patient seen in ▶ Fig. 9.1, who was 5 weeks status post right hepatic arterial embolization. Note "gas bubbles" in the large segment 7 lesion.

should be considered a side effect and not a complication of embolotherapy. The severity of the syndrome varies between patients and between different treatments in the same patient. In its mildest form the syndrome lasts no longer than 24 hours, and patients can even be managed as outpatients with oral medication for pain relief. In more severe forms, patients cannot tolerate oral medication and require intravenous hydration, antiemetics, and pain relief medication. PES is less frequently seen after RAE than after conventional HAE procedures (HAE or TACE). In general, RAE is better tolerated compared to HAE or TACE, with the most common complaints being abdominal pain, weakness, mild nausea, and mild fever that do not require hospitalization.

Occasionally, in patients with functional carcinoid metastases, HAE can precipitate a massive acute release of vasoactive peptides resulting in a carcinoid crisis. Carcinoid crisis is a potentially life-threatening event manifested by hypotension or hypertension, severe flushing, bronchospasm, arrhythmia, and acidosis. Treatment of carcinoid crisis includes fluid expansion and high-dose intravenous octreotide.

Liver abscess is a rare complication of hepatic embolization, and the typical postembolization appearance of a low-density lesion with scattered gas bubbles should not be confused with a liver abscess (▶ Fig. 9.5). We avoid scanning patients in the immediate postembolization period to avoid raising the issue of liver abscess. Similar to postsurgical patients, liver abscess does not usually occur earlier than 7 to 10 days after embolization. It is seen most commonly in patients who have undergone bilioenteric bypass or who for any reason (e.g., sphincterotomy) do not have an intact sphincter of Oddi.[53] Patients who develop a liver abscess will appear ill and have an elevated white blood cell count and fever.

Nontarget embolization is one of the most dreaded complications of hepatic embolotherapy but occurs infrequently when strict attention is paid to arterial anatomy. The gallbladder is probably the most commonly involved nontarget organ. Inadvertent embolization of the gallbladder can result in prolonged PES with fever, pain, and nausea/vomiting but rarely requires surgical intervention. In our practice, despite some inflammatory, thick-walled gallbladders, few patients have required intervention. Rarely, a cholecystostomy catheter is placed that can be removed in 2 to 3 weeks.

Very rarely, more severe consequences of nontarget embolization are seen, such as pancreatitis or gastric or duodenal ulceration. Transient deterioration in liver function or even frank liver failure may occur, more commonly following embolization of the whole liver or when > 75% of the liver volume is involved by tumor.

Cardiotoxicity, a known risk of anthracycline chemotherapy, is decreased with TACE compared to systemic administration, and is possibly even lower with doxorubicin-eluting beads embolization. Because these patients often require multiple embolizations the cumulative dose of doxorubicin should be tracked. This is a complication not seen after HAE.

RAE has demonstrated a better toxicity profile than conventional TACE. Serious complications have been reported, such as gastritis and duodenitis that result from inadvertent administration of ^{90}Y microspheres into branches supplying the gastrointestinal tract. Such complications can in theory be prevented by careful preprocedural planning as previously discussed. Radiation-induced liver disease, radiation pneumonitis, and pancreatitis are very rarely seen.

9.8 Clinical Data and Outcomes

In many retrospective nonrandomized studies, transarterial therapies have demonstrated excellent results in palliating symptoms related to hormonal excess and tumor bulk in patients with unresectable hepatic neuroendocrine metastases.[3,6,21,23,37,38,40,41,43,44,45,47,48,49,50,57,58,59] Median survival of 13 to 80 months and 5-year survival rates between 32 and 75% have been reported for patients with NETs after HAE/TACE.[6,21,22,23,24,37,38,39,40,41,42,44,57,58,59] Similar overall survival times have been observed after RAE (median survival 14–70 months, 5-year survival rates up to 55%).[59,60,61,62,63,64,65,66,67,68] A common finding of most series of HAE or TACE, and more recently of RAE, for the management of NET is a morphological response as documented by imaging. Partial or complete response rates have been reported ranging from 7.7 to 95% for HAE or TACE treatment.[43,47,69,70,71] These rates have been reported to be improved in patients treated with RAE, ranging from 12.5 to 100%.[59,60,61,62,63,64,66,67,68] Nevertheless, a recent retrospective study compared clinical outcomes of patients with metastatic NETs treated with HAE, TACE, and RAE at a single institution and found

no significant difference in overall survival and radiographic response between the three treatment groups.[59] With regard to DEB-TACE, a limited number of studies showed rates of morphological response at short-term and intermediate-term follow-up similar to those of HAE/TACE (up to 95% and up to 65% radiological response, respectively),[35,70] but, given the DEB-TACE hepatotoxicity profile, the fact that the response is comparable should probably be used to favor HAE or TACE.

Better prolonged overall survival times after HAE and TACE have been reported in patients with carcinoid tumor metastatic to the liver compared to patients with pNET.[3,11,22,38,41] Similarly, radiological response was reportedly greater in patients with carcinoid, with significantly longer hepatic progression-free survivals in comparison to patients with pNET.[22,38,41] Prior series by Gupta et al[22] suggested that HAE may be more effective than TACE for carcinoid.

Few studies have investigated factors affecting outcomes after transarterial therapies.[22,58,66,72] Unresected primary tumor, liver involvement with metastasis of > 75%, and the presence of extrahepatic disease were predictors of poorer outcome in patients with pNET metastases in one of these studies.[22] In patients who had carcinoid tumors, only male gender was predictive for decreased survival. Compared to carcinoid, pNET alone is associated with a shorter overall survival.[22] Hur et al[72] demonstrated that bilioenteric communication, hepatic tumor burden, and extrahepatic metastasis before the first TACE were associated with poor overall survival. A more recent study by Sofocleous et al[58] including patients treated with only HAE demonstrated that metastatic disease involving > 50% of the liver and the presence of extrahepatic metastasis were independent predictors for shorter survival. Additionally, they reported that patients who were embolized urgently for exacerbated symptomatology refractory to medical management were twice as likely to die compared with those embolized electively.[58] For patients treated with RAE, low hepatic tumor burden, female gender, well-differentiated tumor, and absence of extrahepatic metastasis were associated with improved survival.[66]

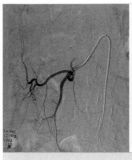 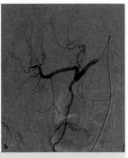

Fig. 9.6 Common hepatic artery (CHA) angiograms obtained at (a) the time of the second hepatic arterial embolization and then (b) 5½ years later at the time of eighth treatment. Note the preservation of branch arteries.

The main controversy with regard to TAT for primary and secondary hepatic malignancies revolves around the use of chemotherapeutic agents. Although the concept of delivering high-dose chemotherapy to the tumor or tumors is interesting, there is a paucity of evidence-based findings supporting the routine use of chemoembolization. This would be particularly important in tumors such as NET that are not responsive to the chemotherapeutic agents typically used for TACE. Because TACE is not standardized, adds the expense of chemotherapy, has the potential for systemic side effects, and may have a higher incidence of postembolization vessel occlusion[73] (▶ Fig. 9.6), there are barriers to its routine use. If indeed the primary effect of TACE, as currently practiced, is one that is caused by ischemia, particle embolization makes more sense, would be less expensive, would not have any risk of side effects from chemotherapy, and might be more readily practiced in the community setting.

To date, there are contradictory data regarding the added toxicity of chemotherapy in patients treated with TACE. Some investigators did not experience a higher degree of toxicity,[74] whereas others reported severe complications[27,36] in the management of NETs. A recent study using doxorubicin DEB-TACE reported a very high rate of biliary complications when compared to traditional TACE.[36] This paper suggests that the addition of chemotherapy to spherical particles (DEB-TACE) may cause terminal capillary blockade and deliver high local doses of doxorubicin, which may increase the risk of complications when compared to traditional TACE or HAE with particles only.

Most studies conclude that outcomes are inversely related to the degree of liver replacement by tumor. Patients with > 75% of the liver replaced by tumor are poor candidates for embolization in general. Poor outcomes and response rates have been documented in this population. In contrast, patients with < 50% involvement have a trend for longer survival. A large percentage of (and in some series all) patients with > 75% involvement died within 30 days to 6 months after TAE or TACE. Some practitioners undertake embolization of patients with > 50% tumor load as a palliative treatment only, especially when severe symptomatology impedes quality of life. In these high-risk patients, embolization should be performed in stages, with only a part of the vascular tumor embolized at each session, frequently not more than one sector at a time.[38,51] Using this approach, one series[38] treated patients with > 75% replacement of the liver and reported response rates of 43 and 25% and overall survival of 20.1 and 16 months for patients with carcinoid tumor and pNET, respectively. The issue of pain relief in patients with metastatic NET was addressed directly in a series of HAE procedures where it was noted that more extensive tumor burden is likely to be present when the primary symptom is pain rather than symptoms of hormonal excess. This series also reported that symptomatic relief of pain was of shorter duration than control of hormonal symptoms and that 40% of patients treated for pain alone died within an average follow-up period of 13.7 months, whereas only 6% of patients treated for hormonal symptoms died within an average follow-up period of 24 months,[38] findings that would be expected in patients with greater tumor burden. It is likely that pain develops in patients who are farther along in the natural history of the disease with a larger volume of tumor in the liver, explaining the poorer results of treatment in this subgroup.

Pearls

- Make sure the patient has a tissue diagnosis so that the tumor is properly classified and graded. Patients with a poorly differentiated high-grade tumor should be considered for systemic therapy.
- If newly diagnosed, do not offer TAT until the patient has had a trial of SSA unless the tumor burden is already excessive or borderline for treatment. SSA not only controls hormonal symptoms but has been demonstrated to be cytostatic as well, and patients may live for years with a stable hepatic tumor.
- Always begin with a multiphase cross-sectional imaging study and look carefully at the tumor distribution, hepatic arterial anatomy, prominent nonhepatic vessels that may be supplying tumor (phrenic, internal mammary, intercostals), and any evidence of cirrhosis/portal hypertension (even though uncommon).
- Give 250 µg of SSA subcutaneously prior to embolization, even to patients who have octreotide long-acting release on board, and have another 250 µg in the room, which can be used for unexplained hyper- or hypotension that might occur during procedure.
- Be prepared for impressive PES for 24 to 48 hours with marked increase in liver function tests. These typically peak on the second post-embolization day and then return to baseline within a month.
- If the plan includes embolization of the contralateral side to complete treatment there is no need to image in between unless something unusual is suspected.
- After treatment is completed see the patient with multiphase imaging within 1 month. If there is clearly persistent tumor in territory that was not treated (e.g., phrenic territory), then bring the patient back to complete and touch up other areas as needed.
- Use caution when asked to perform urgent embolization to treat patients admitted in the hospital for refractory symptoms. Educate these patients and referral physicians about poor clinical outcomes in this population.
- Consider administration of prophylactic biliary-secreting antibiotics when treating patients with biliary enteric anastomosis or prior manipulation of the sphincter of Oddi.

References

[1] Jackson J, Hemingway A, Allison D. Embolization of liver tumors. In: Blumgart L, Fong Y, eds. Surgery of the Liver and Biliary Tract. Vol 2. London: Saunders; 2000:1521–1544

[2] Moertel CG. Karnofsky memorial lecture. An odyssey in the land of small tumors. J Clin Oncol 1987; 5(10): 1502–1522

[3] Moertel CG, Johnson CM, McKusick MA et al. The management of patients with advanced carcinoid tumors and islet cell carcinomas. Ann Intern Med 1994; 120(4): 302–309

[4] Tsikitis VL, Wertheim BC, Guerrero MA. Trends of incidence and survival of gastrointestinal neuroendocrine tumors in the United States: a seer analysis. J Cancer 2012; 3: 292–302

[5] Frilling A, Li J, Malamutmann E, Schmid KW, Bockisch A, Broelsch CE. Treatment of liver metastases from neuroendocrine tumours in relation to the extent of hepatic disease. Br J Surg 2009; 96(2): 175–184

[6] Chamberlain RS, Canes D, Brown KT et al. Hepatic neuroendocrine metastases: does intervention alter outcomes? J Am Coll Surg 2000; 190(4): 432–445

[7] Chen H, Hardacre JM, Uzar A, Cameron JL, Choti MA. Isolated liver metastases from neuroendocrine tumors: does resection prolong survival? J Am Coll Surg 1998; 187(1): 88–92, discussion 92–93

[8] Mayo SC, de Jong MC, Pulitano C et al. Surgical management of hepatic neuroendocrine tumor metastasis: results from an international multi-institutional analysis. Ann Surg Oncol 2010; 17(12): 3129–3136

[9] Sarmiento JM, Heywood G, Rubin J, Ilstrup DM, Nagorney DM, Que FG. Surgical treatment of neuroendocrine metastases to the liver: a plea for resection to increase survival. J Am Coll Surg 2003; 197(1): 29–37

[10] Di Bartolomeo M, Bajetta E, Bochicchio AM et al. A phase II trial of dacarbazine, fluorouracil and epirubicin in patients with neuroendocrine tumours. A study by the Italian Trials in Medical Oncology (I.T.M.O.) Group. Ann Oncol 1995; 6(1): 77–79

[11] Moertel CG. Treatment of the carcinoid tumor and the malignant carcinoid syndrome. J Clin Oncol 1983; 1(11): 727–740

[12] Oberg K, Norheim I, Lundqvist G, Wide L. Cytotoxic treatment in patients with malignant carcinoid tumors. Response to streptozocin—alone or in combination with 5-FU. Acta Oncol 1987; 26(6): 429–432

[13] Saltz L, Kemeny N, Schwartz G, Kelsen D. A phase II trial of alpha-interferon and 5-fluorouracil in patients with advanced carcinoid and islet cell tumors. Cancer 1994; 74(3): 958–961

[14] Wang SC, Fidelman N, Nakakura EK. Management of well-differentiated gastrointestinal neuroendocrine tumors metastatic to the liver. Semin Oncol 2013; 40(1): 69–74

[15] Schnirer II, Yao JC, Ajani JA. Carcinoid—a comprehensive review. Acta Oncol 2003; 42(7): 672–692

[16] Soga J, Yakuwa Y, Osaka M. Carcinoid syndrome: a statistical evaluation of 748 reported cases. J Exp Clin Cancer Res 1999; 18(2): 133–141

[17] Rinke A, Müller HH, Schade-Brittinger C et al. PROMID Study Group. Placebo-controlled, double-blind, prospective, randomized study on the effect of octreotide LAR in the control of tumor growth in patients with metastatic neuroendocrine midgut tumors: a report from the PROMID Study Group. J Clin Oncol 2009; 27(28): 4656–4663

[18] Strosberg J, Gardner N, Kvols L. Survival and prognostic factor analysis of 146 metastatic neuroendocrine tumors of the mid-gut. Neuroendocrinology 2009; 89(4): 471–476

[19] Carrasco CH, Charnsangavej C, Ajani J, Samaan NA, Richli W, Wallace S. The carcinoid syndrome: palliation by hepatic artery embolization. Am J Roentgenol 1986; 147(1): 149–154

[20] Clouse ME, Perry L, Stuart K, Stokes KR. Hepatic arterial chemoembolization for metastatic neuroendocrine tumors. Digestion 1994; 55 Suppl 3: 92–97

[21] Drougas JG, Anthony LB, Blair TK et al. Hepatic artery chemoembolization for management of patients with advanced metastatic carcinoid tumors. Am J Surg 1998; 175(5): 408–412

[22] Gupta S, Johnson MM, Murthy R et al. Hepatic arterial embolization and chemoembolization for the treatment of patients with metastatic neuroendocrine tumors: variables affecting response rates and survival. Cancer 2005; 104(8): 1590–1602

[23] Hajarizadeh H, Ivancev K, Mueller CR, Fletcher WS, Woltering EA. Effective palliative treatment of metastatic carcinoid tumors with intra-arterial chemotherapy/chemoembolization combined with octreotide acetate. Am J Surg 1992; 163 (5): 479–483

[24] Hanssen LE, Schrumpf E, Kolbenstvedt AN, Tausjø J, Dolva LO. Recombinant alpha-2 interferon with or without hepatic artery embolization in the treatment of midgut carcinoid tumours. A preliminary report. Acta Oncol 1989; 28(3): 439–443

[25] Meij V, Zuetenhorst JM, van Hillegersberg R et al. Local treatment in unresectable hepatic metastases of carcinoid tumors: Experiences with hepatic artery embolization and radiofrequency ablation. World J Surg Oncol 2005; 3: 75

[26] Stokes KR, Stuart K, Clouse ME. Hepatic arterial chemoembolization for metastatic endocrine tumors. J Vasc Interv Radiol 1993; 4(3): 341–345

[27] Winkelbauer FW, Niederle B, Pietschmann F et al. Hepatic artery embolotherapy of hepatic metastases from carcinoid tumors: value of using a mixture of cyanoacrylate and ethiodized oil. Am J Roentgenol 1995; 165(2): 323–327

[28] Dodd GD, III, Soulen MC, Kane RA et al. Minimally invasive treatment of malignant hepatic tumors: at the threshold of a major breakthrough. Radiographics 2000; 20(1): 9–27

[29] Sullivan KL. Hepatic artery chemoembolization. Semin Oncol 2002; 29(2): 145–151

[30] Ahlman H, Nilsson O, Olausson M. Interventional treatment of the carcinoid syndrome. Neuroendocrinology 2004; 80 Suppl 1: 67–73

[31] Soulen MC. Chemoembolization of hepatic malignancies. Oncology (Williston Park) 1994; 8(4): 77–84, discussion 84, 89–90 passim

[32] Aliberti C, Benea G, Tilli M, Fiorentini G. Chemoembolization (TACE) of unresectable intrahepatic cholangiocarcinoma with slow-release doxorubicin-eluting beads: preliminary results. Cardiovasc Intervent Radiol 2008; 31(5): 883–888

[33] Lewis AL, Gonzalez MV, Lloyd AW et al. DC bead: in vitro characterization of a drug-delivery device for transarterial chemoembolization. J Vasc Interv Radiol 2006; 17(2 Pt 1): 335–342

[34] Varela M, Real MI, Burrel M et al. Chemoembolization of hepatocellular carcinoma with drug eluting beads: efficacy and doxorubicin pharmacokinetics. J Hepatol 2007; 46(3): 474–481

[35] Gaur SK, Friese JL, Sadow CA et al. Hepatic arterial chemoembolization using drug-eluting beads in gastrointestinal neuroendocrine tumor metastatic to the liver. Cardiovasc Intervent Radiol 2011; 34(3): 566–572

[36] Guiu B, Deschamps F, Aho S et al. Liver/biliary injuries following chemoembolisation of endocrine tumours and hepatocellular carcinoma: lipiodol vs. drug-eluting beads. J Hepatol 2012; 56(3): 609–617

[37] Ajani JA, Carrasco CH, Charnsangavej C, Samaan NA, Levin B, Wallace S. Islet cell tumors metastatic to the liver: effective palliation by sequential hepatic artery embolization. Ann Intern Med 1988; 108(3): 340–344

[38] Brown KT, Koh BY, Brody LA et al. Particle embolization of hepatic neuroendocrine metastases for control of pain and hormonal symptoms. J Vasc Interv Radiol 1999; 10(4): 397–403

[39] Carrasco CH, Chuang VP, Wallace S. Apudomas metastatic to the liver: treatment by hepatic artery embolization. Radiology 1983; 149(1): 79–83

[40] Dominguez S, Denys A, Madeira I et al. Hepatic arterial chemoembolization with streptozotocin in patients with metastatic digestive endocrine tumours. Eur J Gastroenterol Hepatol 2000; 12(2): 151–157

[41] Eriksson BK, Larsson EG, Skogseid BM, Löfberg AM, Lörelius LE, Oberg KE. Liver embolizations of patients with malignant neuroendocrine gastrointestinal tumors. Cancer 1998; 83 (11): 2293–2301

[42] Kim YH, Ajani JA, Carrasco CH et al. Selective hepatic arterial chemoembolization for liver metastases in patients with carcinoid tumor or islet cell carcinoma. Cancer Invest 1999; 17(7): 474–478

[43] Kress O, Wagner HJ, Wied M, Klose KJ, Arnold R, Alfke H. Transarterial chemoembolization of advanced liver metastases of neuroendocrine tumors—a retrospective single-center analysis. Digestion 2003; 68(2–3): 94–101

[44] Loewe C, Schindl M, Cejna M, Niederle B, Lammer J, Thurnher S. Permanent transarterial embolization of neuroendocrine metastases of the liver using cyanoacrylate and lipiodol: assessment of mid- and long-term results. Am J Roentgenol 2003; 180(5): 1379–1384

[45] Mavligit GM, Pollock RE, Evans HL, Wallace S. Durable hepatic tumor regression after arterial chemoembolization-infusion in patients with islet cell carcinoma of the pancreas metastatic to the liver. Cancer 1993; 72(2): 375–380

[46] Mitty HA, Warner RR, Newman LH, Train JS, Parnes IH. Control of carcinoid syndrome with hepatic artery embolization. Radiology 1985; 155(3): 623–626

[47] Perry LJ, Stuart K, Stokes KR, Clouse ME. Hepatic arterial chemoembolization for metastatic neuroendocrine tumors. Surgery 1994; 116(6): 1111–1116, discussion 1116–1117

[48] Roche A, Girish BV, de Baère T et al. Trans-catheter arterial chemoembolization as first-line treatment for hepatic metastases from endocrine tumors. Eur Radiol 2003; 13(1): 136–140

[49] Ruszniewski P, Rougier P, Roche A et al. Hepatic arterial chemoembolization in patients with liver metastases of endocrine tumors. A prospective phase II study in 24 patients. Cancer 1993; 71(8): 2624–2630

[50] Therasse E, Breittmayer F, Roche A et al. Transcatheter chemoembolization of progressive carcinoid liver metastasis. Radiology 1993; 189(2): 541–547

[51] Madoff DC, Gupta S, Ahrar K, Murthy R, Yao JC. Update on the management of neuroendocrine hepatic metastases. J Vasc Interv Radiol 2006; 17(8): 1235–1249, quiz 1250

[52] Brown DB, Geschwind JF, Soulen MC, Millward SF, Sacks D. Society of Interventional Radiology position statement on chemoembolization of hepatic malignancies. J Vasc Interv Radiol 2006; 17(2 Pt 1): 217–223

[53] Mezhir JJ, Fong Y, Fleischer D et al. Pyogenic abscess after hepatic artery embolization: a rare but potentially lethal complication. J Vasc Interv Radiol 2011; 22(2): 177–182

[54] Brown KT. Re: Fatal pulmonary complications after arterial embolization with 40–120-microm tris-acryl gelatin microspheres. J Vasc Interv Radiol 2004; 15(8): 887–888

[55] Strosberg JR, Cheema A, Kvols LK. A review of systemic and liver-directed therapies for metastatic neuroendocrine tumors of the gastroenteropancreatic tract. Cancer Contr 2011; 18(2): 127–137

[56] Sofocleous CT, Garcia AR, Pandit-Taskar N et al. Phase I trial of selective internal radiation therapy for chemorefractory colorectal cancer liver metastases progressing after hepatic arterial pump and systemic chemotherapy. Clin Colorectal Cancer 2014; 13(1): 27–36

[57] Hanssen LE, Schrumpf E, Jacobsen MB et al. Extended experience with recombinant alpha-2b interferon with or without hepatic artery embolization in the treatment of midgut carcinoid tumours. A preliminary report. Acta Oncol 1991; 30(4): 523–527

[58] Sofocleous CT, Petre EN, Gonen M et al. Factors affecting periprocedural morbidity and mortality and long-term patient survival after arterial embolization of hepatic neuroendocrine metastases. J Vasc Interv Radiol 2014; 25(1): 22–30, quiz 31

[59] Engelman ES, Leon-Ferre R, Naraev BG et al. Comparison of transarterial liver-directed therapies for low-grade metastatic neuroendocrine tumors in a single institution. Pancreas 2014; 43(2): 219–225

[60] Kennedy AS, Dezarn WA, McNeillie P et al. Radioembolization for unresectable neuroendocrine hepatic metastases using resin 90Y-microspheres: early results in 148 patients. Am J Clin Oncol 2008; 31(3): 271–279

[61] Lacin S, Oz I, Ozkan E, Kucuk O, Bilgic S. Intra-arterial treatment with 90yttrium microspheres in treatment-refractory and unresectable liver metastases of neuroendocrine tumors and the use of 111in-octreotide scintigraphy in the evaluation of treatment response. Cancer Biother Radiopharm 2011; 26(5): 631–637

[62] Murthy R, Kamat P, Nunez R et al. Yttrium-90 microsphere radioembolotherapy of hepatic metastatic neuroendocrine carcinomas after hepatic arterial embolization. J Vasc Interv Radiol 2008; 19(1): 145–151

[63] Rajekar H, Bogammana K, Stubbs RS. Selective internal radiation therapy for gastrointestinal neuroendocrine tumour liver metastases: a new and effective modality for treatment. Int J Hepatol 2011; 2011: 404916

[64] Rhee TK, Lewandowski RJ, Liu DM et al. 90Y Radioembolization for metastatic neuroendocrine liver tumors: preliminary results from a multi-institutional experience. Ann Surg 2008; 247(6): 1029–1035

[65] Sato KT, Lewandowski RJ, Mulcahy MF et al. Unresectable chemorefractory liver metastases: radioembolization with 90Y microspheres—safety, efficacy, and survival. Radiology 2008; 247(2): 507–515

[66] Saxena A, Chua TC, Bester L, Kokandi A, Morris DL. Factors predicting response and survival after yttrium-90 radioembolization of unresectable neuroendocrine tumor liver metastases: a critical appraisal of 48 cases. Ann Surg 2010; 251(5): 910–916

[67] Shaheen M, Hassanain M, Aljiffry M et al. Predictors of response to radio-embolization (TheraSphere®) treatment of neuroendocrine liver metastasis. HPB (Oxford) 2012; 14(1): 60–66

[68] Whitney R, Vàlek V, Fages JF et al. Transarterial chemoembolization and selective internal radiation for the treatment of patients with metastatic neuroendocrine tumors: a comparison of efficacy and cost. Oncologist 2011; 16(5): 594–601

[69] Bloomston M, Al-Saif O, Klemanski D et al. Hepatic artery chemoembolization in 122 patients with metastatic carcinoid tumor: lessons learned. J Gastrointest Surg 2007; 11 (3): 264–271

[70] de Baere T, Deschamps F, Teriitheau C et al. Transarterial chemoembolization of liver metastases from well differentiated gastroenteropancreatic endocrine tumors with doxorubicin-eluting beads: preliminary results. J Vasc Interv Radiol 2008; 19(6): 855–861

[71] Varker KA, Martin EW, Klemanski D, Palmer B, Shah MH, Bloomston M. Repeat transarterial chemoembolization (TACE) for progressive hepatic carcinoid metastases provides results similar to first TACE. J Gastrointest Surg 2007; 11(12): 1680–1685

[72] Hur S, Chung JW, Kim HC et al. Survival outcomes and prognostic factors of transcatheter arterial chemoembolization for hepatic neuroendocrine metastases. J Vasc Interv Radiol 2013; 24(7): 947–956, quiz 957

[73] Erinjeri JP, Salhab HM, Covey AM, Getrajdman GI, Brown KT. Arterial patency after repeated hepatic artery bland particle embolization. J Vasc Interv Radiol 2010; 21(4): 522–526

[74] Ruutiainen AT, Soulen MC, Tuite CM et al. Chemoembolization and bland embolization of neuroendocrine tumor metastases to the liver. J Vasc Interv Radiol 2007; 18(7): 847–855

Chapter 10

Cholangiocarcinoma: Ablation and Intra-arterial Therapies

10

10 Cholangiocarcinoma: Ablation and Intra-arterial Therapies

Matthew Brown, Paul J. Rochon, Rajan K. Gupta, and Charles E. Ray, Jr.

10.1 Introduction

Cholangiocarcinoma is an aggressive neoplasm originating from the bile duct epithelium. Historically, cholangiocarcinomas have been described as rare tumors, but they represent the second most common primary hepatic tumor after hepatocellular carcinoma. A variety of conditions can predispose to the development of cholangiocarcinoma (▶ Table 10.1). The incidence of cholangiocarcinoma appears to be on the rise.[1] Prognosis and treatment options are variable depending on location and tumor biology but have historically been poor, with survival from time of diagnosis ranging from 3 to 11 months in the face of best available therapy.[2,3,4]

Cholangiocarcinomas are classified by their location; this has important treatment and prognostic implications. They can occur anywhere along the bile tract, from small intrahepatic ductules to the ampulla. The hilar variant or Klatskin tumor is the most common, with extrahepatic and gallbladder variants. Up to 10% of tumors are solely intrahepatic.[5]

The mainstay of therapy for cholangiocarcinoma of any type remains surgical resection, with cure rates ranging from 28 to 40%. Unfortunately, many patients are deemed unresectable at presentation, likely owing to the multifocal nature of cholangiocarcinoma and proximity to hilar structures.[6] Transplantation is another surgical option, with a recent series showing a 5-year survival of 38% in transplanted patients, which increased to 68% in those treated with neoadjuvant chemotherapy. These results are tempered by strict patient selection criteria and a limited supply of organs.[7,8]

Optimal second-line therapy for cholangiocarcinoma has not been determined. Systemic chemotherapy, external beam radiation, localized photodynamic therapy, and brachytherapy have all been used, most with limited success and high levels of toxicity. Given the fact that no single nonsurgical therapy is particularly effective, the intrahepatic variant of cholangiocarcinoma represents an enticing potential target for liver-directed therapy. Furthermore, malignant tumors of the liver and the biliary ducts theoretically derive their blood supply preferentially from the hepatic arterial circulation, in contrast to normal hepatocytes, which are preferentially supplied by the portal vein. Liver-directed therapy is largely limited to treating the intrahepatic variant; however, extrahepatic cholangiocarcinoma metastatic to the liver also represents a potential target.[9]

10.2 Indications

The main indications for percutaneous therapy of patients with intrahepatic cholangiocarcinoma fall into a few major categories: primarily unresectable (due to anatomy/location), poor performance status precluding surgery, recurrent disease after resection, or extrahepatic cholangiocarcinoma metastatic to the liver. Palliation of mass symptoms and refractory biliary obstruction are other potential indications for locoregional therapy. An emerging indication for percutaneous treatment is to downstage initially unresectable patients for possible resection or transplantation.

10.3 Contraindications

Absolute contraindications are a life-threatening anaphylaxis to contrast or any other medications used and an uncorrectable coagulopathy. Poor performance status is a strong relative contraindication, because most studies have excluded patients with an Eastern Cooperative Oncology Group (ECOG) score > 2 or a short life expectancy (< 6

Table 10.1 Conditions predisposing to cholangiocarcinoma

Definite predisposing factors	Possible predisposing factors
Primary sclerosing cholangitis	Hepatitis C
Chronic liver fluke infection	Cirrhosis
	Toxins
Hepatolithiasis	Biliary-enteric anastomotic procedures
Biliary malformations (choledochal cyst)	

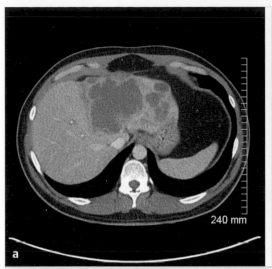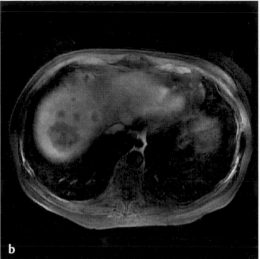

Fig. 10.1 (a) Contrast-enhanced computed tomographic image of liver demonstrates low-attenutation masses with peripheral enhancement on early arterial phase. (b) Contrast-enhanced magnetic resonance image of liver demonstrates low-attenuation masses with peripheral enhancement on early arterial phase.

months). Poor liver function reserve also represents a relative contraindication to therapy, given the potential of locoregional therapy to damage normal liver. Patients with extrahepatic metastatic disease are unlikely to benefit from treating only some of their metastatic burden. Prior biliary enteric anastomoses or an incompetent sphincter of Oddi are relative contraindications to percutaneous therapy given the high risk of infectious complications. Uncorrected anemia and leukopenia are contraindications to chemotherapy. Platelet levels should be reviewed to insure they are at levels adequate for hemostasis for both arterial and solid organ punctures.

10.4 Patient Consideration and Workup

As in any interventional oncology procedure, initial patient selection is crucial to success. The initial workup and treatment planning process are centered around a meticulous review of the patient's medical history, oncological history, and diagnostic imaging. Oncological clinical decision making is complex and is best performed in a multidisciplinary setting combining surgical specialists, medical specialists, diagnostic radiologists, interventional radiologists, and radiation therapy specialists.

Surgical therapy has demonstrated superior survival benefit with respect to all other treatment modalities in the treatment of intrahepatic cholangiocarcinoma, and the initial concern is whether complete resection can be achieved (i.e., R0 resection). The scope of surgical decision making is beyond the scope of this text, but the imaging findings pertinent to surgical planning significantly overlap those used in locoregional therapy planning. Imaging is reviewed, with specific attention paid to the location of the tumor, proximity to/encasement of adjacent vascular structures, centricity/number of tumors, arterial supply, and possible percutaneous approaches (▶ Fig. 10.1a, b). The relative conspicuity of the tumor on imaging modalities can be useful to determine the optimal method of image guidance for ablation. Determination of portal venous and biliary patency is important because these are associated with an increased risk of complication. Lastly, accurate determination of the stage is important given that extrahepatic metastatic disease is a relative contraindication to liver-directed therapy.

Laboratory and clinical data are also reviewed for relevant contraindications. ECOG score is a useful assessment of performance status. Patients appropriate for therapy typically have an ECOG score < 3 because patients with higher scores are less likely to derive benefit from therapy due to coexisting morbidity. Complete blood counts, chemistries, and liver function tests are routinely obtained to evaluate for possible procedural contraindications. Elevated bilirubin values in this

Table 10.2 Ablative versus transarterial therapy

Transarterial therapy	Ablation
Multicentric disease	Focal disease
Infiltrative tumor type	Mass forming type
Central location	Peripheral location
Adjacent to diaphragm	

population must be interpreted with caution as biliary obstruction may falsely give the impression of poor hepatocyte function. Lastly, baseline tumor markers (usually CA 19–9 and CA-125) are obtained and, if initially elevated in a patient with proven cholangiocarcinoma, they have some value for following the efficacy of therapy. Caution must be used because biliary system infection (sometimes subclinical) can spuriously elevate these values. A complete blood count is obtained to ensure adequate platelet numbers and cell counts prior to the patient receiving any chemotherapy.

10.5 Selection of Therapy

The clinical superiority of one percutaneous treatment modality over another has not been determined in any randomized, controlled clinical trial. Determining which treatment to pursue focuses largely on technical considerations, theoretical considerations, individual patient factors, and operator/institutional experience.

A comparison of patient factors favoring ablative or transarterial therapy is shown in ► Table 10.2. Ablative therapy tends to favor smaller, oligocentric disease. The best results have been seen in tumors < 3 cm and intermediate results in tumors < 5 cm, and emerging literature suggests acceptable recurrence rates in tumors up to 7 cm.[10] Central tumors, diffuse/infiltrative morphology, and mutilfocality are more feasibly treated with transarterial therapy. Despite historical concerns over arterial chemoembolic therapy in the presence of portal vein thrombosis, recent data suggest that this is safe.[11] If downstaging to resectability/transplantation is a consideration, consultation with the surgical team may also provide insight into optimal therapy.

10.5.1 Technique

Considerable individual and institutional variation exists in the particular techniques used for both hepatic chemoembolization and percutaneous ablation. The techniques described hereafter are given as examples.

10.5.2 Preprocedure

Informed consent is obtained, with special attention paid to the risks of the particular procedure at hand. Prophylactic antibiotics are necessary given the possibility of bacteremia, infected biloma formation, and systemic sepsis after both transarterial therapy and ablation, particularly in this patient population with an increased incidence of prior biliary instrumentation. Multiple prophylactic antibiotic regimens have been described; it is important that the selected regimen cover typical skin flora as well as gram-negative organisms likely to colonize the biliary tract (**see the following list**).[12] Continuation of antibiotics is left to the discretion of the operator after evaluation of individual patients, with courses of 3 to 7 days being common and courses up to 14 days used in patients at particularly high risk. A bowel preparation regimen may reduce the risk of biliary infection.[13]

Possible Prophylactic Antibiotic Regimens

- 1.5 to 3 g intravenous (IV) ampicillin/sulbactam
- 1 g cefazolin IV + 500 mg metronidazole IV
- 1 gm ceftriaxone IV
- Levofloxacin 500 mg IV or ciprofloxacin 500 mg IV + 500 mg metronidazole IV (penicillin allergic)

Drugs Commonly Used to Treat Postembolization Pain, Nausea, and Malaise

- Dexamethasone 10 mg IV every 8 hours (pain and nausea)
- Ondansetron (Zofran, GlaxoSmithKline) 4 to 8 mg IV every 4 hours (nausea)
- Patient-controlled analgesic pumps
- Ofirmev (Cadence Pharmaceuticals) (acetaminophen 1 g) IV—*use with caution in liver disease*

Preprocedure imaging and laboratory values are again reviewed. IV hydration is administered in a standard fashion for the prophylaxis of contrast-induced nephropathy, and conscious sedation is administered as necessary. Given the high incidence of postembolization syndrome (> 80%), some advocate preprocedural administration of IV steroids, analgesics, and antiemetics, whereas others treat symptoms as needed. Refer to the following list for commonly used drugs and dosages extrapolated from systemic chemotherapeutic experience.

10.5.3 Transarterial Therapy

The equipment necessary is similar to diagnostic hepatic angiography and embolization performed for other tumors (**see** text box). Before the procedure begins, the team determines a plan of which liver locations to treat, level of injection (lobar, superselective, etc.), a drug, and a drug vehicle. Last-minute review of the patient's most recent imaging is invaluable to identify anomalous vessel origin, accessory arteries, parasitic arterial supply, and other arterial anomalies.

Equipment List For Hepatic Chemoembolization

Standard

- Ultrasound with high-frequency linear transducer
- Micropuncture (22 gauge) access set, with 0.018 wire and 3/5F transitional dilator.
- Power injector and tubing, loaded with low/iso-osmolar contrast
- 5F vascular sheath with pressurized heparinized saline flush and tubing (2 U/mL typically)
- 5F angiographic catheters—commonly used shapes include Cobra 2 (Terumo Manufacturing Corporation), SOS Omni (AngioDynamics)
- 0.035 to 0.038 in guidewires, Amplatz and Benson are typical choice
- Separate Mayo stand and tray with color-coded 3 mL injection syringes for chemotherapy
- Embolic material loaded with appropriate chemotherapy

Optional

- Microcatheter and microwire for tortuous hepatic arterial anatomy, small parasitic vessels, or subselective injection
- Femoral arterial closure device

Lobar versus more subselective injection remains at the discretion of the operator. The hypovascular nature, multicentricity, and infiltrative nature of the disease mean that lobar injection may be preferred for feasibility reasons in any event.

Transfemoral arterial access is obtained in the standard fashion, and the proper hepatic artery is selected with a 5F diagnostic catheter of the operator's choice. Microcatheter systems are typically reserved for more distal embolization or challenging anatomy. Angiography is performed as needed for confirmation of proper vessel selection and tumor identification and to ensure the catheter is placed beyond any potential sources of nontarget embolization. If one chooses subselective injection, correlation with preprocedural cross-sectional imaging and in-room cone beam computed tomography (CT) are helpful to ensure the appropriate arterial branch has been selected because lesions are often angiographically occult. Once the appropriate artery has been selected and the catheter/microcatheter is appropriately positioned, preparation for injection of chemotherapeutic drugs is begun (▶ Fig. 10.2**a, b**).

No chemotherapeutic agent is specifically approved by the Food and Drug Administration (FDA) for intra-arterial therapy of cholangiocarcinoma; usage of all current drugs is off label, and the optimal chemotherapeutic regimen has not been determined through randomized, controlled trials. Operators should refer to the manufacturer's instructions and be knowledgeable about the contraindications/toxicities regarding each chemotherapeutic drug before administration.

A variety of chemotherapeutic agents have been reported, including platinum agents, 5-fluorouracil (5-FU), gemcitabine, doxorubicin, and others, often in combination. Drug-eluting beads are a typical vehicle, with polyvinyl alcohol (PVA) and Gelfoam also being used. The following list provides a summary of recently reported drugs and dosages adapted from Ray et al.[14]

Chemotherapeutic Regimens Previously Described in Transarterial Therapy

- Irinotecan 200 mg.
- Mitomycin C 2 to 15 mg.
- Cisplatin 50 mg, 45 to 50 mg/m^2, 2 mg/kg.
- Oxaliplatin 50 mg, 85 to 100 mg/m^2.
- Doxorubicin 50 to 150 mg, 50 mg/m^2.
- 5-FU 450 mg/m^2.
- Gemcitabine 1,000 to 2,250 mg/m^2.

Adapted from Ray, et al.

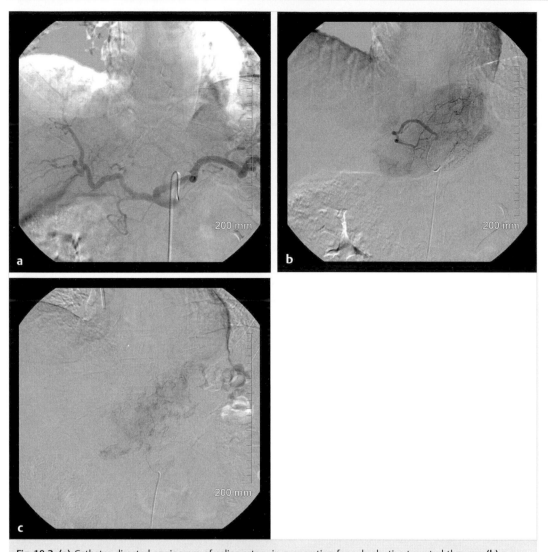

Fig. 10.2 (a) Catheter-directed angiogram of celiac artery in preparation for subselective-targeted therapy. **(b)** Catheter-directed angiogram of replaced left hepatic artery off the left gastric artery demonstrates tumor blush. **(c)** Postembolization angiogram after therapy with drug-eluting beads demonstrates relatively gentle embolization staining.

Ideally, if drug-eluting beads are used as a vehicle, they will have been soaked in the chemotherapeutic preparation for at least 2 to 4 hours. The supernatant is removed, and the beads are reconstituted with a 50/50 mix of saline and contrast to maximize bead suspension. Handling protocols for chemotherapeutic drugs will vary institutionally; however, most use a separate tray, syringe set, and gloves to avoid cross contamination, with proper disposal of agents in a designated waste container.

Injection is performed slowly under intermittent fluoroscopy to avoid reflux and subsequent nontarget embolization. Injection continues until one of two end points, either complete injection of the planned chemotherapeutic dose, or 2- to 5-beat stasis (► Fig. 10.2c). Some authors have cautioned against complete stasis in hepatic chemoembolization, due to concern for increased risk of necrosis and collateral liver damage.

Radioembolization is performed in a similar manner, with pretreatment planning and determination of shunt fraction by lobar injection of technetium-99 m macroaggregated serum albumin (^{99m}Tc-MAA) injection into the hepatic artery, and subsequent gamma camera imaging. Nontarget embolization has more serious consequences with radioembolization, as such collateral branches are typically permanently embolized with coils prior to the MAA study. Radioembolization is typically performed in a lobar fashion, with bilobar disease being treated in separate sessions and sequential fashion.

10.5.4 Ablative Therapy

In percutaneous ablative therapy, the target lesion and the device must both be readily visible to ensure a complete ablation and avoidance of collateral damage. CT and ultrasound (US) guidance can both be used. Given the variability, it seems prudent that the procedure be performed in the CT suite with an ultrasound machine, so that both modalities can be used. Multiple methods for tumor ablation are currently FDA approved, including radiofrequency, microwave, cryoablation, and, most recently, irreversible electroporation. No technique has been shown to be superior to any others; however, the largest experience in the literature is radiofrequency ablation (RFA). Regardless of the modality, the operator should be proficient with the apparatus and probe selection. A probe or array of probes should be selected that is sufficient to ablate the tumor itself and an adjacent area of at least 0.5 cm, preferably 1 cm adjacent tissue while avoiding normal structures. After local anesthesia, conscious sedation, and a skin incision, the apparatus is advanced to the planned location. If the tumor and adjacent structures are poorly visible, using an alternative imaging modality can be helpful, or under CT a single contrast injection can be used, assuming minimum subsequent patient movement. When optimal probe position is obtained, the device is activated as necessary. Tract ablation during probe removal is also sometimes performed as a prophylactic measure against seeding the tract with tumor cells. The latter also helps preclude bleeding complications. A postprocedure scan is obtained with a focus on possible complications and the adequacy of the ablation zone.

10.6 Postprocedure Management

Routine postsedation recovery followed by overnight admission in the hospital is standard for symptomatic management and evaluation for complications; however, outpatient management is being proposed with radioembolization.[15] Medical consultations are obtained as necessary. Barring any immediate complications, patients are typically discharged in the next day with clinic follow up in 1 to 2 weeks, with repeat laboratory work.

Follow-up imaging is typically obtained in 4 to 6 weeks, with imaging typically performed after the final session, if multiple treatment sessions are planned. Additional therapy sessions are planned based on tumor response and patient tolerance of therapy, with studies showing good tolerance to subsequent therapy.

10.7 Side Effects and Complications

Liver-directed therapy has a low morbidity and mortality rate; nevertheless, complications do occur, and meticulous preprocedure patient selection can help to minimize these. Complications and side effects of liver-directed therapy for cholangiocarcinoma are similar to those performed for other indications.

Abscess formation in patients with preexisting biliary enteric anastomoses is high; patient instructions and vigilant postprocedural care should reflect this.[16] When they occur, abscesses/infected bilomas are treated with percutaneous drainage and systemic antibiotic therapy, typically with good results.

As with any embolic therapy, nontarget embolization is a risk, with postembolization cholecystitis, pleural effusions resulting from diaphragm embolization, and gastritis all having been reported.[17] These conditions are typically managed successfully with conservative measures, but early clinical detection is paramount. Other complications reported include arterial dissection, injury, puncture site complications, and, rarely, portal venous thrombosis.

10.8 Clinical Data and Outcomes

Liver-directed therapy for cholangiocarcinoma is a relatively new treatment modality, and progress is constant. Several observational studies of transarterial chemotherapy and radioembolization have been performed, with comparison to historical survival data.

10.8.1 Chemoembolization

Chemoembolization for intrahepatic cholangiocarcinoma has been the most studied liver-directed treatment modality. The body of literature is promising, but studies have been limited to small enrollments, variable drugs, and varying patient populations.

A recent meta-analysis by Ray et al included 542 patients from 2005 to 2012, with 76.8% having stable disease or response by imaging criteria posttreatment, and conferring an estimated survival benefit of 2 to 7 months versus historical controls using only systemic chemotherapy.[14] A multicenter retrospective review from Hyder et al that included 198 patients from five major hepatobiliary centers also demonstrated stable disease or response by imaging in about 75% of patients with an overall survival of 13 months, increased from historical controls of systemic therapy.[18]

10.8.2 Radioembolization

Radioembolization shows promise in the treatment of intrahepatic cholangiocarcinoma. A recent retrospective study included 46 patients with up to 15.6-month survival in certain patient subtypes, with an additional 11% (5 of 46) becoming resectable.[4]

Pearls

- *Patient selection is crucial.* Careful history, determination of performance status, and a careful review of imaging can go a long way toward determining optimal therapy and minimizing complications.
- *Set appropriate patient expectations.* A variety of liver-directed therapies have shown promise in prolonging survival and achieving local tumor control; however, none has been shown to be a "magic bullet" or cure.
- *Follow the patient clinically.* Clinic visits are crucial to assess for early complications, develop relationships with patients and providers, and plan future treatment.
- *Carefully review diagnostic imaging.* Variant anatomy readily visible by cross-sectional imaging can be difficult or impossible to identify angiographically.
- *Patients with a biliary enteric anastomosis have high rates (≥ 25%) of infected biloma formation.* Antibiotic prophylaxis and bowel preparation may reduce this risk.

10.8.3 Ablation

Various ablative methods have been used as treatment of intrahepatic cholangiocarcinoma. Of the modalities, the most studied is radiofrequency ablation. Several small (< 10) retrospective studies have been performed at multiple institutions and suggest an increased survival, with median survival up to 33 months.[19]

References

[1] Amini N, Ejaz A, Spolverato G, Kim Y, Herman JM, Pawlik TM. Temporal trends in liver-directed therapy of patients with intrahepatic cholangiocarcinoma in the United States: a population-based analysis. J Surg Oncol 2014; 110(2): 163–170

[2] Valle J, Wasan H, Palmer DH et al. ABC-02 Trial Investigators. Cisplatin plus gemcitabine versus gemcitabine for biliary tract cancer. N Engl J Med 2010; 362(14): 1273–1281

[3] Okusaka T, Nakachi K, Fukutomi A et al. Gemcitabine alone or in combination with cisplatin in patients with biliary tract cancer: a comparative multicentre study in Japan. Br J Cancer 2010; 103(4): 469–474

[4] Mouli S, Memon K, Baker T et al. Yttrium-90 radioembolization for intrahepatic cholangiocarcinoma: safety, response, and survival analysis. J Vasc Interv Radiol 2013; 24(8): 1227–1234

[5] Razumilava N, Gores GJ. Classification, diagnosis, and management of cholangiocarcinoma. Clin Gastroenterol Hepatol 2013; 11(1): 13–21.e1, quiz e3–e4

[6] Khan SA, Davidson BR, Goldin RD et al. British Society of Gastroenterology. Guidelines for the diagnosis and treatment of cholangiocarcinoma: an update. Gut 2012; 61(12): 1657–1669

[7] Robles R, Sánchez-Bueno F, Ramírez P, Brusadin R, Parrilla P. Liver transplantation for hilar cholangiocarcinoma. World J Gastroenterol 2013; 19(48): 9209–9215

[8] Rea DJ, Heimbach JK, Rosen CB et al. Liver transplantation with neoadjuvant chemoradiation is more effective than resection for hilar cholangiocarcinoma. Ann Surg 2005; 242 (3): 451–458, discussion 458–461

[9] Park SY, Kim JH, Won HJ, Shin YM, Kim PN. Radiofrequency ablation of hepatic metastases after curative resection of extrahepatic cholangiocarcinoma. Am J Roentgenol 2011; 197 (6): W1129–34

[10] Haidu M, Dobrozemsky G, Schullian P et al. Stereotactic radiofrequency ablation of unresectable intrahepatic cholangiocarcinomas: a retrospective study. Cardiovasc Intervent Radiol 2012; 35(5): 1074–1082

[11] Chern M-C, Chuang VP, Liang C-T, Lin ZH, Kuo T-M. Transcatheter arterial chemoembolization for advanced hepatocellular carcinoma with portal vein invasion: safety, efficacy, and prognostic factors. J Vasc Interv Radiol 2014; 25(1): 32–40

[12] Venkatesan AM, Kundu S, Sacks D et al. Society of Interventional Radiology Standards of Practice Committee. Practice guidelines for ault antibiotic prophylaxis during vascular and interventional radiology procedures. Written by the Standards of Practice Committee for the Society of Interventional Radiology and Endorsed by the Cardiovascular Interventional Radiological Society of Europe and Canadian In-

terventional Radiology Association [corrected]. J Vasc Interv Radiol 2010; 21(11): 1611–1630, quiz 1631

[13] Patel S, Tuite CM, Mondschein JI, Soulen MC. Effectiveness of an aggressive antibiotic regimen for chemoembolization in patients with previous biliary intervention. J Vasc Interv Radiol 2006; 17(12): 1931–1934

[14] Ray CE, Jr, Edwards A, Smith MT et al. Metaanalysis of survival, complications, and imaging response following chemotherapy-based transarterial therapy in patients with unresectable intrahepatic cholangiocarcinoma. J Vasc Interv Radiol 2013; 24(8): 1218–1226

[15] Gates VL, Marshall KG, Salzig K, Williams M, Lewandowski RJ, Salem R. Outpatient single-session yttrium-90 glass microsphere radioembolization. J Vasc Interv Radiol 2014; 25 (2): 266–270

[16] Kim W, Clark TW, Baum RA, Soulen MC. Risk factors for liver abscess formation after hepatic chemoembolization. J Vasc Interv Radiol 2001; 12(8): 965–968

[17] Clark TWI. Complications of hepatic chemoembolization. Semin Intervent Radiol 2006; 23(2): 119–125

[18] Hyder O, Marsh JW, Salem R et al. Intra-arterial therapy for advanced intrahepatic cholangiocarcinoma: a multi-institutional analysis. Ann Surg Oncol 2013; 20(12): 3779–3786

[19] Fu Y, Yang W, Wu W, Yan K, Xing BC, Chen MH. Radiofrequency ablation in the management of unresectable intrahepatic cholangiocarcinoma. J Vasc Interv Radiol 2012; 23 (5): 642–649

Chapter 11

Bone Tumors: Ablation

11 Bone Tumors: Ablation

Matthew R. Callstrom, and A. Nicholas Kurup

11.1 Introduction

Approximately 70% of the 1 million people that die each year in the United States due to cancer have breast, lung, or prostate cancer, and approximately one-half of these, or 350,000 people, will die with bone metastases.[1] Although bone metastases can indicate a poor prognosis with a median survival of 3 years or less, many patients now live many years with metastatic cancer, with 5 to 40% of patients alive at 5 years, dependent on tumor histology and burden.[2,3] Quality of life is an important consideration for patients, and unfortunately bone-related cancer pain is often undertreated, with nearly 80% of patients experiencing severe pain before a sufficient palliative treatment plan is initiated.[4]

A multidisciplinary team that can offer optimal analgesic therapy, radiation therapy (RT), surgery, hormonal and chemotherapies, and focal image-guided ablation therapies provides the most effective management of patients with painful skeletal metastases. The front-line therapy for treatment of painful metastatic skeletal disease is external beam radiation therapy (EBRT). This treatment is at least partially effective for 50 to 80% of patients, with complete pain response in 50 to 60%.[5] Although many patients experience complete or partial relief of pain following RT, the time to pain relief can be extended, with the median relief of pain achieved in 3 to 7 weeks.[6] Although RT results in an initial reduction in pain for the majority of patients, at least for a period of weeks, 20 to 30% of patients do not experience pain relief, and a majority that had complete or partial response experience pain recurrence.[7,8,9,10,11,12] Retreatment is possible for many patients, but for many patients that experience minimal or transient relief of pain following EBRT, further treatment is not offered due to lack of response or due to limitations in normal tissue tolerance.

Surgery is generally reserved for lesions at great risk for fracture or following fracture, or for spinal metastases causing neurological compromise. Systemic therapies, including chemotherapy, hormonal therapy, radiopharmaceuticals, and bisphosphonates, in combination with opioid and nonsteroidal analgesics, can be effective treatment for widespread skeletal metastases. However, these are not generally offered for focal painful metastases because pain due to metastatic skeletal disease is often refractory. Radiopharmaceuticals are often effective in patients with diffuse painful bony metastases, but are not considered standard of care for patients with isolated, painful lesions. For many patients with focal painful metastatic disease that have failed EBRT, analgesics remain the only alternative treatment option that is typically offered. Many patients will limit their use of these medications due to significant side effects, such as constipation, nausea, and sedation.

Increasingly minimally invasive, percutaneous thermal ablation techniques have found clinical effectiveness for palliation for patients with limited skeletal metastases. These treatments use image guidance to place ablative devices into focal metastatic tumors. These ablation methods include the use of radiofrequency ablation (RFA), cryoablation, laser ablation, microwave ablation, and magnetic resonance–guided focused ultrasound (MRgFUS). In addition, patients at risk for fracture due to metastases in axially loaded locations (e.g., vertebral bodies and the periacetabular region) may benefit from percutaneous cementoplasty. Of these minimally invasive methods, RFA and cryoablation have been the most studied.

More recently, percutaneous ablation has been used to achieve local tumor control in patients with limited metastatic disease involving the musculoskeletal system. These patients with oligometastatic disease benefit from cost-effective minimally invasive treatments while avoiding the morbidity of surgery and, if new disease presents, retreatment is possible.[13,14,15]

11.2 Indications

Patients that benefit from focal ablative therapy for painful metastatic disease report moderate or severe pain, typically ≥ 4 of 10 for the worst pain in a 24-hour period. Patients with lower reported pain scores are not usually treated because it is difficult to improve on mild pain, and type of pain can usually be managed by oral analgesics. An important consideration is that pain should be limited to one or two sites, and the pain should correlate with a corresponding abnormality evident with cross-sectional imaging. For patients with multiple painful tumors or otherwise diffuse disease, identifying critical sites for treatment can be difficult, and it is also not practical to treat more than two or three sites in a typical treatment session. Often, multiple painful tumors are better treated with a systemic rather than focal approach. Tumors that are well suited to ablative therapy are most typically osteolytic or mixed osteolytic/ osteoblastic in nature or otherwise composed of soft tissue. Osteoblastic lesions can also be treated, and this is commonly encountered in limited breast or prostate cancer. Treatment of osteoblastic disease requires the use of bone access devices or drills for access to the target tumor, and the ablation system used should be able to penetrate the sclerotic bone effectively. Adjacent critical structures, such as motor nerves or bowel, should be displaced using fluid or other displacement maneuvers to avoid collateral injury. Typically, a 1 cm margin between the target tumor and nearest critical structure is preferred, although operator experience and neural monitoring can allow safe treatment of tumors in closer proximity to these normal tissues. Patients at risk for fracture or risk for progression of fracture due to skeletal metastatic disease should be considered for surgery. If the tumor in question is in an axially loading location, augmentation with cement following ablation may also be helpful.

11.3 Contraindications

The most common technical contraindication for treatment of metastases involving bone or soft tissue is inaccessibility of the target tumor from a percutaneous approach. Close proximity of adjacent normal critical structures may also preclude ablation treatment. Safe treatment of tumors near normal critical structures can be achieved, although careful device placement, tissue displacement or other protective maneuvers, neural monitoring, and careful ablation monitoring are necessary. Absolute contraindications include uncorrectable bleeding diatheses and patient incompatibility with the level of anesthesia required to perform the procedure. Active infection is a strong relative contraindication, given the potential to seed necrotic, ablated tissue with circulating micro-organisms. Relative contraindications include widespread skeletal metastases, for which a systemic approach would be more appropriate, and mildly painful metastases, which are more suitable for analgesic medication and inconsistently respond to ablation.

11.4 Patient Selection and Preprocedural Workup

Patient history and preprocedural imaging are important to characterize the target tumors and to correlate with a patient's symptoms. Imaging acquired at the time of presentation allows deliberate consideration of the potential risks versus the benefits of ablation. This imaging is also useful for planning adjunctive maneuvers or additional monitoring that may be of benefit during the procedure. The type of preprocedural imaging employed is dependent on the extent and site of disease. For patients that present with focal painful metastatic disease, computed tomography (CT) is often the modality of choice to determine technical feasibility. Because CT is frequently used to guide and monitor the ablation procedure, it is useful to demonstrate the target tumor and adjacent structures in treatment planning. Patients with disease involving the spine often benefit from the use of magnetic resonance imaging (MRI) to determine the full extent of disease, such as volume of disease within a vertebral body, involvement of adjacent vertebral bodies, and the presence of epidural or perineural involvement that may not be evident with CT imaging. MRI is also helpful in treatment of patients with oligometastatic disease because MRI more closely approximates the clinical, rather than the gross, extent of tumor burden.[16] Positron emission tomography (PET) with CT (PET-CT) offers the added benefit of demonstrating metabolic activity, which can add value for targeting tumors that have ill-defined borders on CT or previously treated/irradiated tumors that show surrounding bony changes (sclerosis or lucency) related to treatment effect rather than tumor infiltration. PET-CT is also helpful for staging patients with oligometastatic disease, and treatment goals are impacted by unexpected metastatic disease not previously identified.

11.5 Technique

11.5.1 Radiofrequency Ablation

RFA is the most commonly used percutaneous thermal tumor ablation method and also the most used method for treatment of painful metastatic disease involving bone. RFA can be performed with either general anesthesia or, with experience, moderate conscious sedation. A general anesthetic is more commonly used because the level of focal pain during the RFA treatment using monopolar systems can be greater than most patients can tolerate, even with moderate conscious sedation, and because the procedures can be long, lasting more than an hour depending on the size of the target lesion. More recently available bipolar systems used in treatment of metastatic skeletal disease do not cause pain during ablation, and moderate sedation is well tolerated. However, the use of general anesthesia allows the procedure to be performed without the additional necessity of providing supportive care for the patient as is required with conscious sedation. Less complex lesions (i.e., superficial, small, easily accessible, predominantly osteolytic or soft tissue lesions remote from normal vital structures) may be readily treated with patients under moderate sedation with sufficient local analgesia. Epidural spinal anesthesia or focal nerve blocks are often helpful to ease the pain during the immediate postablation period. If an epidural catheter is employed, the duration of use is typically for a 12- to 24-hour period following the RFA treatment using a monopolar system. Prior to removal of the catheter, it is helpful to halt the medication delivery for a trial period of several hours. If the patient's pain has returned to the pretreatment level or is improved, the catheter can be removed. Most patients are observed overnight in the hospital to provide adequate pain control or to allow transition and modification of oral analgesic medication dosage. The patient is usually discharged with oral opioid analgesics for mild to moderate discomfort or pain.

For treatment of patients with tumors adjacent to important neural structures, intravenous conscious sedation permits intraprocedural focused neurological physical examination as a means of monitoring vulnerable neural structures. With the use of bipolar RFA systems, the patient can provide feedback when the ablation zone approaches neural structures because focal pain precedes nerve injury. Alternatively, use of intravenous anesthesia allows evoked potential monitoring for nerve monitoring with cases adjacent to motor nerves or the spinal cord.[16] Following ablation, instillation of long-acting local anesthetic along the periosteum may diminish postprocedural pain.

RFA procedures should be performed under appropriate cross-sectional imaging guidance and monitoring. Fluoroscopy may be useful for portions of the procedure, in particular for tumors contained in vertebral bodies. Fluoroscopy may also be used for treatment of patients with bipolar RFA systems as the end-point of the procedure is time and temperature patient pain, and thus not dependent on imaging. However, cross-sectional imaging is usually beneficial to carefully avoid critical structures and to estimate the treatment coverage for complex tumors. Ultrasound (US) may be used for superficial, predominantly soft tissue lesions, particularly in the chest wall or extremities. CT is the most commonly used modality for guidance, given its widespread availability for most practices and typical excellent delineation of the target tumor and surrounding structures. MRI possibly provides the best imaging for ablation monitoring with superior tumor depiction in bone; however, the MRI suite is a difficult environment for most procedures. Also, MRI-compatible devices remain limited, and when they are available, artifacts associated with devices can obscure the target tumor. Treatment of tumors involving bone or tumors adjacent to bone require percutaneous placement of RFA electrodes into the target tumor. RFA electrodes may be placed directly into soft tissue metastases or osteolytic skeletal metastases with destroyed or thin overlying cortex. To penetrate osteoblastic metastases or to access tumors deep to intact cortical bone, bone access devices may be required. These include manually operated bone biopsy needles or powered bone drills.

The targeted area of ablation includes the bone–tumor interface or the entire tumor, rather than simply targeting the central portions of the mass. Treatment of the tumor boundary is necessary in order to achieve destruction of likely sites of origin of the pain, including nerve endings and involved periosteum (▶ Fig. 11.1). Monopolar multitined electrodes or cool-tip electrodes, or bipolar electrode systems can be used, depending on physician preference and experience and device availability. A single ablation is typically performed for lesions < 3 cm in diameter, and the time of ablation is typically 5 to 10 minutes at the target temperature of 100°C, or until tissue impedance limits energy delivery to the target tissue. For larger lesions, overlapping ablations are performed with the goal of treating the entire bone–tumor interface, with the time of ablation again typically 5 to 10 minutes at the target temperature of 100°C or until tissue impedance limits energy delivery to the target tissue.

The target tumor should be isolated or adjacent critical structures displaced from the anticipated ablation zone to avoid injury. Multiple methods can be used to reduce the risk of collateral thermal damage of adjacent normal structures. This can typically be accomplished through careful patient positioning or displacement of tissues using fluid (hydrodisplacement), balloons, or gas (carbon dioxide). For example, sterile water (usually 5% dextrose in water [D5W] with the use of RFA to prevent the risk of conduction of energy with buffered fluids) can be injected through a needle to displace loops of bowel away from a target lesion (▶ Fig. 11.2). The fluid can be used with or without the addition of dilute iodinated contrast contrast

material (1:50). Thermal monitoring provides feedback during an RFA procedure with placement of a temperature-sensing probe adjacent to a critical structure (▶ Fig. 11.3). Because the margin of the RF ablation cannot be accurately visualized with CT or US imaging (MRI may allow visualization), this thermal monitoring avoids unexpected elevations of temperature and potential injury to adjacent normal structures.

11.5.2 Cryoablation

Cryoablation has emerged as an exceptional treatment method for palliation of painful metastatic disease involving bone and soft tissue outside of the liver and lung.[17,18,19,20,21,22] Although cryoablation has a long history of successful treatment of neoplasms in various locations in the body, including prostate, kidney, liver, and lung, early systems were not insulated and could only be used in an intraoperative setting. With the advent of well-insulated cryoprobes and the use of Joule–Thomson ports using room-temperature, high-pressure argon gas as a cooling source, percutaneous systems became possible. As the argon gas passes from approximately 3,000 psi in a thin tube within sealed cryoprobes to the relatively larger sealed chamber at the tip of the probe at atmospheric pressure, the gas undergoes rapid cooling to achieve temperatures < −100°C. At the cellular level, intracellular and extracellular fluid freezes, and tissue destruction results from cell membrane disruption by ice crystals, cellular dehydration, and vascular thrombosis. Temperatures below −20 to −40°C are necessary to achieve complete cell death, usually present within 3 to 5 mm of the

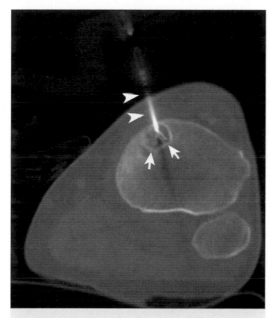

Fig. 11.1 Noncontrast computed tomography demonstrating an osteolytic tumor involving the anterior tibia. A multitined radiofrequency ablation electrode *(arrowheads)* is deployed along the bone tumor interface *(arrows)*.

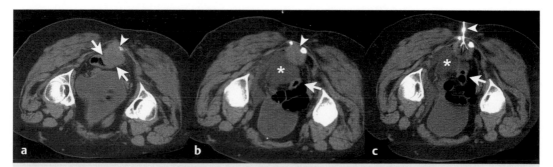

Fig. 11.2 **(a)** Prone contrast-enhanced computed tomographic (CT) image showing a soft tissue osteolytic tumor *(arrowhead)* involving the low sacrum with tumor abutting *(arrows)* the adjacent rectum. **(b)** Prone noncontrast CT image with 5% dextrose in water *(asterisk)* displacing the rectum *(arrow)* from the target tumor *(arrowhead)*. **(c)** Prone noncontrast CT image with a multitined radiofrequency ablation electrode *(arrowhead)* deployed in the sacral tumor with the rectum *(arrow)* adequately displaced with the use of water *(asterisk)*.

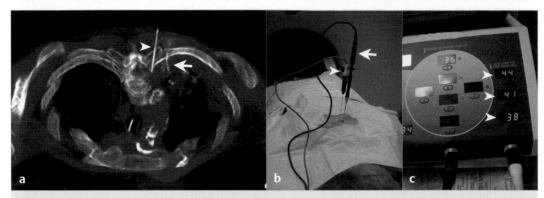

Fig. 11.3 **(a)** Thick-section prone noncontrast computed tomographic (CT) image showing a metastatic tumor involving the vertebral body with soft tissue extension along the adjacent rib. A thermocouple *(arrowhead)* is placed adjacent to the involved pedicle, and a multitined radiofrequency ablation (RFA) electrode placed into a portion of the tumor located in the soft tissue deep to the rib with tines deployed *(arrow)*. **(b)** Photo of a thermocouple (arrowhead) and RFA electrode *(arrow)* at the time of a paraspinal ablation procedure. **(c)** RFA controller with maximal temperatures along the thermocouple *(arrowheads)*.

edge of the ice ball.[23,24] Current generation systems can generate an ice ball, using a single probe, of ~ 3.5 cm diameter. Infusion of helium gas into the cryoprobes, which has a Joule–Thomson coefficient opposite that of argon gas, results in tissue heating. Multiple cryoprobes are used simultaneously to generate confluent ice, with the size dependent on the number of cryoprobes, with > 8 cm diameter ice balls readily achieved. The shape of the ablation zone can be controlled through varied geometry of probe placement. Although a freeze–thaw–freeze cycle is necessary to ensure complete cell death, the overall procedure times are not prohibitively long because large or complex tumors can be treated without the time-consuming overlapping ablations needed with other ablation techniques. In addition, in consideration of achieving local tumor control, synchronous ablation with several cryoprobes eliminates residual disease at the ablation interfaces that can result from performing overlapping sequential ablations.[25]

Fortunately, the ablation zone that is generated with cryoablation is visualized as a discrete low-attenuation area with noncontrast CT imaging or as a low-signal area with MRI. The edge of the ice ball corresponds to 0°C, and tissue outside this boundary is not at risk for injury.[26] The CT environment is readily available for intervention in most practices, and wide-bore systems are also becoming more common, allowing placement of ablation devices while retaining the ability to image patients without great difficulty. It is

possible to image thermal changes with MRI, and some practices are overcoming challenges of performing ablation procedures in this environment while benefiting from improved tumor conspicuity for guidance and ablation monitoring.

Two cryoablation manufacturers produce clinical systems, the Endocare Cryocare System (HealthTronics, Inc.) and the Visual-ICE or SeedNet Cryoablation System (Galil Medical, Inc.). The Endocare System uses two different sizes of insulated cryoprobes measuring 2.4 mm (13-gauge) and 1.7 mm (16-gauge) in diameter. The Galil system employs 1.5 mm (17-gauge; insulated IceRod + and uninsulated IceSphere and IceSeed) cryoprobes (similar MRI-compatible cryoprobes are available) as well as 2.4 mm IceEdge cryoprobes. The Endocare system has 8 separately controlled channels (8 total), whereas the Galil system has 10 separately controlled channels with two ports on each channel (20 total). These systems generate ice balls of various geometries; for example, the Endocare Perc-24 produces an ice ball up to 3.7 cm in diameter and 5.7 cm in length along the probe shaft.

Using typical sterile preparation, cryoprobes are introduced through a skin nick under CT, US, or MRI guidance. Operator experience is necessary to prescribe the placement of cryoprobes, although a general guideline is to place probes within 1 cm of the tumor boundary and at an interprobe spacing of 2 cm within the target tumor. A single freeze–thaw–freeze cycle is performed for each lesion, with typical times for these cycles of 10 minutes–

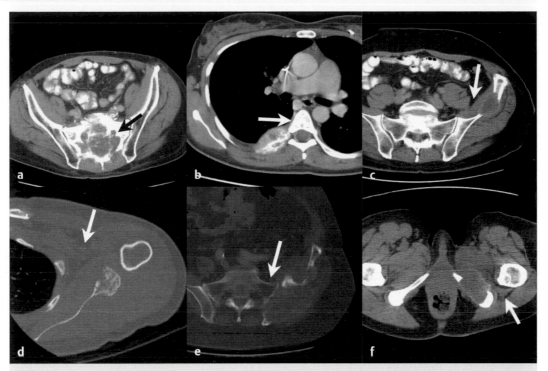

Fig. 11.4 Common anatomical areas of concern for ablation of bone and soft tissue metastases. **(a)** Destructive tumor involving the sacrum extending along the posterior aspect of the left S1 neural foramen *(arrow)*. **(b)** Paravertebral mass ablations that extend along the lateral margin of the vertebral body may encompass the segmental artery *(arrow)* and potentially the feeding vessel of the artery of Adamkiewicz. **(c)** Computed tomographic image with a tumor involving the left ilium. The femoral nerve is located along the posterolateral aspect of the psoas muscle *(arrow)*. **(d)** Mixed osteolytic and osteoblastic tumor involving the scapula with the brachial plexus visualized anteriorly *(arrow)*. **(e)** A metastasis involves the left iliac bone extending near to the adjacent lumbar plexus located along the anterior aspect of the sacrum *(arrow)*. **(f)** A metastasis in the left inferior pubic ramus in close proximity to the sciatic nerve *(arrow)*.

8 minutes–10 minutes, respectively. Shorter or longer times are often used for the freezing portions of the cycle, depending on the adequacy of coverage of the lesion and the proximity of adjacent critical structures. The rate of ice-ball growth can also be controlled by reducing the percentage of time that gas flows through the probes from 100% to as low as 20%. Most commonly, noncontrast CT imaging is performed approximately every 2 to 4 minutes throughout the freezing portions of the cycle, with body window and level settings (W400, L40) to monitor the growth of the ice ball. Typically, the cryoprobes are placed along the long axis of the tumor and at an angle to allow slow growth of the ice in the direction of adjacent critical structures. Identification of adjacent critical structures at the time of the procedure and employment of protective maneuvers is commonly performed. Understanding the path of major motor nerves and the artery of Adamkiewicz is helpful for the

performance of safe ablation procedures.[16] As illustrated in ► Fig. 11.4, these structures can be clearly identified and avoided at the time of the ablation procedure. An example of the use of cryoablation in the proximity of the obturator nerve is shown in ► Fig. 11.5. A soft tissue and bony metastasis involving the pubic bone was treated with four cryoprobes placed through the tumor to generate ice that matched the shape of the complex tumor. The evolution of the ice ball showed complete coverage of the tumor while avoiding the adjacent obturator nerve.

Following completion of the second freeze cycle, cryoprobes are warmed by switching to helium gas until temperatures within the treated tissue are > 20°C. The cryoprobes can be withdrawn at this point, although continued warming of the probes over a period of approximately 10 minutes may result in a reduced risk of hematoma formation.

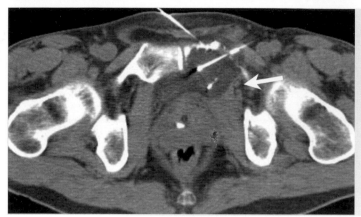

Fig. 11.5 Cryoablation of a renal cell metastasis adjacent to the obturator nerve. Multiple cryoprobes placed in the pubic bone with ice encompassing the target tumor avoiding the obturator nerve *(arrow)*.

11.5.3 Cementoplasty for Metastatic Disease

Vertebroplasty of benign vertebral body fractures is usually performed with fluoroscopy. This approach allows careful monitoring of the distribution of the cement to avoid cement leakage into veins, epidural space, and neural foramina. Similar considerations are important when cementoplasty is performed outside the spine. CT fluoroscopy allows rapid placement of bone biopsy needles into the targeted tumor via access sites from the previously performed ablation procedure. In order to address the need for careful monitoring of the spread of cement into often large, treated tumors while avoiding leakage, it is necessary to modify the CT data acquisition parameters to provide more rapid and broader monitoring for administration of the bone cement. Typical parameters employed include the use of CT body windows with CT fluoroscopy slice thickness of 4.8 mm and a step of 5 mm.

In order to avoid leakage of cement through bone access sites generated during the ablation portion of the procedure, the same number of bone biopsy needles is used to access the tracts used in the ablation procedure. The tumor site can be accessed with 13- or 11-gauge Osteo-Site M2 needles (Cook Medical) or an 11-gauge AVAflex curved injection needle (Cardinal Health) can be used to access the tumor site. Ten or 20 mL of Ava-Tex Radiopaque Bone Cement (Cardinal Health) is then prepared and administered within 12 to 15 minutes using a vertebroplasty injector set (Duro-Ject, Cook Medical) with intermittent monitoring with CT fluoroscopy. The cement is anchored into intact medullary bone either deep to the tumor or when withdrawing the cement delivery system. It may be of benefit to withdraw the inner stylet of needles not used for injecting cement to allow venting of necrotic tumor during the delivery of cement. For example, a patient with an osteolytic lung metastasis involving the right periacetabular ilium was treated with cryoablation followed by cementoplasty (▶ Fig. 11.6). The cementoplasty procedure was performed 3 days following the cryoablation. Although the cementoplasty can be performed following the ablation procedure once the ice ball has melted, thawing of the ice ball takes time as a function of the size of the ablation volume, and waiting for tumor necrosis may be of benefit for the cementoplasty procedure. Following the combination treatment, the patient had relief of pain and improved quality of life with improved ambulation.

11.6 Postprocedure Management and Follow-up Evaluation

Immediate postprocedural pain is typically treated with IV fentanyl (Sublimaze, Abbott Laboratories) and midazolam (Versed, American Pharmaceutical Partners). For patients with persistent pain, oral analgesics or a patient-controlled analgesia unit can be used and the dose titrated to provide adequate pain relief.

For patients with metastatic musculoskeletal disease, the need for posttreatment imaging is based on the indications for treatment. For patients that are treated for palliation of pain or to prevent fracture through the combined use with cementoplasty, pain response and clinical performance status are the most important parameters to monitor. Follow-up imaging for these patients is typically not necessary unless pain

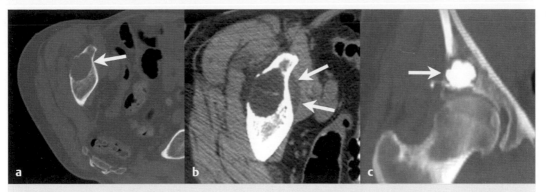

Fig. 11.6 Cryoablation and cementoplasty of an osteolytic lung metastasis involving the right periacetabular ilium. **(a)** Noncontrast axial computed tomography (CT) demonstrates an osteolytic metastasis *(arrow)* involving the right supraperiacetabular ilium. **(b)** Axial noncontrast CT image obtained immediately following removal of the cryoprobes demonstrates an ice ball encompassing the tumor with extension into the adjacent soft tissues *(arrows)*. **(c)** Coronal reformatted noncontrast CT following cementoplasty shows adequate filling of the osteolytic metastasis *(arrow)*.

symptoms or clinical performance change during the follow-up. If there is recurrent pain, CT or MRI can be performed to correlate with focal findings and to determine the need for repeat ablation treatment.

For patients that are treated with the goal of local tumor control in the presence of oligometastases, the necessary frequency of imaging following image-guided ablation is related to the natural history of the treated metastases and anticipated rates of progression. The patient should undergo a contrast-enhanced CT or MRI examination immediately following ablation and approximately 3 months after the treatment to document ablation of all viable tumor. Typically it is appropriate to perform CT or MRI at 3- to 6-month intervals in subsequent follow-up. PET-CT imaging may also be employed if appropriate, based on tumor histology and clinical indication. Clinical factors may influence the choice of imaging (e.g., pacemaker precluding MRI or contrast agent allergy or renal insufficiency precluding CT).

11.6.1 Follow-up Clinical Status

Evaluation of each patient's clinical status should be performed with at least the same frequency as follow-up imaging. These assessments should record the patient's general medical condition, including clinical and functional status. Pain relief, such as measured by the Brief Pain Inventory (BPI), and analgesia usage should be documented. The BPI is a validated numeric scale for the evaluation of pain in cancer patients.[27,28] In the BPI, patients are asked to rate their worst, least, and average pain in the past 24 hours, with allowed responses ranging from 0 to 10 (0 = no pain, 10 = pain as bad as you can imagine). Relief of pain secondary to the RFA procedure or to pain medications is scored on a scale of 0% (no relief) to 100% (complete relief). Pain interference with daily living is evaluated with questions concerning general activity, mood, walking ability, normal work, relations with other people, sleep, and enjoyment of life, also on a 0 to 10 scale (0 = no interference, 10 = completely interferes). Physical exam findings, such as muscle atrophy, should be documented and compared to pretreatment findings. Any late complications possibly related to image-guided ablation, including fracture, infection, nerve damage, transient bowel or bladder incontinence, and skin burn should be captured.

11.7 Side Effects and Complications

Complications from ablation of musculoskeletal tumors include the most common injuries also experienced from other types of ablation, including infection and bleeding. The most common serious complications specific to musculoskeletal ablation are related to thermal injury of adjacent neural structures.[16] Nerve injury may result from exposure of the nerve to temperatures of 44 to 45° C or higher when using heat-based ablation systems or 10°C or lower when using cryoablation. Ablation of a sensory nerve can result in altered sensation, such as dysesthesia or paresthesia, or lack of sensation in the distribution of the affected

Table 11.1 Patients treated with radiofrequency ablation in two prospective multicenter trials

Trial	Goetz et al[30,31]	Dupuy et al[32]
No. patients	62	55
Female/male	22/40	26/29
Age, mean (range)	64 (range 28–88)	62 (range 34–85)
Tumor type (number)		
Renal cancer	14	10
Colorectal cancer	12	10
Lung cancer	4	17
Breast cancer	4	4
Other	28	14
Tumor Size (longest diameter, cm)	6.3 cm (range 1–18 cm)	5.2 cm (range 2–8 cm)
Tumor location		
Pelvis	31	22
Chest wall	6	20
Vertebrae	4	8
Other	21	5

nerve. These sensory nerve injuries can be symptomatic, and patients may benefit from oral medications, including gabapentin. Injury of a motor nerve may lead to paresis or even paralysis. These injuries can be temporary or permanent, and maneuvers to avoid injury are critical to employ when these structures are at risk.[29]

11.8 Clinical Data and Outcomes

11.8.1 Radiofrequency Ablation Pain Palliation Outcomes

RFA has proven effective for palliation of focal cancer-related pain in two prospective clinical trials.[30,31,32] These trials involved similar cohorts of patients, and both studies found that RFA provides significant and durable pain relief for patients that have failed or refused EBRT (▶ Table 11.1). The cohort of patients in these prior RFA trials are similar, although the measure of treatment response was different with the Goetz et al study, using the BPI, a visual analog scale of 0 to 10, whereas Dupuy et al used a modified Memorial Pain Assessment Card (a visual analog scale of 0–100%).

In the Goetz et al study, 62 patients at five centers in the United States and Europe with painful metastatic lesions that had failed or refused conventional radiation treatment were treated, typically using general anesthesia, with RFA using a multitined electrode.[17,30] Patients in this study had moderate to severe pain (≥ 4 of 10 worst pain over a 24-hour period) from ≤ 2 painful sites of metastasis, with tumors measuring 6.3 cm on average and ranging from 1 to 18 cm in diameter. Following treatment, 59 of 62 (95%) patients experienced a clinically significant decrease in pain (≥ 2 point drop in worst pain in a 24-hour period). Pain scores for worst pain using the BPI were 7.9 of 10 points prior to treatment, and 1, 4, 8, and 24 weeks following RFA treatment were reduced to 5.8, 4.5, 3, and 1.4 of 10, respectively. Similar improvements in pain and quality of life were observed with measures of the BPI (▶ Fig. 11.7). Six patients experienced complications, with three experiencing exacerbation of preexisting tumor cutaneous fistulae in the perineum within 1 to 2 weeks of the procedure due to generation of a large volume of necrotic tissue following RFA. One patient each developed transient bowel and bladder incontinence following treatment of a previously irradiated leiomyosarcoma metastasis involving the

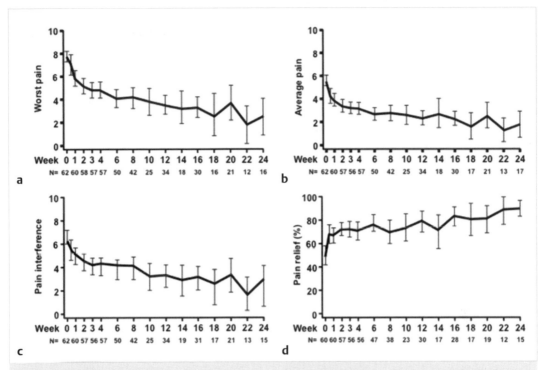

Fig. 11.7 Mean Brief Pain Inventory pain scores over time for patients treated with radiofrequency ablation (RFA). **(a)** Worst pain. **(b)** Average pain. **(c)** Interference of daily activities. **(d)** Pain relief from RFA and medications. Error bars represent the 95% confidence intervals. N = the number of patients completing BPI at each time point. (Reproduced from Callstrom et al with kind Permission from Springer Science and Business Media.[31])

upper sacrum; an acetabular fracture 6 weeks following RFA of a breast cancer metastasis with significant involvement of the ilium, ischium, and acetabulum; and a second-degree skin burn at a grounding pad site.

Dupuy and colleagues, across six centers, used the American College of Radiology Imaging Network (ACRIN), to treat 55 patients with a single painful (>50 on a 1–100 point scale) osseous metastasis using a single 17-gauge or cluster cooltip radiofrequency (RF) electrode with conscious sedation.[32] Mean treated tumor size was 5.2 cm in diameter, ranging in size from 2 to 8 cm. Prior to treatment, patients reported a mean pain score of 54 of 100 points with a range of 51 to 91 of 100 points. These patients reported an average decrease in pain at the 1-month follow-up of 27 of 100 points, and at the 3-month follow-up, a decrease of 14 of 100 points. Immediately following RFA, 27% of patients reported pain greater than the baseline pain score. In order to use sensorimotor testing during the procedure, moderate conscious sedation, rather than general anesthesia,

was used for the procedure. Twenty-seven of 55 patients had tumors that were treated within 3 cm of a major neurovascular bundle. With the use of sensorimotor monitoring, only one patient suffered a motor nerve deficit, and three other patients developed neuropathic pain, developing as late as 35 days post-RFA. Complications with grade 3 toxicities were reported in 3 of 55 patients (5.4%), including 1 patient with foot drop, 1 patient with increased pain, and 1 patient with neuropathic pain. Although prior studies found a benefit from both EBRT and RFA, this trial did not find a benefit from prior RT for a reduction in pain intensity.[33]

The degree of pain relief following the ACRIN study was not as great as that reported by Goetz and colleagues, most notably at the 3-month time point, with a scaled reduction in pain of 1.4 of 10 points in the ACRIN study and a corresponding reduction of 2.8 of 10 points in the Goetz et al study, although these pain reductions are likely within statistical error of the studies. The durability of pain relief was not assessed beyond the

3-month time point in the ACRIN study; however, continued decreases in pain scores were reported by patients in the Goetz et al study with reductions in pain of 5.3 of 10 points at the week 24 follow-up evaluation.

There are several differences between the Goetz et al and Dupuy et al studies that may explain the relatively decreased pain relief realized in the ACRIN study. A majority of patients in the Goetz et al trial had mostly exhausted conventional treatments, with 74% receiving RT prior to ablation treatment, while in the ACRIN study, only 24% had received RT prior to treatment. Although this is a substantial difference in treatment history, neither study found that prior treatment with RT had an impact on the pain response. However, in a separate report, the combination of RFA and RT did help a subset of patients treated with metastatic disease involving chest wall masses.[33] Different ablation electrodes were used in the two trials, and it is possible that differences in response were due to the use of an expandable RF electrode (Starburst XL, RITA Medical Systems, Angiodynamics) in the Goetz et al trial versus the use of a straight electrode (Cool-tip, Radionics, Covidien) in the ACRIN trial. It is possible that the total volume of tissue destruction could be different between the two studies due to more aggressive tumor destruction accomplished with general anesthesia used in the Goetz et al trial versus pain limiting treatment in some patients in the ACRIN trial that used conscious sedation for a majority of cases. Finally, it is possible that the differences in treatment response could be due to differences in types of tumors treated; however, the majority of tumor histology and location of tumors were the same in both studies, including lung, colon, and renal metastases, and no difference in pain response was observed for tumor type. It is unlikely that a comparative trial of these two methods could be conducted to determine a possible difference in patient response to these treatments because the differences, if present, would likely be small and of doubtful clinical significance.

11.8.2 Cryoablation Pain Palliation Outcomes

There is increasing use of MRI for guidance and monitoring of interventional procedures. Percutaneous cryoablation is also effective in treating painful primary and secondary bone tumors. An advantage of cryoablation is excellent visibility of the ice ball during the ablation with both CT and MRI. MRI monitoring of the cryoablation procedure offers the ability to visualize complex structures, such as important motor nerves, in multiple imaging planes, although the MRI environment restricts devices that can be used. Tuncali and colleagues reported the use of MRI-guided and monitored cryoablation for treatment of patients with refractory or painful metastatic tumors in bone and soft tissue adjacent to critical structures.[34] Partial or complete pain palliation was achieved in 17 of 19 patients (89%), with complete pain relief in 6 of the 17 patients. Importantly, the visibility of the ice ball with MRI monitoring allowed the visualization of critical normal structures, and, with the use of additional measures to reduce the risk of injury, including warming urethral catheters, intramedullary rod placement, and skin warming, no immediate complications were noted as a result of immediate thermal injury. One patient suffered a femoral neck fracture 6 weeks after cryoablation of a metastatic renal cell carcinoma in this location that had not been treated with an intramedullary rod.

The cryoablation procedure can be performed with methods to monitor and avoid potential neural injury. Lessard and colleagues reported the use of somatosensory-evoked potentials to monitor the S1 nerve during ablation of a painful recurrent Ewing sarcoma in the mid and upper right hemisacrum. This treatment resulted in pain palliation and avoided nerve damage in this distribution. However, the ablation caused incontinence of bowel and bladder, possibly due to ablation injury of the S2–S4 nerve roots bilaterally compounded by prior extensive RT and baseline nerve dysfunction.[35]

Although MRI has significant potential advantages for monitoring of ablation procedures, in most centers, CT interventional rooms are more accessible for ablation procedures and have larger-bore diameters compatible with placement of current ablation devices than are available with most interventional MRI suites. Ullrick and colleagues reported the CT-guided and monitored use of cryoablation for the treatment of three patients with painful metastatic disease involving the pelvis and ribs, with effective pain palliation in two of three patients.[36]

In a multicenter prospective clinical trial using CT guidance and monitoring, 69 painful skeletal metastases were treated with cryoablation in 61 patients.[37] The patients in this cryoablation trial were similar to the cohorts in the previous multi-center RFA trials for pain palliation due to meta-static skeletal disease (▶ Table 11.2). ▶ Fig. 11.8 shows the cryoablation treatment of a painful metastatic paraganglioma contained in a left rib with durable response to treatment throughout the follow-up period. Mean pain scores reported by patients during the trial (worst pain in a 24-hour period using the BPI 10-point scale) were significantly decreased from 7.1 to 5.1, 4, 3.6, and 1.4 at 1, 4, 8, and 24 weeks after treatment, respectively (▶ Fig. 11.9). Thirty-nine of the 47 patients (83%) who were treated with opioid analgesic use prior to the procedure reported a reduction in the use of these medications after the procedure. A single major complication (2%) was observed, which was osteomyelitis occurring at the ablation site.

Twenty-three of 61 patients (38%) patients had not received radiation prior to treatment, and 13 of 61 patients (21%) had received neither radiation treatment nor chemotherapy prior to cryoablation treatment. There was no significant difference in pain scores for patients with respect to RT prior to the cryoablation treatment, and there was no significant difference in pain scores throughout the follow-up period. Postprocedure pain control was managed with patient controlled IV opioid analgesia for 12 of 61 patients (20%) in the immediate posttreatment recovery period. Hospitalization length of stay averaged 1.5 days, with a range from 0 to 6 days. No events of injury to a major motor nerve or neuropathic pain were observed following the cryoablation procedure.

It is difficult to compare patient pain palliation outcomes from the RFA and cryoablation trials despite the similar cohorts of patients. However, the clinical response rates and magnitude of pain palliation are similar. There are a few conclusions that can be drawn from these studies. Despite similar clinical outcomes, cryoablation can be performed more confidently on tumors in close proximity to critical structures due to the visibility of the ice ball with noncontrast CT imaging. This observation is supported by the fact that no patients suffered an injury to a major motor nerve or reported neuropathic pain following the cryoablation procedures as has been observed with RFA treatment. Although the overall complication rate using RFA for treatment of painful metastases

Table 11.2 Patients treated with cryoablation in a prospective multicenter trial

No. patients	
Female	22/39
Age, mean (range)	61 (range 21–95)
Tumor type, number (%)	
Lung	16 (31%)
Renal	10 (20%)
Colorectal	7 (14%)
Melanoma	4 (8%)
Prostate	4 (8%)
Squamous cell (nonlung)	3 (6%)
Transitional cell	2 (4%)
Paraganglioma	2 (4%)
Breast	2 (4%)
Other (1 each)	11 (22%)
Tumor size (longest diameter)	4.8 cm (range 1–11 cm)
Tumor location, number (%)	
Rib/chest wall	33 (48%)
Iliac/ischium/pubic bones	20 (29%)
Scapula/clavicle/sternum	7 (10%)
Sacrum	5 (7%)
Extremity	2 (3%)
Vertebral body	1 (1%)
Mastoid	1 (1%)

is low, 2 of 55 patients (4%) suffered neurological injuries in a clinical trial.[32] Although not explicitly evident in the methods reported in these clinical trials, pain management following RFA can be difficult, often requiring regional anesthetic blocks or epidural catheters for effective pain control, whereas postprocedural pain with cryoablation is readily managed with IV or oral opioid analgesia when necessary.[38]

11.8.3 Emerging Bone Ablation Technologies Clinical Outcomes

Several recent reports have described the use of MRgFUS for the pain palliation of skeletal

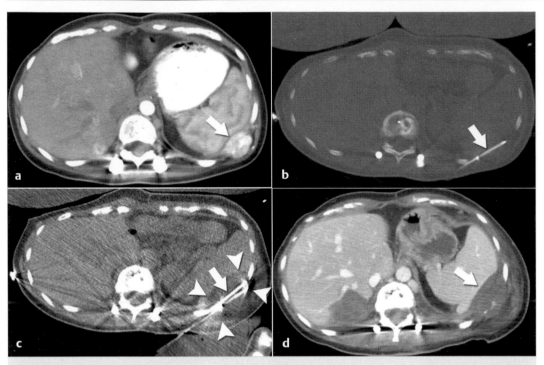

Fig. 11.8 Treatment of a painful metastatic paraganglioma contained in a rib. Prior to treatment, the patient had 5 of 10 points worst pain, which was reduced to 2 of 10 points by week 4 and 0 of 10 by week 8. Patient reported 0 of 10 points pain at latest follow-up of 24 weeks. **(a)** Contrast-enhanced computed tomographic (CT) image of the upper abdomen with body windows demonstrates an enhancing osteolytic metastasis in the left 10th rib *(arrow)*. **(b)** Noncontrast CT image of the upper abdomen with bone windows demonstrates a cryoprobe *(arrow)* placed in the metastasis. **(c)** Noncontrast CT image of the upper abdomen with body windows demonstrates an ice ball, visible as a low-attenuation area *(arrowheads)* surrounding the cryoprobe *(arrow)* and tumor. **(d)** Contrast-enhanced CT image of the upper abdomen with body windows performed following the ablation procedure shows no residual enhancement of the mass contained in the left 10th rib *(arrow)*. (Reproduced from Callstrom et al with permission from John Wiley and Sons. [38])

metastases.[39,40,41] MRI guidance is used to direct FUS energy at the target, with focal tissue heating and the resulting tissue destruction. This approach exploits excellent tumor and soft tissue delineation available with MRI, thermal feedback for treatment monitoring, and ablation margin estimation, and it has the advantage of being a noninvasive treatment. The MRgFUS procedure is best managed with conscious sedation with the use of regional blocks or epidural catheter analgesia where appropriate.[41] An advantage of this approach for treatment of skeletal metastases is that the high acoustic absorption energy at the bone interface results in efficient transfer of heat into the targeted tumor.[42,43] A direct US acoustic pathway to the target tumor is necessary for safe treatment, because bowel or neurological structures intervening between the skin and skeletal

tumor are at potential risk of injury. A prospective randomized clinical trial for palliation of painful skeletal metastases using MRgFUS was conducted that was also designed to measure the placebo effect.[44] This involved a 3:1 randomization to MRgFUS treatment for 112 patients with a sham arm of 35 patients. The treatment arm was statistically superior to the placebo arm, with a drop in average worst pain from 7 of 10 points at presentation to 3.4 of 10 points following treatment versus a drop to 6.1 of 10 points for the placebo arm at the 3-month time point. Treatment pain related to sonication (32.1% of patients) ranged from mild, to moderate, to severe in 6.2%, 10.7%, and 15.2%, respectively. Adverse events included two fractures (one likely unrelated to the procedure), one patient with neuropathy, and one third-degree skin burn.

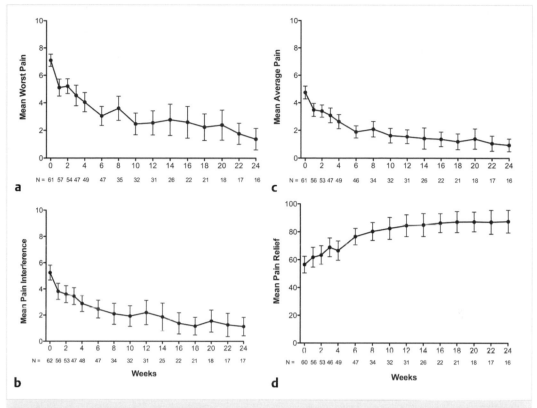

Fig. 11.9 Mean Brief Pain Inventory (BPI) scores over time for patients treated with percutaneous cryoablation for **(a)** worst pain, **(b)** average pain, **(c)** pain interference, and **(d)** pain relief. Error bars represent the 95% confidence intervals. N = the number of patients completing BPI at each time point. (Reproduced from Callstrom et al with permission from John Wiley and Sons.[38])

Additional thermal and nonthermal ablative technologies beyond RFA, cryoablation, and MRgFUS have been applied to the treatment of painful tumors and skeletal metastases in limited series. Ethanol, laser ablation (or laser interstitial thermal therapy), and microwave ablation are effective for palliation of painful metastases.[23,45,46] Microwave ablation is a heat-based technique similar to RFA, using image-guided placement of antennae into target tumors. These antennae transmit microwave energy (915 MHz or 2.45 GHz) with oscillation of water molecules about the antennae with localized heating reaching cytotoxic temperatures faster than RFA and likely penetrating into intact bone more effectively.[24] Laser ablation uses flexible small-caliber neodymium: yttrium-aluminum-garnet (Nd-YAG) or diode laser fibers placed through a thin guide needle. Most experience with laser ablation in bone has been in the treatment of osteoid osteomas.[47]

11.8.4 Ablation for Local Control of Oligometastatic Disease

The musculoskeletal system is the third most common site of metastatic disease, following liver and lung.[48] Strategies are evolving regarding the treatment of patients with oligometastatic disease with the goal of complete local control of all clinically detectable metastases.[48,49,50,51,52] The use of device-based image-guided thermal ablation to eradicate oligometastases in bone and nonvisceral soft tissue has only recently been reported.[13,14,15,53] Cryoablation is an excellent technology for this application, with accurate ablation zone monitoring to avoid injury of adjacent normal tissues and achieving effective penetration of bone.

Outcomes using cryoablation for treatment of metastatic renal cell carcinoma tumors involving bone and soft tissue beyond liver and lung are encouraging, with cost-effective treatments with local control rates of ~ 95%.[14,53] Similar outcomes have been found for the treatment of non–small cell carcinoma.[13] Although there are limited reports for the use of focal therapies for treatment of oligometastatic disease, the outcomes are encouraging.

Pearls

- Safe, effective treatment can be achieved using multiple different ablative therapies. The choice of ablative system by the individual proceduralist should be based on (1) experience of the proceduralist with the ablation systems available, (2) determination of the technical limitations of the ablation system relative to the risk of injury to adjacent tissues, (3) availability of support staff (sedation nurse vs. anesthesiologist) to provide pain control during the procedure, and (4) availability of monitoring systems to provide a greater safety margin for the treatment.
- Treatment goals of the procedure should be clearly understood and related to the patient. If the goal of treatment is palliation of pain, the description of the typical response to therapy (e.g., 80% response to treatment with those that respond experiencing a 2-point drop in pain in 1 to 2 weeks and gradual improvement of pain over 1 month) is valuable to set expectations for the patient postprocedure.
- If the goal of the treatment is local tumor control for oligometastatic disease, it is first critical to determine if this can be achieved technically. Although the impact of achieving local control of oligometastatic disease on patient mortality is yet to be defined, there is clearly no benefit of partial treatment.
- If aggressive treatment is expected to result in local control, sufficient imaging to define the extent of focal disease and to exclude the potential for remote disease should be performed. Although imaging is helpful to define the area of treatment, for patients with metastatic disease, it should be recognized that imaging represents the gross tumor volume, that the clinical volume likely extends beyond the evident disease on imaging, and that this microscopic disease can be covered only by extending the ablation margin beyond the area evident on imaging.
- In patients with complex disease, combination therapy of image-guided thermal ablation and RT may be of benefit.

11.8.5 Bone Ablation and Cementoplasty Clinical Outcomes

Cementoplasty has been used for treatment of patients with metastatic disease involving the axial skeleton.[54,55,56,57,58,59,60,61,62,63] More recently, this strategy has been used in the treatment of periacetabular metastases.[64] Patients with periacetabular metastases can be managed surgically, but it is often complex and recovery can be difficult for patients. Combination treatment with cryoablation and cementoplasty has been effective in patients with cortical disruption with possible avoidance of subsequent fracture. Pain relief is likely derived by a direct effect on nociceptors as well as stabilization of painful microfractures within metastases.[18]

References

[1] Mundy GR. Metastasis to bone: causes, consequences and therapeutic opportunities. Nat Rev Cancer 2002; 2(8): 584–593

[2] Coleman RE. Skeletal complications of malignancy. Cancer 1997; 80(8) Suppl: 1588–1594

[3] Tubiana-Hulin M. Incidence, prevalence and distribution of bone metastases. Bone 1991; 12 Suppl 1: S9–S10

[4] Janjan N. Bone metastases: approaches to management. Semin Oncol 2001; 28(4) Suppl 11: 28–34

[5] Lutz S, Berk L, Chang E et al. American Society for Radiation Oncology (ASTRO). Palliative radiotherapy for bone metastases: an ASTRO evidence-based guideline. Int J Radiat Oncol Biol Phys 2011; 79(4): 965–976

[6] Tong D, Gillick L, Hendrickson FR. The palliation of symptomatic osseous metastases: final results of the Study by the Radiation Therapy Oncology Group. Cancer 1982; 50(5): 893–899

[7] Massie MJ, Holland JC. The cancer patient with pain: psychiatric complications and their management. J Pain Symptom Manage 1992; 7(2): 99–109

[8] Spiegel D, Sands S, Koopman C. Pain and depression in patients with cancer. Cancer 1994; 74(9): 2570–2578

[9] Jeremic B, Shibamoto Y, Acimovic L et al. A randomized trial of three single-dose radiation therapy regimens in the treatment of metastatic bone pain. Int J Radiat Oncol Biol Phys 1998; 42(1): 161–167

[10] Price P, Hoskin PJ, Easton D, Austin D, Palmer SG, Yarnold JR. Prospective randomised trial of single and multifraction radiotherapy schedules in the treatment of painful bony metastases. Radiother Oncol 1986; 6(4): 247–255

[11] Cole DJ. A randomized trial of a single treatment versus conventional fractionation in the palliative radiotherapy of painful bone metastases. Clin Oncol (R Coll Radiol) 1989; 1 (2): 59–62

[12] Gaze MN, Kelly CG, Kerr GR et al. Pain relief and quality of life following radiotherapy for bone metastases: a randomised trial of two fractionation schedules. Radiother Oncol 1997; 45(2): 109–116

[13] Bang HJ, Littrup PJ, Currier BP et al. Percutaneous cryoablation of metastatic lesions from non-small-cell lung carcino-

ma: initial survival, local control, and cost observations. J Vasc Interv Radiol 2012; 23(6): 761–769

[14] Bang HJ, Littrup PJ, Goodrich DJ et al. Percutaneous cryoablation of metastatic renal cell carcinoma for local tumor control: feasibility, outcomes, and estimated cost-effectiveness for palliation. J Vasc Interv Radiol 2012; 23(6): 770–777

[15] McMenomy BP, Kurup AN, Johnson GB et al. Percutaneous cryoablation of musculoskeletal oligometastatic disease for complete remission. J Vasc Interv Radiol 2013; 24(2): 207–213

[16] Kurup AN, Morris JM, Schmit GD et al. Neuroanatomic considerations in percutaneous tumor ablation. Radiographics 2013; 33(4): 1195–1215

[17] Callstrom MR, Atwell TD, Charboneau JW et al. Painful metastases involving bone: percutaneous image-guided cryoablation—prospective trial interim analysis. Radiology 2006; 241(2): 572–580

[18] Sabharwal T, Katsanos K, Buy X, Gangi A. Image-guided ablation therapy of bone tumors. Semin Ultrasound CT MR 2009; 30(2): 78–90

[19] Sabharwal T, Salter R, Adam A, Gangi A. Image-guided therapies in orthopedic oncology. Orthop Clin North Am 2006; 37(1): 105–112

[20] Callstrom MR, Kurup AN. Percutaneous ablation for bone and soft tissue metastases—why cryoablation? Skeletal Radiol 2009; 38(9): 835–839

[21] Callstrom MR, York JD, Gaba RC et al. Technology Assessment Committee of Society of Interventional Radiology. Research reporting standards for image-guided ablation of bone and soft tissue tumors. J Vasc Interv Radiol 2009; 20 (12): 1527–1540

[22] Rybak LD. Fire and ice: thermal ablation of musculoskeletal tumors. Radiol Clin North Am 2009; 47(3): 455–469

[23] Groenemeyer DH, Schirp S, Gevargez A. Image-guided percutaneous thermal ablation of bone tumors. Acad Radiol 2002; 9(4): 467–477

[24] Brace CL. Radiofrequency and microwave ablation of the liver, lung, kidney, and bone: what are the differences? Curr Probl Diagn Radiol 2009; 38(3): 135–143

[25] Dodd GD, III, Frank MS, Aribandi M, Chopra S, Chintapalli KN. Radiofrequency thermal ablation: computer analysis of the size of the thermal injury created by overlapping ablations. Am J Roentgenol 2001; 177(4): 777–782

[26] Chosy SG, Nakada SY, Lee FT, Jr, Warner TF. Monitoring renal cryosurgery: predictors of tissue necrosis in swine. J Urol 1998; 159(4): 1370–1374

[27] Cleeland CS, Gonin R, Hatfield AK et al. Pain and its treatment in outpatients with metastatic cancer. N Engl J Med 1994; 330(9): 592–596

[28] Daut RL, Cleeland CS, Flanery RC. Development of the Wisconsin Brief Pain Questionnaire to assess pain in cancer and other diseases. Pain 1983; 17(2): 197–210

[29] Kurup AN, Morris JM, Boon AJ et al. Motor evoked potential monitoring during cryoablation of musculoskeletal tumors. J Vasc Interv Radiol 2014; 25(11): 1657–1664

[30] Goetz MP, Callstrom MR, Charboneau JW et al. Percutaneous image-guided radiofrequency ablation of painful metastases involving bone: a multicenter study. J Clin Oncol 2004; 22 (2): 300–306

[31] Callstrom MR, Charboneau JW, Goetz MP et al. Image-guided ablation of painful metastatic bone tumors: a new and effective approach to a difficult problem. Skeletal Radiol 2006; 35(1): 1–15

[32] Dupuy DE, Liu D, Hartfeil D et al. Percutaneous radiofrequency ablation of painful osseous metastases: a multicen-

ter American College of Radiology Imaging Network trial. Cancer 2010; 116(4): 989–997

[33] Grieco CA, Simon CJ, Mayo-Smith WW, Dipetrillo TA, Ready NE, Dupuy DE. Image-guided percutaneous thermal ablation for the palliative treatment of chest wall masses. Am J Clin Oncol 2007; 30(4): 361–367

[34] Tuncali K, Morrison PR, Winalski CS et al. MRI-guided percutaneous cryotherapy for soft-tissue and bone metastases: initial experience. Am J Roentgenol 2007; 189(1): 232–239

[35] Lessard AM, Gilchrist J, Schaefer L, Dupuy DE. Palliation of recurrent Ewing sarcoma of the pelvis with cryoablation and somatosensory-evoked potentials. J Pediatr Hematol Oncol 2009; 31(1): 18–21

[36] Ullrick SR, Hebert JJ, Davis KW. Cryoablation in the musculoskeletal system. Curr Probl Diagn Radiol 2008; 37(1): 39–48

[37] Callstrom MR, Dupuy DE, Solomon SB et al. Percutaneous image-guided cryoablation of painful metastases involving bone: multicenter trial. Cancer 2013; 119(5): 1033–1041

[38] Thacker PG, Callstrom MR, Curry TB et al. Palliation of painful metastatic disease involving bone with imaging-guided treatment: comparison of patients' immediate response to radiofrequency ablation and cryoablation. Am J Roentgenol 2011; 197(2): 510–515

[39] Liberman B, Gianfelice D, Inbar Y et al. Pain palliation in patients with bone metastases using MR-guided focused ultrasound surgery: a multicenter study. Ann Surg Oncol 2009; 16(1): 140–146

[40] Napoli A, Anzidei M, Marincola BC et al. Primary pain palliation and local tumor control in bone metastases treated with magnetic resonance-guided focused ultrasound. Invest Radiol 2013; 48(6): 351–358

[41] Napoli A, Anzidei M, Marincola BC et al. MR imaging-guided focused ultrasound for treatment of bone metastasis. Radiographics 2013; 33(6): 1555–1568

[42] Mercadante S, Fulfaro F. Management of painful bone metastases. Curr Opin Oncol 2007; 19(4): 308–314

[43] Ripamonti C, Fulfaro F. Malignant bone pain: pathophysiology and treatments. Curr Rev Pain 2000; 4(3): 187–196

[44] Hurwitz MD, Ghanouni P, Kanaev SV et al. Magnetic resonance-guided focused ultrasound for patients with painful bone metastases: phase III trial results. J Natl Cancer Inst 2014; 106(5)

[45] Gangi A, Kastler B, Klinkert A, Dietemann JL. Injection of alcohol into bone metastases under CT guidance. J Comput Assist Tomogr 1994; 18(6): 932–935

[46] Pusceddu C, Sotgia B, Fele RM, Melis L. Treatment of bone metastases with microwave thermal ablation. J Vasc Interv Radiol 2013; 24(2): 229–233

[47] Gangi A, Alizadeh H, Wong L, Buy X, Dietemann JL, Roy C. Osteoid osteoma: percutaneous laser ablation and follow-up in 114 patients. Radiology 2007; 242(1): 293–301

[48] Eleraky M, Papanastassiou I, Vrionis FD. Management of metastatic spine disease. Curr Opin Support Palliat Care 2010; 4(3): 182–188

[49] Palma DA, Salama JK, Lo SS et al. The oligometastatic state—separating truth from wishful thinking. Nat Rev Clin Oncol 2014; 11(9): 549–557

[50] Weichselbaum RR, Hellman S. Oligometastases revisited. Nat Rev Clin Oncol 2011; 8(6): 378–382

[51] Ollila DW, Gleisner AL, Hsueh EC. Rationale for complete metastasectomy in patients with stage IV metastatic melanoma. J Surg Oncol 2011; 104(4): 420–424

[52] Singh D, Yi WS, Brasacchio RA et al. Is there a favorable sub-set of patients with prostate cancer who develop oligometa-stases? Int J Radiat Oncol Biol Phys 2004; 58(1): 3–10

[53] Welch BT, Callstrom MR, Morris JM et al. Feasibility and on-cologic control after percutaneous image guided ablation of metastatic renal cell carcinoma. J Urol 2014; 192(2): 357–363

[54] Gangi A, Guth S, Imbert JP, Marin H, Dietemann J-L. Percuta-neous vertebroplasty: indications, technique, and results. Radiographics 2003; 23(2): e10

[55] Anselmetti GC, Manca A, Ortega C, Grignani G, Debernardi F, Regge D. Treatment of extraspinal painful bone metastases with percutaneous cementoplasty: a prospective study of 50 patients. Cardiovasc Intervent Radiol 2008; 31(6): 1165–1173

[56] Basile A, Giuliano G, Scuderi V et al. Cementoplasty in the management of painful extraspinal bone metastases: our experience. Radiol Med (Torino) 2008; 113(7): 1018–1028

[57] Belfiore G, Tedeschi E, Ronza FM et al. Radiofrequency abla-tion of bone metastases induces long-lasting palliation in patients with untreatable cancer. Singapore Med J 2008; 49 (7): 565–570

[58] Carrafiello G, Laganà D, Pellegrino C et al. Percutaneous imaging-guided ablation therapies in the treatment of symptomatic bone metastases: preliminary experience. Ra-diol Med (Torino) 2009; 114(4): 608–625

[59] Hoffmann RT, Jakobs TF, Trumm C, Weber C, Helmberger TK, Reiser MF. Radiofrequency ablation in combination with os-teoplasty in the treatment of painful metastatic bone dis-ease. J Vasc Interv Radiol 2008; 19(3): 419–425

[60] Masala S, Manenti G, Roselli M et al. Percutaneous combined therapy for painful sternal metastases: a radiofrequency thermal ablation (RFTA) and cementoplasty protocol. Anti-cancer Res 2007; 27 6C: 4259–4262

[61] Munk PL, Rashid F, Heran MK et al. Combined cemento-plasty and radiofrequency ablation in the treatment of pain-ful neoplastic lesions of bone. J Vasc Interv Radiol 2009; 20 (7): 903–911

[62] Schaefer O, Lohrmann C, Herling M, Uhrmeister P, Langer M. Combined radiofrequency thermal ablation and percutane-ous cementoplasty treatment of a pathologic fracture. J Vasc Interv Radiol 2002; 13(10): 1047–1050

[63] Toyota N, Naito A, Kakizawa H et al. Radiofrequency ablation therapy combined with cementoplasty for painful bone metastases: initial experience. Cardiovasc Intervent Radiol 2005; 28(5): 578–583

[64] Castañeda Rodriguez WR, Callstrom MR. Effective pain palli-ation and prevention of fracture for axial-loading skeletal metastases using combined cryoablation and cemento-plasty. Tech Vasc Interv Radiol 2011; 14(3): 160–169

Chapter 12

Portal Vein Embolization

12 Portal Vein Embolization

Steven L. Hsu, and Sanjeeva P. Kalva

12.1 Introduction

Liver transplantation, surgical resection, and percutaneous ablative approaches are potentially curative treatments for patients with hepatic malignancies. Transplantation criteria have been rigorously designed given the scarcity of available donor livers to ensure patients with the most critical need receive transplants; thus surgical resection and percutaneous ablation are the main curative therapies for liver malignancies. Patients with underlying liver disease or large tumor burden may develop perioperative hepatic failure following hepatic resection. Portal vein embolization (PVE) is a procedure that takes advantage of the regenerative properties of the liver by redirecting portal venous blood flow from liver segments to be resected to the future liver remnant (FLR) for induction of hepatic hypertrophy. PVE has been shown to improve the postoperative outcomes of patients following hepatic resection, and therefore has become an established standard of care prior to major hepatectomies.[1,2]

12.2 Indications

Portal vein embolization is indicated when the future liver remnant is deemed insufficient to provide adequate hepatic function following hepatic resection.[3]

12.3 Contraindications

One absolute contraindication to PVE is the presence of extensive portal venous tumor thrombi. Large tumor thrombi divert portal venous blood to the future liver remnant, and attempts to perform additional PVE can result in deleterious nontarget embolization of the FLR.[4]

A second absolute contraindication to PVE is clinically evident portal hypertension, which is considered a contraindication to hepatic resection. However, many investigators have demonstrated similar postoperative course and survival benefits following hepatic resection in patients with and without portal hypertension; thus hepatectomy in this group of patients remains a topic of debate.[4,5,6,7]

Relative contraindications to PVE are uncorrectable coagulopathy, renal insufficiency, intrahepatic biliary dilation in the FLR, and extrahepatic metastatic disease.

12.4 Patient Selection and Preprocedural Workup

The formation of a multidisciplinary team of hepatologists, medical oncologists, surgical oncologists, radiologists, and interventional radiologists is of immense importance in the selection of appropriate patients for PVE and subsequent hepatic resection.

The preprocedural workup includes evaluating the patient for baseline liver function, acquiring volumetric cross-sectional examination of the liver, and determining the extent of liver resection. Traditionally, computed tomographic (CT) examinations of the liver have been used for assessment of FLR and estimated total liver volume. However, magnetic resonance imaging (MRI) examination of the liver can also be used to compute hepatic volumes (► Fig. 12.1).

Computer software designed for manipulation of volumetric data can permit the calculation of FLR volume and the total liver volume. The FLR volume is calculated by tracing the FLR on each axial image. The total estimated liver volume (TELV) can be computed by tracing the entire liver border on each axial image, with or without subtracting the outline of the tumor(s). Alternatively, the total liver volume can be estimated using the following formula: Total Estimated Liver Volume = − 791.41 + 1,267.28 × Body Surface Area.[8] A standardized FLR (sFLR) is the ratio of the FLR volume to the TELV expressed as a percentage.

In patients with normal hepatic function, an sFLR of > 20% is associated with reduced length of hospital stay and reduced postoperative complications following hepatic resection.[9,10] Accordingly, PVE is recommended for patients with normal hepatic function and an sFLR of < 20%.[11]

In patients with hepatotoxic liver injury resulting from chemotherapy, PVE is recommended when the sFLR is < 30%.[10,12] Similar to systemic hepatotoxic chemotherapy, hepatic steatosis is typically a diffuse hepatic parenchymal process resulting in hepatic injury and dysfunction;

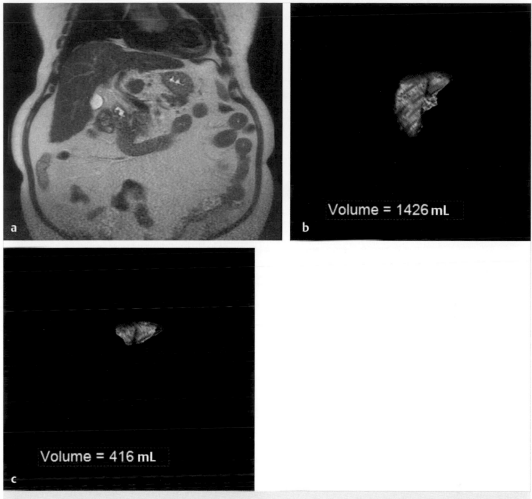

Fig. 12.1 Preprocedural magnetic resonance imaging (MRI) evaluation of the liver. **(a)** Coronal MRI of the abdomen. **(b)** The calculated estimated total liver volume was 1,426 mL. **(c)** The calculated left hepatic lobe volume was 416 mL, resulting in a marginal standardized future liver remnant of 29.2%.

therefore, PVE is recommended when the sFLR is also < 30%.

Patients with chronic liver disease, such as cirrhosis and retained hepatic function, with good functional status can be considered for hepatic resection. PVE is recommended for cirrhotic patients when the sFLR is < 40%.[10,12]

12.5 Technique

The procedure is usually performed under conscious sedation and sometimes with general anesthesia. Portal venous access is established via an ipsilateral or contralateral percutaneous transhepatic approach.[4,13,14,15] The ipsilateral approach involves access into the hepatic lobe containing the tumor(s). Two advantages of the ipsilateral approach are avoidance of injury to the FLR with needle access, sheath placement, and catheter manipulations and ease of selection of segment 4 branches, assuming a right portal venous access for a planned extended right hepatectomy. The main disadvantage of the ipsilateral approach relates to the selection of the right portal veins, which can be difficult given the acute angulation of right portal veins with respect to the site of access.

The contralateral percutaneous transhepatic approach involves an initial access in the FLR. The main advantage of the contralateral approach is

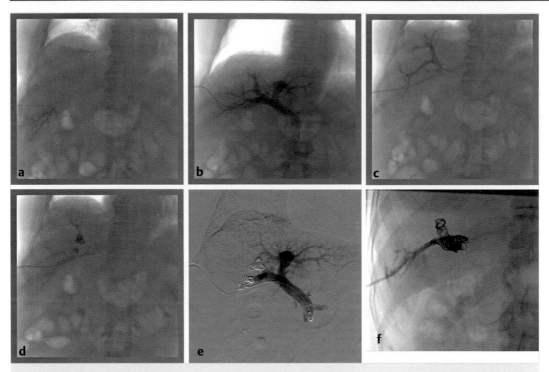

Fig. 12.2 Ipsilateral transhepatic right portal vein embolization using 100 to 700 μm triacryl gelatin microspheres followed by coil embolization. **(a)** Ultrasound-guided access of a right-sided peripheral portal vein branch using a 21-gauge Chiba needle. Contrast injection confirms appropriate portal venous access. **(b)** Anteroposterior flush portography using a 5 French flush pigtail catheter demonstrates patent bilateral portal venous branches. **(c, d)** Selective right portal venograms using a reverse-curve Simmons 1 catheter. **(e)** Postembolization portal venogram demonstrates successful particle and coil embolization of the right portal venous branches. **(f)** Single anteroposterior fluoroscopic image demonstrating contrast-stained Gelfoam in the liver parenchyma from tract embolization.

the ease in which right portal venous branches can be selected, and the shorter catheter lengths required, thus reducing the amount of catheter dead space. Limiting the catheter dead space is particularly important when using N-butyl cyanoacrylate (NBCA) and Lipiodol (Guerbet) mixture for embolization. The main disadvantage of the contralateral approach is potential for injury to the FLR. The ipsilateral and contralateral techniques described here specifically discuss the use of particles and coils for PVE; however, other embolic agents may also be employed.

The ipsilateral approach involves access into a right-sided peripheral portal venous branch using a 21- or 22-gauge Chiba needle (▶ Fig. 12.2). This may be performed under fluoroscopy using landmarks, or under direct ultrasound guidance. The access is usually along the right midaxillary line. Appropriate needle access into the peripheral portal venous branch can be confirmed with injection of contrast through the needle. At this time, a

0.018 in wire is inserted into the needle and advanced under fluoroscopic guidance into the main portal vein. Applying the Seldinger technique, a 5 or 6 French vascular sheath is advanced into the right portal vein to permit introduction of catheters. Initially, an anteroposterior flush portal venogram using a 5 French flush catheter is performed to delineate the portal venous anatomy. Rotational angiography with three-dimensional (3D) reconstruction of the portal venous system can also be performed as a convenient reference during the procedure.

When embolization involves segment 4, some authors advocate segment 4 embolization first given the potential difficulty of catheter exchanges and possible dislodgment of embolic agents following embolization of the right-sided portal venous system.[10,12] Segment 4 can be selected using a 0.035 in hydrophilic guidewire (Glidewire, Terumo Medical Corp.) and several 5 French catheters (i.e., Kumpe catheter, Cook Medical; Glidecath,

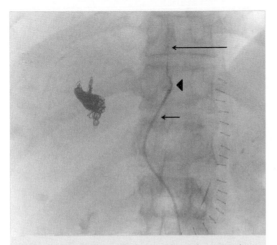

Fig. 12.3 Portal vein embolization from the contralateral approach. Through a 6 French sheath *(short arrow)*, a 5 French Kumpe catheter *(arrowhead)* has been inserted and used to select the segment 4a branch. A 3 French Renegade Hi-Flo microcatheter *(long arrow)* has been coaxially inserted through the Kumpe catheter to obtain more distal access for delivery of embolic particles.

Terumo Medical Corp.). Then a microcatheter (i.e., 3 French Renegade Hi-Flo catheter, Boston Scientific; 2.8 French Progreat catheter, Terumo Medical Corp.) is advanced coaxially through the 5 French catheter more distally into segment 4 branch for delivery of embolic agents (▶ Fig. 12.3). Some authors embolize the portal veins with particles of increasing size, ranging from 100 to 700 μm in diameter, until stasis, followed by coil embolization of the proximal segment 4 vein to further reinforce portal venous flow diversion. Attention is then directed to the rest of the right portal venous branches. The 5 French catheter is exchanged for a 5 French reverse-curve catheter to select the right portal venous branches (Simmons 1, AngioDynamics, Simmons 2, Cook Medical, Bloomington, IL. Sos Omni 2, AngioDynamics). Through the reverse-curve catheter, a microcatheter is advanced more distally where particle embolization is performed until stasis, followed by coil embolization. Finally, the reverse-curve catheter is exchanged for a flush catheter for a flush portal venogram to confirm occlusion of the embolized branches. The catheter and sheath are subsequently removed, and the access tract is occluded with Gelfoam or coils.

The contralateral percutaneous transhepatic approach involves an initial access in the FLR. Access is achieved into a peripheral branch of the left hepatic lobe, usually segment 3, using a 21- or 22-gauge Chiba needle under ultrasound guidance. Selection of the right and segment 4 portal venous branches can be achieved using a standard 5 French catheter (Kumpe catheter, Cook Medical) and a coaxially inserted microcatheter (Renegade Hi-Flo, Boston Scientific) without an associated sheath.

There are many embolic agents and combinations of embolic agents that have been employed for PVE, including gelatin sponge, fibrin glue, NBCA glue, thrombin, polyvinyl alcohol particles, Amplatzer vascular plugs (St. Jude Medical), embolization coils, and Lipiodol. As mentioned previously, the techniques for PVE are the same regardless of the embolic agent used. It is worth stating that some studies report that the use of NBCA results in a greater volume of FLR increase.[16,17]

12.6 Postprocedural Management and Follow-up Evaluation

PVE is a well-tolerated procedure. Patients can be discharged the same day after 4 to 6 hours of observation, but some may require 1 to 2 days of hospital stay. Prophylactic antibiotics are usually administered at the time of the procedure only. Nausea and vomiting are controlled with antiemetics and intravenous hydration. Intravenous pain medications can be provided to alleviate associated postprocedural discomfort, which will require oral transition prior to discharge. A time interval of 4 to 5 weeks following PVE is typically sufficient for induction of adequate hepatic hypertrophy for surgical resection.[18] A follow-up volumetric CT or MRI scan of the liver is required for evaluation of hepatic hypertrophy. Although a longer time period of 5 weeks permits greater volume expansion of the FLR, hepatic hypertrophy has been shown to peak during the 2 weeks following PVE and plateaus following 3 weeks (▶ Fig. 12.4).[16,19,20,21,22,23] The timing of the follow-up cross-sectional examination should also take into consideration the presence or absence of chronic liver disease. Patients with chronic liver disease have impaired regenerative ability of the liver, thus follow-up CT or MRI in these individuals can be performed 4 to 5 weeks following

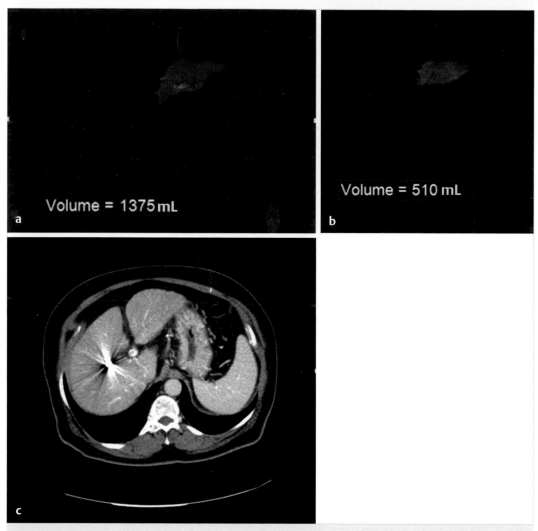

Fig. 12.4 Volumetric computed tomography (CT) of the liver with hepatic volumes following portal vein embolization (PVE). **(a)** Total estimated liver volume was 1,375 mL following PVE. **(b)** Future liver remnant (FLR) volume was 510 mL following PVE, resulting in a standardized FLR of 37.1% **(c)** Contrast-enhanced axial CT image of the abdomen demonstrates streak artifacts resulting from the coils placed during PVE and hypertrophy of the left hepatic lobe.

PVE, whereas individuals with normal livers should obtain their cross-sectional examination 3 to 4 weeks following PVE.

12.7 Side Effects and Complications

There are complications in PVE that are specific to the procedure, and there are complications which generally apply to all percutaneous transhepatic procedures. General complications include sepsis, hemobilia, subcapsular hematoma, pseudoaneurysm, hemoperitoneum, and pneumothorax. Complications specific to PVE include portal hypertension, which may result in variceal hemorrhage, nontarget embolization, complete main portal vein thrombosis, and recanalization of embolized branches.[24,25] The rate of complications comparing the ipsilateral approach to the contralateral approach is not statistically significant.[24]

12.8 Clinical Data and Outcomes

In a recent literature review of outcomes of PVE,[16] the technical success rate of performing PVE was 99.3%. The clinical success rate, measured by adequate FLR hypertrophy following PVE, was 96.1%. Major complications from PVE were reported to be approximately 2.5%, with a mortality rate of 0.1%. The mean increase in FLR volume was 37.9 ± 0.1%. Of the total planned liver resections, 20% were canceled following PVE. In the studies that reported etiologies for the cancellations, 6.1% were attributed to local hepatic tumor progression or development of metastases in the FLR, 8.1% were attributed to extrahepatic tumor metastases, and 4.5% were attributed to miscellaneous causes, such as PVE-specific complications resulting in nonresectability, patients' refusal of further procedures, and lack of sufficient FLR expansion.

Pearls ◻

- PVE is a technically safe and efficacious treatment with a high clinical success rate.[16]
- Major complications are low.
- Start first with ultrasound guidance into a peripheral right portal vein before using fluoroscopically guided access.
- Consider using a microcatheter to deliver embolic agents to reduce the volume of catheter dead space, obtain better control and delivery of embolic agents, and secure access into the selected vessel.
- Schedule follow-up CT or MRI expeditiously (3 to 4 weeks for patients with normal hepatic function, 4 to 5 weeks for patients with impaired hepatic function).

References

[1] Farges O, Belghiti J, Kianmanesh R et al. Portal vein embolization before right hepatectomy: prospective clinical trial. Ann Surg 2003; 237(2): 208–217

[2] Abulkhir A, Limongelli P, Healey AJ et al. Preoperative portal vein embolization for major liver resection: a meta-analysis. Ann Surg 2008; 247(1): 49–57

[3] Beal IK, Anthony S, Papadopoulou A et al. Portal vein embolisation prior to hepatic resection for colorectal liver metastases and the effects of periprocedure chemotherapy. Br J Radiol 2006; 79(942): 473–478

[4] Madoff DC, Abdalla EK, Vauthey JN. Portal vein embolization in preparation for major hepatic resection: evolution of a new standard of care. J Vasc Interv Radiol 2005; 16(6): 779–790

[5] Jarnagin W, Chapman WC, Curley S et al. American Hepato-Pancreato-Biliary Association. Society of Surgical Oncology. Society for Surgery of the Alimentary Tract. Surgical treatment of hepatocellular carcinoma: expert consensus statement. HPB (Oxford) 2010; 12(5): 302–310

[6] Cucchetti A, Ercolani G, Vivarelli M et al. Is portal hypertension a contraindication to hepatic resection? Ann Surg 2009; 250(6): 922–928

[7] Ishizawa T, Hasegawa K, Aoki T et al. Neither multiple tumors nor portal hypertension are surgical contraindications for hepatocellular carcinoma. Gastroenterology 2008; 134 (7): 1908–1916

[8] Vauthey JN, Abdalla EK, Doherty DA et al. Body surface area and body weight predict total liver volume in Western adults. Liver Transpl 2002; 8(3): 233–240

[9] Abdalla EK, Barnett CC, Doherty D, Curley SA, Vauthey JN. Extended hepatectomy in patients with hepatobiliary malignancies with and without preoperative portal vein embolization. Arch Surg 2002; 137(6): 675–680, discussion 680–681

[10] May BJ, Madoff DC. Portal vein embolization: rationale, technique, and current application. Semin Intervent Radiol 2012; 29(2): 81–89

[11] Memon K, Riaz A, Madoff DC, et al. Colorectal metastases: intra-arterial therapies (chemoembolization/radioembolization) and portal vein embolization. In: Geschwind JF, Dake MD, ed. Abrams' Angiography Interventional Radiology. Philadelphia, PA: Lippincott Williams & Wilkins; 2014:126–128

[12] Avritscher R, de Baere T, Murthy R, Deschamps F, Madoff DC. Percutaneous transhepatic portal vein embolization: rationale, technique, and outcomes. Semin Intervent Radiol 2008; 25(2): 132–145

[13] Nagino M, Nimura Y, Kamiya J, Kondo S, Kanai M. Selective percutaneous transhepatic embolization of the portal vein in preparation for extensive liver resection: the ipsilateral approach. Radiology 1996; 200(2): 559–563

[14] de Baere T, Roche A, Vavasseur D et al. Portal vein embolization: utility for inducing left hepatic lobe hypertrophy before surgery. Radiology 1993; 188(1): 73–77

[15] Azoulay D, Castaing D, Krissat J et al. Percutaneous portal vein embolization increases the feasibility and safety of major liver resection for hepatocellular carcinoma in injured liver. Ann Surg 2000; 232(5): 665–672

[16] van Lienden KP, van den Esschert JW, de Graaf W et al. Portal vein embolization before liver resection: a systematic review. Cardiovasc Intervent Radiol 2013; 36(1): 25–34

[17] de Baere T, Roche A, Elias D, Lasser P, Lagrange C, Bousson V. Preoperative portal vein embolization for extension of hepatectomy indications. Hepatology 1996; 24(6): 1386–1391

[18] de Baere T, Denys A, Madoff DC. Preoperative portal vein embolization: indications and technical considerations. Tech Vasc Interv Radiol 2007; 10(1): 67–78

[19] Nagino M, Kamiya J, Nishio H, Ebata T, Arai T, Nimura Y. Two hundred forty consecutive portal vein embolizations before extended hepatectomy for biliary cancer: surgical outcome and long-term follow-up. Ann Surg 2006; 243 (3): 364–372

[20] Ribero D, Abdalla EK, Madoff DC, Donadon M, Loyer EM, Vauthey JN. Portal vein embolization before major hepatectomy and its effects on regeneration, resectability and outcome. Br J Surg 2007; 94(11): 1386–1394

[21] Madoff DC, Hicks ME, Vauthey JN et al. Transhepatic portal vein embolization: anatomy, indications, and technical considerations. Radiographics 2002; 22(5): 1063–1076

[22] Abdalla EK, Hicks ME, Vauthey JN. Portal vein embolization: rationale, technique and future prospects. Br J Surg 2001; 88 (2): 165–175

[23] Madoff DC, Hicks ME, Abdalla EK, Morris JS, Vauthey JN. Portal vein embolization with polyvinyl alcohol particles and coils in preparation for major liver resection for hepatobiliary malignancy: safety and effectiveness—study in 26 patients. Radiology 2003; 227(1): 251–260

[24] Kodama Y, Shimizu T, Endo H, Miyamoto N, Miyasaka K. Complications of percutaneous transhepatic portal vein embolization. J Vasc Interv Radiol 2002; 13(12): 1233–1237

[25] May BJ, Talenfeld AD, Madoff DC. Update on portal vein embolization: evidence-based outcomes, controversies, and novel strategies. J Vasc Interv Radiol 2013; 24(2): 241–254

Chapter 13

Emerging Technologies in Interventional Oncology

13 Emerging Technologies in Interventional Oncology

Omar Zurkiya and Rahmi Oklu

13.1 Introduction

Interventional oncology (IO) is a rapidly expanding field with continuous emergence of new concepts and approaches to both percutaneous and intravascular treatment of neoplasms. These approaches offer minimally invasive treatments targeting both primary and metastatic lesions. Although the modalities discussed earlier in the book are well entrenched in oncology treatment, numerous new approaches are under investigation. This chapter discusses promising new technologies in IO.

13.2 Interventional Navigational Systems

The concept behind an interventional navigational system (INS) is to provide a real-time, intraprocedural display of the spatial positions of various instruments. This typically involves integrating the real-time patient position and instrument data with preoperative imaging data.[1,2] INS has been successfully used in neurosurgery, otolaryngology, and orthopedic surgery.[3] In IO, INS is increasingly being used to co-locate the intraprocedural position of a needle or probe within the patient with previously obtained imaging data delineating a lesion of interest.

Preoperative images, usually from computed tomography (CT) or magnetic resonance imaging (MRI), are loaded into a control unit of the INS. The target lesion or location is mapped with three-dimensional (3D) coordinates; fiducial markers or standard anatomical landmarks are used for purposes of registration. These images may be used for surgical planning, including determining the entry point on the skin surface and the trajectory. During the procedure, the critical task of the INS is to track the 3D position of the surgical instrument with respect to the patient and to register this information superimposed on the preprocedure imaging. The performance of the INS is therefore dependent on a robust tracking system.

Tracking systems must be able to follow the location of the surgical instrument in real time because it is used to direct the operator. These systems generally fall into three main categories: optical, electromagnetic, and magnetic gradient tracking.

An optical tracking system requires two components—a position sensor and tracking markers. The position sensor will emit infrared light into a specified volume containing the surgical instrument to be tracked. The tracking markers are physically located on the instrument itself and may consist of passive or active markers. In the case of passive markers, a reflective coating redirects the infrared light back to the position sensor. The position of the instrument may then be calculated using various approaches, such as geometric triangulation and time-of-flight calculation. With active markers, the position sensor emits infrared light, which then triggers the marker to activate and emit its own infrared signal. The position sensor detects this signal and again calculates the position and orientation of the instrument. The information is transmitted to a host computer, which analyzes and displays the data. The information may be fused with the preoperative imaging displaying the real-time relationship of the instrument to a target of interest.

Despite improvements in accuracy and speed of processing, the main drawback of optical detection is that a line of sight must be maintained between the position sensor and the tracking marker. Any object, including the physician, disrupting this line of sight will disable the system. Additionally, accuracy of the system is decreased by any deformation of the instrument. With longer probes, a slight bending can occur with repositioning, causing the accuracy of the system to decrease during the procedure with repeated manipulation of the probe.

The principle of an electromagnetic (EM) tracking system is to localize the surgical instruments by detection of ferromagnetic probes within a magnetic field.[4] Rather than using light, the EM field is used for tracking. Instruments are fitted with sensor coils that move within a magnetic field created by an EM generator. This generates an electrical current according to Faraday's law of electromagnetic induction. The magnitude of the induced voltage is used to calculate the position in Cartesian coordinates. At this point, the system is similar to optical systems where the information is passed to a host computer for analysis and data display. The advantage of EM is that the device does not require a direct line of sight. The sensor may in fact be within the patient's body, allowing for direct tracking of the needle tip. This would theoretically reduce inaccuracies caused by bending of the needle/probe. A drawback of EM tracking is that the working space is smaller (< 1 m^3). Metallic artifacts from objects such as tables and X-ray sources or detectors are also a problem, though to a lesser extent in newer-generation technologies.

INS has been developed for multiple imaging modalities (► Fig. 13.1). Computed tomography (CT) is generally the preferred imaging modality due to its spatial resolution, ability to provide quantitative information on the density and geometry, and widespread availability. Regardless of the tracking system, optical or EM, respiratory motion and deformation of the target organ remain as problems. Some of these inaccuracies can be reduced by tracking reference points and applying geometric transformation methods.

Ultrasound imaging has the advantages of being real time, low cost, and portable, as well as delivering nonionizing radiation. Again, optical and EM tracking has been explored, with some systems overlaying real-time ultrasound images with virtual images of the target.

Magnetic resonance imaging (MRI) systems contain a built-in gradient field, which may be used to implement EM tracking.[5] Three pairs of orthogonal coils are located in the hand piece of the sensor, which detect the gradient field of the MRI scanner. The location and orientation of the sensor are calculated by comparing the measured signals to stored maps of the gradient fields of the MRI scanner. The scan plane is prescribed in reference to the position and orientation of the tracking point by the tracking system. MRI has unique advantages, including superb soft tissue contrast and highly flexible image plane control. MRI-based navigation has been used in thermal ablation of liver tumors since 2000.[5] Real-time MRI scans are collected and overlaid with tracking coordinates from an optical or MRI gradient-based tracking system. However, the high cost and the large space and resource requirement are major impediments to wider adoption.

Different imaging modalities may also be combined. Preoperative imaging may be obtained on MRI while the procedure is performed by CT. If real-time visualization is desired, preoperative cross-sectional imaging from MRI or CT may be used with intraoperative ultrasound. In these systems, the tracking is again performed via optical or EM approach to localize the instrument. The data are then fused with the preoperative imaging to give a real-time display of the instrument position with respect to the target identified preoperatively (► Fig. 13.1). The ability to take advantage of multiple modalities may allow INS to use the best features of each modality, such as the soft tissue contrast of MRI with the real-time feedback of ultrasound.

INSs remain an area of great interest, with improvement in technology continually increasing accuracy, speed, and ease of use. These systems are poised to play an increasing role in interventional radiology.

13.3 Immunoembolization

Immunoembolization uses biological response modifiers or immunologic agents in combination with embolization to enhance the antitumor response, specifically in liver malignancies. It is a transcatheter intra-arterial treatment that consists of infusion of an immunologic agent into the hepatic artery followed by embolization.

The rationale behind the procedure is that, in normal liver, immune response is naturally suppressed despite the abundant presence of macrophages (Kupffer cells), antigen-presenting cells and cell populations part of innate immunity. This suppression is thought to be necessary to avoid overactivation of the immune system by persistent exposure to antigens from the gastrointestinal tract.

Immunoembolization, bland embolization, or chemoembolization initially leads to tumor destruction but also serves to provide tumor antigens to the local immune system. Concurrent use of biological response modifiers would then induce an inflammatory response, which improves the antigen presentation to the local immune system. Local stimulation of the immune system would then result in development of a systemic immune response against tumor cells suppressing the growth of untreated tumors and circulating cancer cells.

Kanai et al first described the use of OK-432 (Picibanil, Chugai Pharmaceutical Co., Ltd.) for immunoembolization in hepatocellular carcinoma patients.[6] OK-432 is a freeze-dried biological product prepared from *Streptococcus pyogenes* (group A) by treatment with benzylpenicillin and heat. It has been used as an anticancer agent in Japan since 1975 and has been reported to induce multiple cytokines, including interleukin (IL)-1, IL-2,

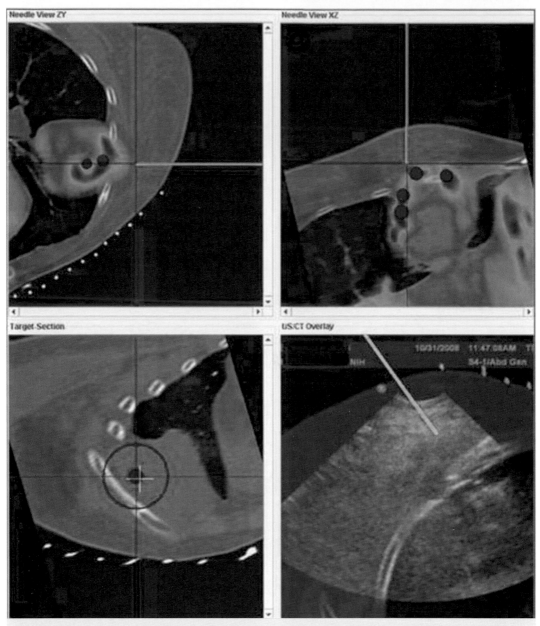

Fig. 13.1 Patient with recurrent tumor and multiple recent nondiagnostic computed tomographically (CT)-guided biopsies. Graphical user interface showing metabolic activity *(blue dots)* on positron emission tomographic (PET) scan targeted with navigation to sample a viable part of the tumor. PET data were registered to procedural multiplanar reconstructed CT and procedural ultrasound for real-time feedback. A virtual needle is represented by the blue line. Multiplanar/multimodality navigation is displayed, as well as a view down the needle shaft *(lower left)*. (Reproduced from Wood et al[1] with permission.)

interferon (IFN)-gamma, tumor necrosis factor (TNF)-alpha, IL-6, IL-8, granulocyte colony–stimulating factor (G-CSF), granulocyte-macrophage colony–stimulating factor (GM-CSF), IL-12, and IL-18.[7] Initially, protocols involved transcatheter arterial administration of the OK-432 compound followed by bland embolization with fibrinogen, thrombin, and lipiodol.[8] Various protocols have been reported since its first use, with the central concept being transcatheter arterial administration of an immunologic agent, followed by embolization or chemoembolization.

The approach has been pursued for patients with metastatic uveal melanoma predominantly using GM-CSF, a glycoprotein secreted by immune cells that increases myeloid cell production, stimulates macrophages, increases cytotoxicity of monocytes toward tumor cell lines, and promotes maturation of dendritic cells. Intra-arterial GM-CSF with Ethiodol was shown to be safe in a phase 1 trial in which 34 of the 39 patients in the study had metastatic uveal melanoma. All were considered unresectable. Patients underwent lobar hepatic artery embolization every 4 weeks using an escalating dose of GM-CSF with Ethiodol, followed by Gelfoam. CT of the chest/abdomen/pelvis and MRI of the liver were performed to assess results using Response Evaluation Criteria in Solid Tumors (RECIST), along with clinical assessment. Two patients had a complete response, 8 patients had a partial response (32% response rate), and 10 patients (32%) had stable disease. The median survival was 33.7 months for those with complete or partial responses compared with 12.4 months for those with stable or progressive disease.

Systemic progression-free survival was also prolonged in patients receiving higher-dose therapy— 12.4 months compared to 5.6 months in patients receiving low-dose immunoembolization ($\geq 1,500$ µg for high dose, $\geq 1,000$ µg for low dose, $p < 0.05$). This suggests that immunoembolization may induce a systemic immune response against the melanoma cells.

During follow-up, six patients underwent resection of extrahepatic metastases with pathology showing signs of immunologic response. Two showed CD4 + and CD8 + T cell and dendritic cell infiltration, and one showed monocyte infiltration with tumor necrosis. Of the 10 patients undergoing administration of 2,000 µg of GM-CSF, there was only one grade 3 toxicity (asymptomatic elevation of liver function tests) and one grade 4 toxicity (respiratory suppression due to narcotic use).

A subsequent randomized, double-blind, phase 2 clinical study in patients with metastatic uveal melanoma included 52 patients randomized to undergo embolization with Ethiodol and Gelfoam, with or without 2,000 µg GM-CSF. Both groups demonstrated induced cytokine production, but it was more prominent in patients receiving immunoembolization. Survival in patients with 20 to 50% tumor involvement was 18.2 months in the immunoembolization group versus 16 months for those in the bland embolization group ($p = 0.047$). Both immunoembolization and bland embolization were well tolerated with low toxicity profiles.

13.4 Chemosaturation with Percutaneous Hepatic Perfusion

Chemosaturation with percutaneous hepatic perfusion (CS-PHP) is a minimally invasive locoregional therapy. The goal is to deliver high-dose chemotherapy to the liver while preventing toxicity to the remainder of the body by extracorporeal filtering hepatic venous blood.[9] The concept of isolating hepatic perfusion involves diverting the venous return of the liver to an external circuit. Therapeutic agents are administered intra-arterially to the liver, and the hepatic venous return is passed to a perfusion circuit. This then returns the blood to the arterial infusion. Therefore, the therapeutic agent is continuously administered to the liver over the period of cycle time, typically on the order of 1 hour. During this period, a veno-venous bypass is also needed to pass the venous return of the lower body to the heart.

Procedures involving the isolation of hepatic perfusion were first described in the surgical literature and involved an extensive operation. The hepatic vasculature is dissected and exposed. The hepatic portion of the inferior vena cava (IVC) is isolated with clamping and directly cannulated to provide venous return to the circuit. The gastroduodenal artery is directly cannulated and the common hepatic artery clamped to ensure arterial flow is isolated to the liver. The right saphenous vein is exposed and cannulated to provide venous return of the lower body to the left axillary vein, also via direct cannulation.

Percutaneous hepatic perfusion is a newer approach using a double-balloon catheter placed percutaneously into the IVC to isolate the hepatic venous blood (▶ Fig. 13.2). High doses of chemotherapy are then infused directly into the hepatic artery accessed percutaneously via the femoral artery. A fenestrated section in the double-balloon catheter allows the isolated hepatic blood to be filtered extracorporeally before being returned to the systemic circulation via percutaneous access of an internal jugular vein.[10]

CS-PHP has been developed commercially (Hepatic CHEMOSAT Delivery System, Delcath Systems

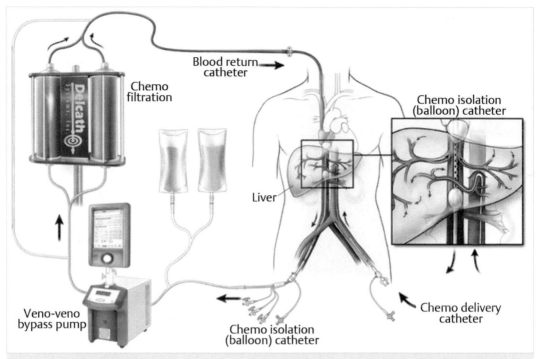

Fig. 13.2 Diagram of the Delcath Hepatic CHEMOSAT Delivery System. The technique of chemosaturation with percutaneous hepatic perfusion is performed via a specialized double-balloon catheter, which occludes the intrahepatic inferior vena cava adjacent to the hepatic venous outflow. This allows extracorporeal filtration of the chemotherapeutic agent in the effluent venous blood, with subsequent return to the systemic circulation via a veno–veno bypass into the internal jugular vein. (Reproduced from Deneve et al[10] with permission.)

Inc.) with clinical trials under way in patients with hepatic metastases from melanoma. The chemotherapeutic agent melphalan was chosen for the clinical trial program because it does not cause significant liver toxicity, even when given at high doses. It has also previously been used in the operative version of isolated hepatic perfusion for treating several primary cancers, including melanoma, hepatocellular carcinoma, colorectal cancer, and neuroendocrine tumor. The phase 1 study established the maximum tolerated dose of melphalan (3 mg/kg) by CS-PHP. Overall response rate (complete and partial response) was reported as 30%, with a response rate of 50% in the subset of patients with metastatic ocular melanoma. A phase 3, multicenter randomized trial of CS-PHP with melphalan versus best alternative care in patients with metastatic ocular or cutaneous melanoma isolated to the liver reported 8 months versus 1.6 months ($P < 0.0001$) hepatic progression-free survival and 6.7 months versus 1.6 months ($P < 0.0001$) overall progression-free survival, respectively.

In a single-center experience of patients with metastatic melanoma or sarcoma to the liver, Forster et al reported 90%[11] of patients experiencing either stable disease or partial response to therapy as evaluated by tumor volume. During the follow-up period, 6 of the 10 patients died of their disease, with a median survival rate from time of diagnosis of hepatic metastasis of 12.6 months.[11] Of the four patients alive at the end of the follow-up period, one has experienced hepatic progression-free survival of 5.5 months and a second of 44.5 months. This compares favorably with a report of the Collaborative Ocular Melanoma Study (CMOS) Group finding a median time from diagnosis of metastasis to death of < 6 months in melanoma metastasis.[12]

The CS-PHP concept does not prescribe a particular chemotherapeutic agent, and clinical trials will be needed to determine factors such as chemotherapy choice, dose, and circulation time individually for each tumor type.

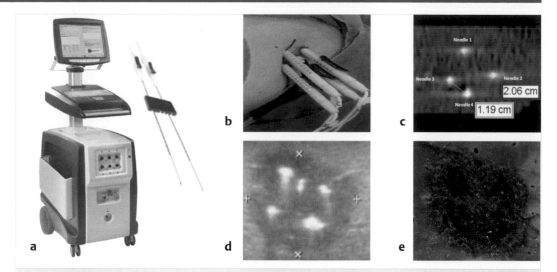

Fig. 13.3 The NanoKnife system and implementation. The NanoKnife generator is pictured with **(a)** two irreversible electroporation probes. **(b)** In vivo ablation of pig liver showing the probes in position. **(c)** Real-time imaging of probe placement by computed tomography. **(d)** Ultrasound immediately postablation showing the hypoechoic ablation zone and **(e)** a macroscopic gross specimen of the ablation zone. (Images courtesy of AngioDynamics.)

13.5 Irreversible Electroporation

Electroporation was initially developed for the laboratory to increase the permeability of cell membranes by exposing it to electrical pulses. This effect can be reversible or irreversible, depending on the electrical field. By temporarily creating "pores" in the cell membrane, various drugs or genes can be transferred rapidly and efficiently to the cell. A procedure known as electrochemotherapy using electroporation to administer chemotherapy drugs, which would otherwise not be taken up by the cell, has also been described. Irreversible electroporation (IRE) can be used to ablate a volume of tissue, without the addition of adjuvant drugs. Moreover, electroporation does not induce the negative thermal effects seen with other modes of ablation. This has led to increasing use of IRE as a primary method of treating tumors, finding its greatest application to date in hepatic lesions.[13]

IRE uses electrodes to apply a high-voltage, low-energy direct current that travels through cells causing the formation of pores. Cells will normally repair these pores, making the effect reversible. However, when the rate of pore creation exceeds the rate of repair, damage to the cell membrane progresses to a critical level, inducing apoptosis.

This is thought to be an advantage to thermal ablation because the latter causes greater leakage of cell contents into the surrounding tissue. This can incite an inflammatory reaction followed by cellular infiltration, and ultimately fibrosis and scarring.[14]

The commercially available system is known as the NanoKnife (AngioDynamics) (▶ Fig. 13.3). Probes are placed percutaneously into the target organ and connected to a generator to create the current. Probes are of similar shape to thermal ablation probes, consisting of a single metallic shaft with a sharp tip. There are two main types of probes, monopolar and bipolar. The monopolar probe requires placement of two probes around the target, each a 19-guage needle with spacing and applied current resulting in of 2 to 3 cm^3, depending on the applied current. The ablative zone can be increased in size by applying up 6 probes. The bipolar probe contains two electrodes spaced in the distal portion. A single 16-gauge bipolar probe can create an ablation zone of approximately $2 \times 2 \times 3$ cm, again with the ability to use multiple probes to increase the ablation zone.

Thomson et al reported the first human experience of IRE[15] describing a single-center prospective, nonrandomized study to investigate the safety of IRE. Thirty-eight patients with advanced

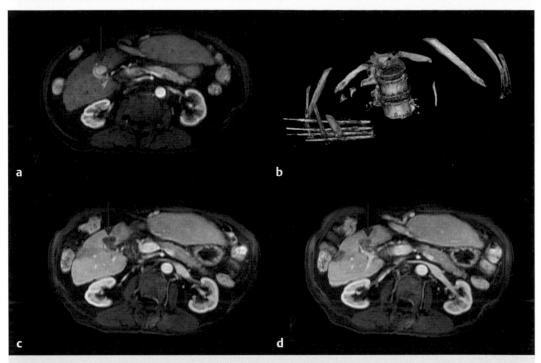

Fig. 13.4 Images from a patient treated with irreversible electroporation for hepatocellular carcinoma. **(a)** Preablation magnetic resonance imaging (MRI) demonstrates an enhancing lesion *(arrow)* just anterior to and abutting the anterior branch of the right portal vein. **(b)** A volume-rendered image from the ablation procedure shows the probes in position. **(c)** Postablation MRI demonstrates the ablation zone *(arrow)* is nonenhancing, with a small amount of expected peripheral hyperemia. **(d)** Portal-phase image from the same postablation MRI *(arrow)* demonstrates that the right portal vein branch remains patent.

liver, kidney, or lung carcinoma unresponsive to standard treatment underwent IRE under general anesthesia. No mortality occurred at 30 days. Transient ventricular arrhythmia occurred in four patients, leading to the use of electrocardiography (ECG) to synchronize delivery in the remaining 30 patients. This study showed that IRE appears safe for clinical use when ECG synchronization is used. The NanoKnife machine uses an ECG trigger monitor to automatically detect the slope of the R wave, which then signals the NanoKnife generator to deliver the energy pulse after a 50 ms delay. The energy is therefore delivered during, or just before, the ventricular refractory period.

The IRE procedure itself involves placing a number of electrodes under CT or ultrasound guidance based on tumor size. Anesthesia depends on preference, though published series have advocated the use of a neuromuscular blockade to counteract the high electrical voltage generated during treatment. Paralyzing agents include cisatracurium besylate or rocuronium bromide. A contrast-enhanced (if renal function permits) postprocedure CT scan is obtained the same or following day to evaluate for any immediate complications and assess if the lesion has been appropriately treated. A successfully treated lesion will show a lack of contrast enhancement in the ablation zone and complete coverage of the lesion by the ablation zone (► Fig. 13.4). Patients are generally admitted overnight for observation and pain control. Narayanan et al retrospectively evaluated pain in IRE versus radiofrequency ablation and found no significant differences.[16]

Initial experiences in IRE have shown promise, including ablation of lesions near vital structures, due to its nonthermal, primarily apoptosis driven, mechanism of action. Cannon et al reported a prospective study of patients undergoing IRE for hepatic tumors over a 2-year period.[17] Primary tumor types included colorectal (45%, $n = 20$), hepatocellular (35%, $n = 14$), non–small cell lung ($n = 2$), breast ($n = 2$), carcinoid/neuroendocrine ($n = 3$), melanoma, renal cell ($n = 1$), and one soft tissue carcinoma ($n = 1$). Forty-six of 46 lesions (100%) were successfully treated. Local recurrence-free survival was 97.4%, 94.6%, and 59.5% at 3, 6, and 12 months, respectively, with a trend toward higher recurrence rates for tumors > 4 cm.

A study performed in 14 patients with pancreatic cancer[18] who were unable to tolerate surgery or had unresectable tumor after standard therapy found no deaths and no evidence of vessel injury on postprocedure scans despite 10 of the patients having > 180-degree encasement of the superior mesenteric artery or hepatic artery. Two patients with unresectable cancer (as a result of celiac axis and common hepatic artery encasement, respectively) went on to undergo margin-negative resections after the IRE procedure. Median event-free survival was 6.7 months, and the median overall survival was not reached in the study period. Overall survival was significantly longer for patients with localized disease versus those with metastatic disease ($p = 0.02$), and event-free survival was significantly longer for patients who went on to resection after IRE ($p = 0.04$). This study shows that IRE may be safely performed in tumors near vascular structures and may provide opportunity for downgrading tumors, allowing for more definitive therapy.

IRE remains a novel technique, though increasing studies indicate safety and efficacy that suggest IRE will become a major tool in IO.

13.6 Viral Oncolytics

Viral oncolysis refers to the use of modified viruses to target tumors.[19] Viral vectors used most commonly for cancer gene therapy are derived from adenovirus, adenoassociated virus, or retrovirus. Several strategies have been developed to render these viruses replication deficient outside of specialized packaging cell lines to minimize the risk toxicity from viral replication or cellular transformation in patients. Such replication-defective viruses have been historically studied as vehicles for delivering genes to cells. However, the direct cytopathic effect caused by viral replication is itself an effective mechanism of tumor destruction (viral oncolysis). This is further enhanced by reinfection of adjacent tumor cells by the progeny virion released from lysed tumor cells. This propagative effect may be used as a novel paradigm for tumor therapy.

Herpes simplex virus 1 (HSV-1) has been examined for its safety and efficacy as an oncolytic virus in several clinical trials. HSV-1 is a double-stranded DNA virus with a capsid and envelope, and is a ubiquitous pathogen that is transmitted by direct mucosal contact. Infection with HSV-1 is common and reported to be 66 to 84% in the United States, although rates vary depending on the population studied. It is generally more prevalent in females than males, increases with age, and is lowest in populations in the developed areas of the world. Skin or mucosal infection of HSV-1 is usually followed by transmission via sensory nerves to the trigeminal ganglia, where lifelong latent infection occurs. Reactivation from ganglionic neurons may occur and results in an epithelial ulcer (e.g., "cold sore") with viral shedding into the oral cavity or epithelia in the trigeminal distribution.

HSV-1 possesses several features that render it well suited to viral oncolytic therapy. It does not integrate into the cellular genome, it has a large transgene capacity of up to 50 kb, and several HSV-1 mutants have been characterized that preferentially replicate in neoplastic cells rather than normal cells. The presence of antibodies against HSV-1 does not attenuate its oncolytic efficacy. Despite the very high prevalence of exposure to HSV-1, it rarely causes severe illness, and effective antiherpetic agents are available to terminate unwanted viral replication.

Several variants of replication-deficient HSV-1 mutants have been created and studied. They follow a similar theme in that their replication is markedly attenuated in normal cells, whereas replication in cancer cells is significantly more robust.[20] Studies have been performed in strains known as G207, NV1020, rRp450, and HSV1716.[19] Each of these mutants is attenuated relative to wild-type HSV-1.

G207 is an HSV-1 mutant under development by Medigene in which both copies of the γ134.5 have been deleted and the UL39 (encodes ICP6) is inactivated by insertion of the β-galactosidase gene. The safety of G207 has been examined in a phase 1 trial in subjects with brain tumors.[21] Although adverse events were noted in some subjects, no toxicity or serious adverse events were unequivocally ascribed to G207. Seropositive and seronegative subjects were included in this study, and no difference in side effects of G207 was observed between the two groups.

NV1020 is an HSV-1 mutant in which the internal repeat domain (joint region) is deleted and replaced by a fragment of the HSV-2 genome. A phase 1, open-label, dose-escalating study of a single 10-minute hepatic arterial infusion of NV1020 has been performed.[22] Adverse events were either mild or moderate in severity and were self-limiting. Only three serious adverse events (one transient rise in serum g-glutamyltransferase, one diarrhea, and one leukocytosis) experienced by three patients were considered to be possibly or probably related to NV1020. There were no deaths during the study, and there was no evidence of disseminated herpes infection.

A multicenter phase 1/2 study evaluated the safety, pharmacokinetics, and antitumor effects of repeated doses of NV1020 in patients with advanced metastatic colorectal cancer (mCRC).[23] Patients with liver-dominant mCRC received four fixed weekly intra-arterial NV1020 doses, followed by two or more cycles of conventional chemotherapy. After infusion at the lowest dose level (3×10^6 pfu) metastases in all three patients showed steady progression. With 1×10^7 pfu, one of three patients showed some stabilization. At the 3×10^7 and 1×10^8 pfu dose levels, three of four and three of three patients, respectively, showed stable disease (SD). One patient at the highest dose also had complete remission of both local pelvic recurrence and pulmonary metastases. After NV1020 treatment at the optimum biological dose, 11 of 22 patients (50%) initially showed SD.

OncoVEXGM-CSF is an HSV-1 mutant expressing GM-CSF, and was administered intratumorally in a phase 1 clinical trial of 30 subjects.[24] Thirteen patients were in a single-dose group, and 17 in a multiple-dose group. Eligibility criteria included seronegative and seropositive patients. In the single-injection group of patients, grade 1 pyrexia, associated constitutional symptoms, local inflammation, and erythema at the site of inoculation into superficial, cutaneous melanoma tumors were more prevalent in the HSV-seronegative individuals compared to the seropositive patients.

In a phase 2 study OncoVEXGM-CSF was injected intratumorally into patients with stage IIIC or IV melanoma.[25] Patients received an initial injection into 1 to 10 tumors followed by a 3-week interval, then continued twice-weekly injections for a total of up to 24 injections. Seropositive and seronegative patients were included in the study. Response rates were similar in seronegative and seropositive patients. The overall response rate by RECIST was 26% (complete response, $n = 8$; partial response, $n = 5$) with overall survival of 58% at 1 year and 52% at 24 months.

Intra-arterial viral oncolysis is a promising new treatment for primary and metastatic liver cancer. Understanding viral oncolytic therapy background and development is important for future applications.

13.7 Conclusion

Interventional oncology has become an established part of cancer treatment. Its role as a standalone therapy or as part of broader treatment plans is not only well rooted but is expanding in many new fronts as discussed in this chapter. Interventional oncologists have a unique opportunity to offer and indeed help develop these new tools as the medical community incorporates IO into standard practices. New approaches are constantly being developed, and it would be impossible to fully address all the avenues of research currently under way. This chapter is an attempt to describe *some* of the emerging technologies entering the IO sphere. The rapid changes in IO may make it challenging to stay current, but such changes are part of the reason that IO is one of the most exciting fields in health care today.

References

[1] Wood BJ, Kruecker J, Abi-Jaoudeh N et al. Navigation systems for ablation. J Vasc Interv Radiol 2010; 21(8) Suppl: S257–S263

[2] Phee SJ, Yang K. Interventional navigation systems for treatment of unresectable liver tumor. Med Biol Eng Comput 2010; 48(2): 103–111

[3] Mirota DJ, Ishii M, Hager GD. Vision-based navigation in image-guided interventions. Annu Rev Biomed Eng 2011; 13: 297–319

[4] Yaniv Z, Wilson E, Lindisch D, Cleary K. Electromagnetic tracking in the clinical environment. Med Phys 2009; 36(3): 876–892

[5] Kurumi Y, Tani T, Naka S et al. MR-guided microwave ablation for malignancies. Int J Clin Oncol 2007; 12(2): 85–93

[6] Kanai T, Monden M, Sakon M et al. New development of transarterial immunoembolization (TIE) for therapy of hepatocellular carcinoma with intrahepatic metastases. Cancer Chemother Pharmacol 1994; 33 Suppl: S48–S54

[7] Ryoma Y, Moriya Y, Okamoto M, Kanaya I, Saito M, Sato M. Biological effect of OK-432 (picibanil) and possible application to dendritic cell therapy. Anticancer Res 2004; 24 5C: 3295–3301

[8] Yoshida T, Sakon M, Umeshita K et al. Appraisal of transarterial immunoembolization for hepatocellular carcinoma: a clinicopathologic study. J Clin Gastroenterol 2001; 32(1): 59–65

[9] Alexander HR, Jr, Butler CC. Development of isolated hepatic perfusion via the operative and percutaneous techniques for patients with isolated and unresectable liver metastases. Cancer J 2010; 16(2): 132–141

[10] Deneve JL, Choi J, Gonzalez RJ et al. Chemosaturation with percutaneous hepatic perfusion for unresectable isolated hepatic metastases from sarcoma. Cardiovasc Intervent Radiol 2012; 35(6): 1480–1487

[11] Forster MR, Rashid OM, Perez MC, Choi J, Chaudhry T, Zager JS. Chemosaturation with percutaneous hepatic perfusion for unresectable metastatic melanoma or sarcoma to the liver: a single institution experience. J Surg Oncol 2014; 109 (5): 434–439

[12] Diener-West M, Reynolds SM, Agugliaro DJ et al. Collaborative Ocular Melanoma Study Group. Development of metastatic disease after enrollment in the COMS trials for treatment of choroidal melanoma: Collaborative Ocular Melanoma Study Group Report No. 26. Arch Ophthalmol 2005; 123 (12): 1639–1643

[13] Narayanan G, Froud T, Suthar R, Barbery K. Irreversible electroporation of hepatic malignancy. Semin Intervent Radiol 2013; 30(1): 67–73

[14] Rubinsky B, Onik G, Mikus P. Irreversible electroporation: a new ablation modality—clinical implications. Technol Cancer Res Treat 2007; 6(1): 37–48

[15] Thomson KR, Cheung W, Ellis SJ et al. Investigation of the safety of irreversible electroporation in humans. J Vasc Interv Radiol 2011; 22(5): 611–621

[16] Narayanan G, Froud T, Lo K, Barbery KJ, Perez-Rojas E, Yrizarry J. Pain analysis in patients with hepatocellular carcinoma: irreversible electroporation versus radiofrequency ablation-initial observations. Cardiovasc Intervent Radiol 2013; 36(1). 176–182

[17] Cannon R, Ellis S, Hayes D, Narayanan G, Martin RC, II. Safety and early efficacy of irreversible electroporation for hepatic tumors in proximity to vital structures. J Surg Oncol 2013; 107(5): 544–549

[18] Narayanan G, Hosein PJ, Arora G et al. Percutaneous irreversible electroporation for downstaging and control of unresectable pancreatic adenocarcinoma. J Vasc Interv Radiol 2012; 23(12): 1613–1621

[19] Kuruppu D, Tanabe KK. Viral oncolysis by herpes simplex virus and other viruses. Cancer Biol Ther 2005; 4(5): 524–531

[20] Chase M, Chung RY, Chiocca EA. An oncolytic viral mutant that delivers the CYP2B1 transgene and augments cyclophosphamide chemotherapy. Nat Biotechnol 1998; 16(5): 444–448

[21] Markert JM, Medlock MD, Rabkin SD et al. Conditionally replicating herpes simplex virus mutant, G207 for the treatment of malignant glioma: results of a phase I trial. Gene Ther 2000; 7(10): 867–874

[22] Kemeny N, Brown K, Covey A et al. Phase I, open-label, dose-escalating study of a genetically engineered herpes simplex virus, NV1020, in subjects with metastatic colorectal carcinoma to the liver. Hum Gene Ther 2006; 17(12): 1214–1224

[23] Geevarghese SK, Geller DA, de Haan HA et al. Phase I/II study of oncolytic herpes simplex virus NV1020 in patients with extensively pretreated refractory colorectal cancer metastatic to the liver. Hum Gene Ther 2010; 21(9): 1119–1128

[24] Hu JC, Coffin RS, Davis CJ et al. A phase I study of OncoVEXGM-CSF, a second-generation oncolytic herpes simplex virus expressing granulocyte macrophage colony-stimulating factor. Clin Cancer Res 2006; 12(22): 6737–6747

[25] Senzer NN, Kaufman HL, Amatruda T et al. Phase II clinical trial of a granulocyte-macrophage colony-stimulating factor-encoding, second-generation oncolytic herpesvirus in patients with unresectable metastatic melanoma. J Clin Oncol 2009; 27(34): 5763–5771

Index